RATIONALE OF BIOLOGICAL RESPONSE MODIFIERS IN CANCER TREATMENT

Rationale of Biological Response Modifiers in Cancer Treatment

Proceedings of the Sixth Symposium on
Rationale of Biological Response Modifiers
in Cancer Treatment
Hakone, Japan
August 31- September 1, 1984

Organizing Committee

Eiro Tsubura (Chairman)
Ichiro Urushizaki
Tadao Aoki

Secretariat

Saburo Sone
Yutaro Kaneko

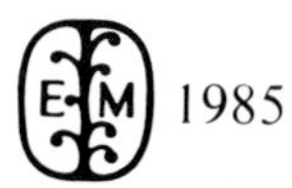
1985

Excerpta Medica, Amsterdam-Princeton-Geneva-Tokyo

International Congress Series No. 690
ISBN Excerpta Medica 4-900392-54-5
ISBN Elsevier Science Publ. Co. 0-444-80700-4

Publisher: Excerpta Medica

Offices: P.O. Box 1126
1000-BC Amsterdam

28, Chemin Colladon
Geneva

P.O. Box 3085
Princeton, N.J. 08540

15-23, Nishi-Azabu 4-chome
Minato-ku, Tokyo

Printed in Japan

CONTENTS

Preface
Eiro Tsubura 1

The use of liposomes as carriers of multiple biological response modifiers for systemic activation of macrophages
Isaiah J. Fidler 3

Anti-metastatic effect of tumor necrosis factor (TNF)
Yoshiro Niitsu, Naoki Watanabe, Hisao Sone, Hiroshi Neda, Naofumi Yamauchi and Ichiro Urushizaki 15

Enhancement of experimental pulmonary metastasis of B16 melanoma in mice with granulocytosis
Makoto Ishikawa, Yutaka Koga, Masuo Hosokawa and Hiroshi Kobayashi 25

The role of macrophages in the therapeutic effect of bleomycin on a rat fibrosarcoma
Kiyoshi Morikawa, Masuo Hosokawa, Jun-ichi Hamada, Michio Sugawara and Hiroshi Kobayashi 33

Therapeutic implications of activation of human monocyte-macrophages to the tumoricidal state by liposomes containing biological response modifiers
Saburo Sone, Seiji Mutsuura, Mitsumasa Ogawara, Teruhiro Utsugi and Eiro Tsubura 44

Macrophage activating factor for cytotoxicity produced by human T cell hybridomas
Toshiaki Osawa and Masahiro Higuchi 53

In vitro activation of human pleural macrophages with *Nocardia rubra* cell wall skeleton (N-CWS)
Mitsunori Sakatani, Tomiya Masuno, Ichiro Kawase, Takeshi Ogura, Susumu Kishimoto and Yuichi Yamamura 62

Generation *in vitro* of human monocyte tumoricidal potential by interferon alpha and beta
Teruhiro Utsugi, Saburo Sone, Seiji Mutsuura, Mitsumasa Ogawara, Toyohiro Shirahama, Kiyoshi Ishii and Eiro Tsubura 74

Neutrophil activating factor (NAF) as a possible mediator in anticancer effector mechanisms
Fujiro Sendo 83

Recombinant human interleukin 2 functions as a differentiative signal in induction of T-lymphocyte cytotoxicity, but does not support long-term T cell growth
Seiko Yamasaki, Keiko Amikura, Shinsuke Taki, Ryota Yoshimoto and Junji Hamuro 87

Anti-Tac antibody does not necessarily recognize the same epitope as that which is defined by specific IL2 binding
Nobuo Kondoh, Michiyuki Maeda, Junji Yodoi and Junji Hamuro 96

Relationships between chemotherapy and immunotherapy: A brief overview
Enrico Mihich 105

Effect of lentinan against allogeneic, syngeneic and autologous primary tumors, and its prophylactic effect against chemical carcinogenesis
Tetsuya Suga, Noriko A. Uchida, Takashi Yoshihama, Tsuyoshi Shiio, Makoto Rokutanda, Jószef Fachet, Yukiko Y. Maeda and Goro Chihara 116

Combination therapy with antitumor polysaccharides in mice
Shigeru Abe, Masatoshi Yamazaki and Den'ichi Mizuno 129

Synergistic effect of lentinan and surgical endocrine therapy on the growth of DMBA-induced mammary tumors of rats and of recurrent human breast cancer
Akio Kosaka, Yuuichi Hattori, Atsuko Imaizumi and Akira Yamashita 138

End-point result of a randomized controlled study on the treatment of gastrointestinal cancer with a combination of lentinan and chemotherapeutic agents
Tetsuo Taguchi, Hisashi Furue, Tadashi Kimura, Tatsuhei Kondo, Takao Hattori, Ichiji Ito and Nobuya Ogawa 151

Lentinan treatment of Japanese cases infected with human T-lymphotropic retroviruses (HTLV-I and -III)
Tadao Aoki, Hideo Miyakoshi, Yoshimaru Usuda, Robert C.Y. Ting and Robert C. Gallo 167

The UV-irradiated mouse as a model for testing biological response modifiers
Margaret L. Kripke 178

Tumor cell xenogenization as a consequence of alterations in gene expression: High frequency induction of heritable immunogenic variants by exposure to strongly or poorly mutagenic compounds
Robert S. Kerbel, Philip Frost, Douglas A. Carlow and Bruce E. Elliott 187

Monoclonal antibody 791T/36 for tumour detection and drug targeting
Michael J. Embleton 200

Tumor cell lysis by antibody-dependent macrophage-mediated cytotoxicity using syngeneic monoclonal antibodies and its augmentation by cell-wall skeleton of *Nocardia rubra*
Ichiro Kawase, Kiyoshi Komuta, Takeshi Ogura, Hiromi Fujiwara, Toshiyuki Hamaoka and Susumu Kishimoto 208

Immune interferon induces mouse IgG2a- and IgG3-dependent cellular cytotoxicity in a human monocytic cell line (U937)
Yukio Akiyama, Michael D. Lubeck, Zenon Steplewski and Hilary Koprowski 223

An approach to cancer chemotherapy by application of monoclonal antibody-modified liposomes
Yoshiyuki Hashimoto 231

Biological response modifiers for the therapy of cancer
Ronald B. Herberman 240

Contributors 259

Preface

This monograph is a collection of contributions presented at the Sixth Symposium on the "Rationale of Biological Response Modifiers in Cancer Treatment", held at the Hakone Prince Hotel in Hakone, Japan, on August 31 and September 1, 1984. This symposium was designed to address the problem of the validity of in vitro and in vivo models for predicting clinical responses during the development and screening of new biological response modifiers (BRMs). Although extensive trials of immunotherapeutic treatment of cancer patients have been carried out in the last 15 years, results have not been satisfactory. Nevertheless, recent progress in the development of new synthetic immunomodulators and in gene technology and engineering have greatly stimulated basic and applied research on new and better BRMs.

In organizing this symposium, particular attention was also directed to the subject of the mechanisms by which BRMs modify the antitumor actions of the host in vivo. The exchange of new information and techniques related to the host's response to cancer and to approaches to the development of new therapeutic modalities was felt to be of major importance; all the participants were asked to address these points.

Scientific interest was great and discussion was lively throughout the two-day conference. I therefore believe that this conference achieved its scientific goals. I hope that this monograph will serve to promote the progress and development of research into BRM treatment of malignant disseminated diseases.

Finally, I wish to offer special thanks to the symposium coordinators, Dr. Saburo Sone, Mr. Yutaro Kaneko and Ms. Mitsuko Mori, who provided invaluable assistance during the meeting. We also owe a special debt of thanks to Ms. Hiroko Ishino, who extensively reviewed and edited all the manuscripts in order to enable rapid publication of the proceedings.

Eiro Tsubura
Department of Internal Medicine
The University of Tokushima
School of Medicine
Tokushima, Japan

The use of liposomes as carriers of multiple biological response modifiers for systemic activation of macrophages

Isaiah J. Fidler

INTRODUCTION

The uncontrolled growth of metastases that are resistant to conventional therapies is a major cause of death from cancer.[1,2] Recent data from our laboratory and others indicate that metastases can arise from the nonrandom spread of specialized malignant cells that pre-exist within a primary neoplasm,[3] that metastases can be clonal in their origin,[4] that different metastases can originate from different progenitor cells,[4] and that, in general, metastatic cells can exhibit a higher rate of spontaneous mutation than benign nonmetastatic cells.[5] These data provide an explanation for the clinical observation that multiple metastases can exhibit different sensitivities to therapeutic modalities.[2] They imply that the successful therapy of disseminated metastases will have to circumvent the problems of neoplastic heterogeneity and the development of resistance to therapy by tumor cells.

Appropriately activated macrophages can fulfill these demanding criteria.[6] Macrophages can be activated to become tumoricidal by interaction with phospholipid vesicles (liposomes) containing various immunomodulators. Tumoricidal macrophages can recognize and destroy neoplastic cells *in vitro* or *in vivo*, while leaving non-neoplastic cells unharmed. Although the exact mechanism by which macrophages discriminate between tumorigenic and normal cells is unknown, it is independent of tumor cell characteristics, such as immunogenicity, metastatic potential, and sensitivity to cytotoxic drugs.[7] Moreover, macrophage destruction of tumor cells is apparently not associated with the development of tumor cell resistance.[6]

There are two major pathways to achieve macrophage activation *in vivo*. Frequently, macrophages are activated as a consequence of their interaction with microorganisms or their products, for example, endotoxins, the bacteria cell wall skeleton, and small components of the bacteria cell wall skeleton such as muramyl dipeptide (MDP).[8–10] *In vivo* activation of macrophages can also take place after their interaction with soluble mediators released by antigen- or mitogen-sensitized lymphocytes. The soluble lymphokine that induces macrophage activation is referred to as macrophage-activating factor (MAF). MAF first binds to a macrophage surface receptor and then is internalized to elicit tumoricidal properties in the macrophages.[11]

In general, attempts to specifically activate macrophages *in vivo* to enhance host defense against metastases have been unsuccessful. Systemic administration of MAF is hindered by the lack of purified preparations of this lymphokine and by the fact that lymphokines injected intravenously have a very short half-life and so do not activate macrophages *in vivo*.[12] The systemic activation of macrophages with microorganisms or their products has also suffered from major drawbacks. For instance, administration of whole bacteria such as Bacillus Calmette-Guerin activates various effector cells and is accompanied by serious toxicity problems such as allergic reaction and granuloma formation.[13] For this reason, little progress was made until the discovery of MDP, a small component of the bacterial cell wall that is capable of activating macrophages.[8,14] However, the use of water-soluble synthetic MDP is limited because, by 60 minutes after parenteral administration, this agent is cleared from the body to be excreted in the urine.[15] This brief period is insufficient to activate macrophages even under ideal *in vitro* conditions.[10]

Advances in liposome technology have provided a mechanism for activating macrophages *in situ* with soluble MAF or MDP or both. Liposomes can be used to carry agents to cells of the reticuloendothelial system, since these cells are responsible for the rapid clearance of particulate material from the circulation.[16–18] There are several advantages to using liposome-encapsulated materials to activate cells of the macrophage-histiocyte series *in vivo*. Many macrophage-activating agents such as bacterial products or lymphokines can be antigenic, and repeated systemic administrations can lead to adverse reactions. Liposomes consisting of natural phospholipids are nonimmunogenic, and thus the elicitation of allergic reactions commonly associated with the systemic administration of other immune adjuvants may be avoided.[18]

Numerous recent studies have shown that both MAF and MDP entrapped in liposomes are very efficient in activating macrophages to become tumoricidal *in vitro*.[6] Unlike free MAF, which requires binding to a macrophage surface receptor,[19] liposome-entrapped MAF enters the cytoplasm via phagocytosis and can activate macrophages that lack receptors for MAF.[20] Moreover, for activators such as MAF and MDP that are ordinarily degraded or cleared from the body too rapidly for effectiveness, encapsulation in liposomes extends their active half-life within the body and enables these agents to activate macrophages *in situ*.[18,21–23]

Recent studies from our laboratory have shown that free or liposome-entrapped MAF and MDP can act synergistically to activate the tumoricidal properties in rat alveolar macrophages (AM) *in vitro*.[24] Since liposomes provide an efficient carrier vehicle for delivery of biologically active materials to macrophages *in vivo*,[25] activation of macrophages can be achieved to enhance host defenses against infections and cancer. In this report, we show that mouse AM can be rendered tumoricidal *in situ* by the intravenous injection of liposomes containing subthreshold doses of MAF and MDP, doses that are without effect when injected individually. Moreover, the repeated administration of these preparations is highly effective in eradicating large, established, spontaneous, pulmonary and lymph node melanoma metastases.

MATERIALS AND METHODS

Tumor culture

The B16BL/6 tumor line was obtained by an *in vitro* selection procedure for invasion.[26] The line originated from the B16 melanoma syngeneic to the C57BL/6 mouse. The cells were grown as monolayer cultures at 37°C in a humidified atmosphere containing 5% CO_2 in Eagle's minimum essential medium supplemented with 5% fetal bovine serum, vitamin solution, sodium pyruvate, L-glutamine, and nonessential amino acids (M.A. Bioproducts, Walkersville, Md). All cultures were free of mycoplasma and pathogenic mouse viruses.

Animals

Eight- to ten-week-old specific pathogen-free male C57BL/6N mice were obtained from the NCI-Frederick Cancer Research Facility's Animal Production Area.

Preparation of MAF

Cell-free supernatant fluids containing MAF activity were harvested from cultures of normal F344 rat lymphocytes incubated *in vitro* for 48 hours with Sepharose-bound concanavalin-A (Pharmacia, Piscataway, NJ), as detailed previously.[18] The cell culture supernatant fluids were centrifuged and filtered through a 0.2 μm Millipore filter. The solution was either used immediately or stored at -20°C.

For convenience and brevity, such supernatant fluids are referred to as MAF throughout the remainder of this report.

Reagents

The MDP was the kind gift of Ciba Geigy, Ltd. (Basel, Switzerland). All reagents used in our studies, such as media, MAF, MDP, and the final liposome preparations did not contain any endotoxins (detection limit of 0.125 ng/ml) as determined by the *Limulus* amebocyte lysate assay (Cape Cod Associates, Mass).

Lipids and preparation of liposomes

Chromatographically pure distearoylphosphatidylcholine (PC) and phosphatidylserine (PS) were purchased from Avanti Biochemicals (Birming ham, Ala). Multilamellar vesicles (MLV) were prepared from a mixture of PC and PS (70/30 mol%). Various dilutions of MAF and MDP were encapsulated within the MLV, as described previously.[17] The liposome preparations were adjusted to a concentration of 12.5 μmol of total lipid/ml in Ca^{++}- and Mg^{++}-free Hanks' balanced salt solution (HBSS) and used within one hour.

Determination of *in vivo* activation of AM

Normal mice were injected intravenously with 2.5 μmol of MLV that contained MAF or MDP, or both. In addition, control groups of mice were injected intravenously with HBSS, or with MLV that contained HBSS within their aqueous interior and that were suspended in HBSS containing free MAF or MDP, or both, at doses comparable to that entrapped within the MLV. Twenty-four hours after injection, the mice were killed, and their AM were harvested by tracheobronchial lavage.[10,24] Differential counts and nonspecific esterase staining revealed that over 95% of the lavaged cells were AM. The cells were plated into wells of Microtest II plates with a surface area of 38 mm² (Falcon Plastics Co., Oxnard, Calif). Nonadherent cells ($<10\%$) were removed by washing with medium 60 minutes after the initial plating.

In vitro AM-mediated cytotoxicity

Macrophage-mediated cytotoxicity against B16 melanoma cells was assessed by a radioactive release assay, as described previously.[10,24] Ten thousand target cells were plated in each culture well to obtain an initial AM: target-cell ratio of 10:1. At this population density, normal (untreated) AM are not cytotoxic to neoplastic cells, whereas activated AM are. All cultures were re-fed 24 hours after the addition of tumor cells. The cultures were then incubated for two additional days. Three-day cultures were washed twice with HBSS, and the remaining adherent viable cells were removed from the wells with 0.1 ml of 0.5 N NaOH. The lysate was then monitored for radiation in a gamma counter. The percent cytotoxicity mediated by activated AM was calculated as follows:

$$\frac{\begin{array}{c}\text{cpm in target cells}\\ \text{cultured with}\\ \text{control AM}\end{array} - \begin{array}{c}\text{cpm in target cells}\\ \text{cultured with}\\ \text{activated AM}\end{array}}{\text{cpm in target cells cultured with control AM}} \times 100$$

The statistical significance of differences among the groups was determined by Student's two-tailed *t*-test.

Treatment of spontaneous metastases by intravenous injection of liposomes containing MAF or MDP

To initiate spontaneous metastases, 2.5×10^4 viable B16BL/6 tumor cells were injected into one hind footpad of a mouse. When the local tumor had reached 10-12 mm in diameter (five to six weeks) the tumor-bearing leg, including the popliteal lymph node, was amputated at the midfemur. Seven days after the surgical removal of the primary tumor, mice with grossly visible spontaneous lung and lymph node metastases were given intravenous injections of liposomes (2.5 μmol of phospholipids suspended in 0.2 ml of HBSS). Each treatment group consisted of 18 to 20 mice. The liposomes contained various dilutions of either MAF or MDP, or both. Liposomes containing HBSS and suspended in HBSS containing MAF and MDP were used as control preparations. An additional control group included mice that received intravenous injections of HBSS alone. The mice were treated twice a week for four weeks and were monitored for up to 250 days. Dead or moribund animals were necropsied.

The Fisher exact test was employed to compare the proportion of survivors in one test group with that in another (control) group. The Cox test was used to compare the survival curve of one test group with that of the controls or other groups.[27]

RESULTS

In vivo activation of AM by liposomes containing two immunomodulators

Mice were injected with control preparations or with MLV containing various agents. Twenty-four hours later, AM were harvested, and their ability to lyse syngeneic tumor cells was assayed *in vitro*. AM harvested from mice injected with HBSS, free MAF, free MDP or a combination of free MAF and MDP did not lyse the B16 melanoma cells (Table 1). In contrast, AM harvested from mice injected with liposomes containing MAF (diluted 1:2 or 1:10 in medium) were significantly cytotoxic against the B16 melanoma cells. When the MAF solution was diluted to 1:20 or 1:50, it did not generate tumoricidal activity in AM. Liposomes containing 6.25 or 0.6 μg of MDP led to a significant cytotoxic activity in AM, but liposomes with less MDP did not generate cytotoxic properties in the AM.

To determine the potential synergistic activation of AM by MAF and MDP encapsulated within the same liposomes, mice were injected intravenously with MLV containing various dilutions of MAF, various dilutions of MDP, combinations of MAF and MDP, or control preparations. AM were harvested 24 hours after treatment, and their tumoricidal properties were determined by the *in vitro* assay. MLV containing either a 1:20 dilution of MAF or a 1:20 dilution of MDP (equivalent to 0.3 μg of entrapped MDP) did not activate the AM. On the other hand, when MLV containing a 1:20 dilution of MAF and a 1:20 dilution of MDP (0.3 μg) were injected, significant *in situ* activation of AM occurred (Table 1).

These data indicate that the encapsulation of subthreshold doses of MAF (1:20 dilution) and MDP ($<$0.3 μg) within the same liposome leads to a significant ($p<0.001$) synergism in the *in situ* activation of AM.

The observed synergistic activation of liposome-entrapped MAF and MDP was dependent upon the delivery of both agents to the same macrophage. We base this conclusion upon the data shown in Table 1, which show that neither 2.5 μmol of MLV containing HBSS injected with a 1:20 dilution of unencapsulated MAF and a 1:20 dilution of unencapsulated MDP nor the injection of two separate liposome preparations (1.25 μmol of liposomes containing a 1:20 dilution of MAF admixed with 1.25 μmol of MLV containing a 1:20 dilution of MDP) activated AM

Table 1 Synergistic activation of tumoricidal properties in murine alveolar macrophages by free MAF or MDP and by liposomes containing MAF or MDP or both

Treatment of AM donors[a]	Percent AM-mediated cytolysis[b,c]
HBSS control	-7%
Free MAF (1:2)	2%
Free MDP (6.25 μg)	1%
Free MAF (1:2) and free MDP (6.25 μg)	-1%
MLV containing MAF (1:2)	48%[d]
MLV containing MAF (1:10)	26%[d]
MLV containing MAF (1:20)	-2%
MLV containing MAF (1:50)	-9%
MLV containing MDP (6.25 μg)	45%[d]
MLV containing MDP (0.62 μg)	41%[d]
MLV containing MDP (0.3 μg)	-1%
MLV containing MDP (0.12 μg)	-3%
MLV containing MAF (1:2) and MDP (6.25 μg)	42%[d]
MLV containing MAF (1:20) and MDP (0.3 μg)	44%[d]
MLV containing MAF (1:20) admixed with MLV containing MDP (0.3 μg)	1%
MLV containing HBSS suspended in MAF (1:20) and MDP (0.3 μg)	1%

[a] At least 3 mice per group. Inoculum dose was 0.2 ml. The injection consisted of either free material or of 2.5 μmol of MLV. AM were harvested 24 hours later.

[b] 10^5 AM were plated into 38 mm² culture wells. One hour later, the nonadherent cells were removed, and 10^4 [^{125}I] IUdR-labeled B16 melanoma cells were added. The values are mean cpm ± SD in viable cells of triplicate cultures terminated after 72 hours of cocultivation.

[c] The percent cytolysis was calculated by comparison with control AM obtained from mice injected with HBSS.

[d] $p<0.001$.

in situ.

Eradication of spontaneous established lung and lymph node metastases by the intravenous injection of liposomes containing MAF or MDP or both

The B16/BL6 melanoma line, which is syngeneic to C57BL/6 mice, was used to determine the effectiveness of liposome-encapsulated immunomodulators in the treatment of metastases. After implantation into the footpad, this tumor metastasizes to lymph nodes and the lungs in over 90% of recipient mice. C57BL/6 mice were given subcutaneous injections of 5×10^4 viable cells in 0.05 ml of HBSS. Four to five weeks later, the tumor-bearing legs and the popliteal lymph nodes were amputated. Intravenous injections of various liposome preparations began seven days after the surgical removal of the primary melanoma. At this time, spontaneous pulmonary and lymph node metastases were well established, with some metastases reaching 1 mm in diameter. Liposomes were injected twice weekly for four weeks.

Practically all the mice receiving HBSS alone and MLV suspended in encapsulated MAF and MDP had died by Day 90 of the experiment (Fig. 1). On the other hand, multiple intravenous injections of liposomes containing either a 1:2 dilution of MAF or 6.25 μg of MDP resulted in long-term survival (>250 days) of 27% of the animals (5/18). Neither liposomes containing MAF at a 1:20 dilution nor liposomes containing MDP at doses lower than 0.6 μg were effective. In contrast, mice treated with liposomes containing both MAF and MDP at individual subthreshold concentrations resulted in enhanced survival rates, with 50% of the mice alive at day 250 ($p=0.0007$).

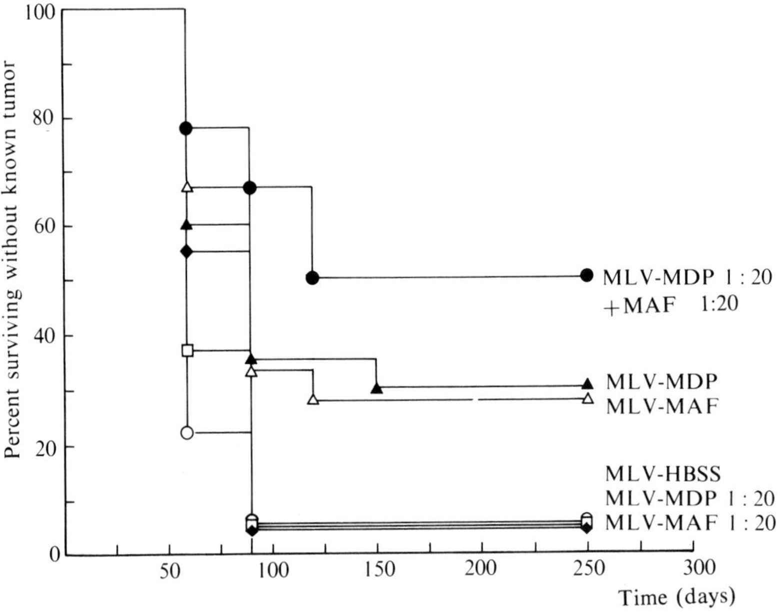

Fig. 1 Treatment of spontaneous melanoma metastases by the systemic administration of liposomes containing immunomodulators. Mice (18-20 mice/group) received two intravenous liposome treatments per week for 4 weeks (8 injections). The difference in survival between the group treated with liposomes containing MAF and MDP and other treatment groups is highly significant ($p<0.0007$).

Time (days)
+MAF 1:20

DISCUSSION

Advances in liposome technology have suggested a way in which immunomodulators might be used to activate macrophages *in vivo*. This involves encapsulating the agent in liposomes. There are several advantages to this approach: First, when injected intravenously, most liposomes localize in phagocytic cells of the reticuloendothelial system, cells responsible for the rapid clearance of particulate matter from the circulation. Second, encapsulation of macrophage activators within liposomes prevents their rapid degradation or clearance. Third, many macrophage-activating agents can be antigenic, and repeated systemic administrations can lead to undesirable side effects. Liposome encapsulation of agents can prevent such consequences.

Synergistic activation of the tumoricidal properties in AM by unencapsulated MAF and MDP has previously been shown to occur *in vitro*.[24] However, neither the intravenous injection of free MAF[18] nor of free MDP[21] led to systemic activation of macrophages *in situ*, whereas the intravenous administration of liposomes containing optimal doses of either MAF or MDP does generate AM tumoricidal properties *in vivo*[18, 21] (Table 1). On the other hand, intravenous administration of liposomes containing a 1:20 dilution of MAF or a 1:20 dilution of MDP did not activate mouse AM to become tumor cytotoxic, although when these two subthreshold doses of MAF and MDP were combined and encapsulated within the same MLV, significant *in situ* activation of AM occurred. Since neither diluted MAF nor diluted MDP entrapped in separate MLV activated AM *in situ*, the results obtained with their combination are evidence for synergistic rather than additive effects.

At the time systemic treatment of lung and lymph node metastasis with liposomes began, some spontaneous metastases were already visible. We deliberately postponed the start of treatment to Day 7 after surgery to allow examination of the hypotheses that MDP and MAF encapsulated within the same liposome would act synergistically to activate macrophages *in situ* and that this activation would increase the capacity of macrophages to destroy tumor cells, thus increasing long-term survival of the mice. Indeed, the results shown in Table 1 support these hypotheses. The intravenous injections of liposomes containing an optimal dose of MAF or MDP led to regression of metastases in at least 33% of the mice treated. Liposomes containing either diluted MAF or diluted MDP had no such effects. Furthermore, the intravenous injections of liposomes containing subthreshold amounts of both MAF and MDP were associated with a significant increase in long-term survival of mice (9 / 18,

$p = 0.0007$).

The mechanisms responsible for the regression of established metastases after the systemic administration of liposomes containing MAF or MDP or both probably involved the activation of macrophages to become tumoricidal. Several lines of evidence tend to support this conclusion.[21] First, administration of macrophage-activating agents encapsulated within liposomes that are not retained in the lung fails to activate lung macrophages and produces no regression of lung metastases. Second, the pretreatment of tumor-bearing animals with agents that are toxic for macrophages (silica, carageenan, hyperchlorinated drinking water) before systemic therapy with liposome-encapsulated lymphokines abrogates the response to liposome therapy, and such animals rapidly die of metastatic disease. Third, intravenous injection of macrophages activated *in vitro* by incubation with liposomes containing MAF effects a reduction in metastatic burden comparable to that achieved by systemic administration of liposome-encapsulated activators.

Although these data strongly suggested that tumoricidal macrophages were involved in the destruction of metastases in this tumor system, their precise role remained unclear. Direct evidence that tumoricidal macrophages are the effector cells responsible for the destruction of established metastases in mice treated systemically with liposome-entrapped MDP was recently obtained.[22] Morphological and functional analysis of macrophages isolated from pulmonary metastases of mice given intravenous injections of liposomes containing an MDP derivative, muramyl tripeptide phosphatidylethanolamine, showed that macrophages containing phagocytosed liposomes infiltrate and localize within pulmonary metastases. Furthermore, once localized, macrophages that have engulfed liposomes containing MDP, but not macrophages that have engulfed liposomes containing a placebo, were rendered cytotoxic against the metastatic tumor cells.

Although the initial results reported from our laboratory regarding the use of macrophages for destruction of metastases are encouraging, it is unlikely that this approach could serve for treatment of large tumor burdens. For example, in a murine melanoma system, the tumor burden in spontaneous metastases that are amenable to treatment by macrophages has been estimated to be less than 10^7 cells. Tumor burdens frequently exceed this level before the disease is even diagnosed. For this reason, potential therapeutic regimens designated to stimulate host immunity must be used in combination with other treatment modalities such as chemotherapy in order to first reduce the tumor burden; the activated macrophages can then lyse tumor cells that have survived destruction by other agents. Nonetheless, the demonstration that the encapsulation of two distinct immunomodulators in the same liposome can lead to synergistic activation of macrophages *in situ* is important. Although this is the first demonstration of such synergism, it suggests that examination of synergism between other biological response modifiers may be rewarding.

REFERENCES

1. Poste, G. and Fidler, I.J. (1979): The pathogenesis of cancer metastasis. *Nature, 283*, 139.
2. Fidler, I.J. and Hart, I.R. (1982): Biological diversity in metastatic neoplasms: Origins and implications. *Science*, *217*, 998.
3. Fidler, I.J. and Kripke, M.L. (1977): Metastasis results from preexisting variant cells within a malignant tumor. *Science*, *197*, 893.
4. Talmadge, J.E., Wolman, S.R. and Fidler, I.J. (1982): Evidence for the clonal origin of spontaneous metastases. *Science*, *217*, 361.
5. Cifone, M.A. and Fidler, I.J. (1981): Increasing metastatic potential is associated with increasing genetic instability of clones isolated from murine neoplasms. *Proc. Natl. Acad. Sci. U.S.A.*, *78*, 6949.
6. Fidler, I.J. and Poste, G. (1982): Macrophage-mediated destruction of malignant tumor cells and new strategies for the therapy of metastatic disease. *Springer Semin. Immunopathol.*, *5*, 161.
7. Fidler, I.J., Robin, R.O. and Poste, G. (1978): *In vitro* tumoricidal activity of macrophages against virus-transformed lines with temperature-dependent transformed phenotypic characteristics. *Cell Immunol.*, *38*, 131.
8. Chedid, L., Carelli, L. and Audibert, F. (1979): Recent developments concerning muramyl dipeptide, a synthetic immunoregulating molecule. *J. Reticuloendothel. Soc.*, *26*, 631.
9. Kleinerman, E.S., Erickson, K.L., Schroit, A.J., Fogler, W.E. and Fidler, I.J. (1983): Activation of tumoricidal properties in human blood monocytes by liposomes containing lipophilic muramyl tripeptide. *Cancer Res.*, *43*, 2010.
10. Sone, S. and Fidler, I.J. (1981): *In vitro* activation of tumoricidal properties in rat alveolar macrophages by synthetic muramyl dipeptide encapsulated in liposomes. *Cell. Immunol.*, *57*, 42.
11. Fidler, I.J. and Raz, A. (1981): The induction of tumoricidal capacities in mouse and rat macrophages by lymphokines. In: *Lymphokines, Vol. 3*, p. 345. Editor: E. Pick. Academic Press, New York.
12. Fidler, I.J. (1984): The MAF dilemma. *Lymphokine Res.*, *3*, 51.
13. Allison, A.C. (1979): Mode of action of immunological adjuvants. *J. Reticuloendothel. Soc.*, *26*, 619.
14. Lederer, E. (1980): Synthetic immunostimulants derived from the bacterial cell wall. *J. Med. Chem.*, *23*, 819.
15. Parant, M., Parant, F., Chedid, L., Yapo, A., Petit, J.F. and Lederer, E. (1979): Fate of the synthetic immunoadjuvant, muramyl dipeptide (^{14}C-labeled) in the mouse. *Int. J. Immunopharmacol.*, *1*, 35.
16. Fidler, I.J., Raz, A., Fogler, W.E., Kirsh, R., Bugelski, P. and Poste, G. (1980): The design of liposomes to improve delivery of macrophage-augmenting agents to alveolar macrophages. *Cancer Res.*, *40*, 4460.
17. Schroit, A.J. and Fidler, I.J. (1982): Effects of liposome structure and lipid composition on the activation of the tumoricidal properties of macrophages by

liposomes containing muramyl dipeptide. *Cancer Res.*, *42*, 1616.
18. Fidler, I.J. and Fogler, W.E. (1982): Activation of tumoricidal properties in macrophages by lymphokines encapsulated in liposomes. *Lymphokine Res.*, *1*, 73.
19. Poste, G., Kirsh, R. and Fidler, I.J. (1979): Cell surface receptors for lymphokines. *Cell. Immunol.*, *44*; 71.
20. Poste, G., Kirsh, R., Fogler, W.E. and Fidler, I.J. (1979): Activation of tumoricidal properties in mouse macrophages by lymphokines encapsulated in liposome. *Cancer Res.*, *39*, 881.
21. Fidler, I.J., Barnes, Z., Fogler, W.E., Kirsh, R., Bugelski, P. and Poste, G.(1982): Involvement of macrophages in the eradication of established metastases following intravenous injection of liposomes containing macrophage activators. *Cancer Res.*, *42*, 496.
22. Key, M.E., Talmadge, J.E., Fogler, W.E., Bucana, C. and Fidler, I.J. (1982): Isolation of tumoricidal macrophages from lung melanoma metastases of mice treated systemically with liposomes containing a lipophilic derivative of muramyl dipeptide. *J. Natl. Cancer Inst.*, *69*, 1189.
23. Fidler, I.J. (1981): The *in situ* induction of tumoricidal activity in alveolar macrophages by liposomes containing muramyl dipeptide is a thymus-independent process. *J. Immunol.*, *127*, 1719.
24. Sone, S. and Fidler, I.J. (1980): Synergistic activation by lymphokines and muramyl dipeptide of tumoricidal properties in rat alveolar macrophages. *J. Immunol.*, *125*, 2454.
25. Schroit, A.J., Hart, I.R., Madsen, J. and Fidler, I.J. (1983): Selective delivery of drugs encapsulated in liposomes: Natural targeting to macrophages involved in various disease states. *J. Biol. Response Modifiers*, *2*, 97.
26. Hart, I.R. (1979): The selection and characterization of an invasive variant of the B16 melanoma. *Am. J. Pathol.*, *97*, 587.
27. Thomas, D.G., Breslow, N. and Gart, J.J. (1977): Trend and homogeneity analyses of proportions and life table data. *Comput. Biomed. Res.*, *10*, 373.

Anti-metastatic effect of tumor necrosis factor (TNF)

Yoshiro Niitsu, Naoki Watanabe, Hisao Sone, Hiroshi Neda, Naofumi Yamauchi and Ichiro Urushizaki

SUMMARY

The anti-metastatic effect of tumor necrosis factor (TNF) on artificial metastasis by B-16 melanoma cells and spontaneous metastasis by Lewis lung carcinoma cells was investigated. The results obtained were as follows:

1) In the experiment on artificial metastasis, tumor necrosis serum (TNS) was administered either 20 minutes or 2 days after B-16 melanoma cell injection. In both cases, TNF showed a high anti-metastatic effect (99%) compared with the control.

2) In the experiment on spontaneous metastasis by Lewis lung carcinoma cells, TNF showed a 60% anti-metastatic effect and the weight of the primary tumor also regressed to 40%.

3) TNF injection did not cause histological changes in normal tissues detectable by microscopic examination.

The above results seem to confirm a highly preventive effect of TNF on metastasis.

INTRODUCTION

Tumor necrosis factor (TNF) was found by Carswell[1] in 1975 in the serum of mice which were treated with BCG and endotoxin. It exerts a cytostatic or cytotoxic effect on tumor cells *in vitro* regardless of the animal species,[2,3,4] and thus is expected to be a biological antitumor substance. The *in vivo* effects of TNF have been described as necrosis of the primary focus of transplanted tumors,[1] and regression of tumors.

In the present study, the anti-metastatic effect of TNF on artificial metastasis by B-16 melanoma cells and spontaneous metastasis by Lewis lung carcinoma cells was examined.

MATERIALS AND METHODS

Induction of TNF

Tumor necrosis serum (TNS) was prepared as follows:
Propionibacterium acnes, 1.5 mg/head, was injected intraperitoneally into Balb/c nu/+ mice as the priming agent. Ten days after the injection, 10 μg/head of lipopolysaccharide (LPS, *E. colli* 055:B5, Difco) was injected at the same site; 1.5 to 2 hours thereafter, whole blood was recovered to isolate TNS.

Assay of TNF activity

L-929 cells, B-16 melanoma cells and Lewis lung carcinoma cells were used as the target cells for the determination of TNF activity. The assay was performed by morphological microassay.[6] TNF activity was express ed by the dilution of TNS showing 50% cytotoxicity.

Examination of TNF clearance from blood

Residual TNF activity in the serum was determined 10, 20, 30, 40 and 60 minutes after injecting 200 μl TNS into the caudal vein of C57BL/6 mice.

Artificial metastasis by B-16 melanoma cells

B-16 melanoma cells ($N=1 \times 10^6$) were injected into the caudal vein; 200 μl of TNS or normal mouse serum (NMS) was injected into the same site 20 minutes later (Exp. 1) or 2 days later (Exp. 2). Three weeks after the injection, pulmonary surface nodules were counted (Fig. 1).

Spontaneous metastasis by Lewis lung carcinoma cells

Lewis lung carcinoma cells ($N=7.5 \times 10^5$) were inoculated into the footpads of C57BL/6 mice, and 50 μl of TNS or NMS was injected intravenously every other day for 7 days from the 5th day, (four times in total). On the 12th day after tumor inoculation, the forelimb of each mouse (including the primary tumor) was amputated. The pulmonary surface nodules were counted on the 21st day (Fig. 2).

RESULTS

Cytotoxic activity of TNF against B-16 melanoma cells and Lewis lung carcinoma cells

The cytotoxic effect of TNF on B-16 melanoma cells and Lewis lung carcinoma cells was examined *in vitro* by a morphological microassay (Table 1).

Both tumor cells showed sensitivity to TNF : TNS showed 50% cytotoxicity for B-16 melanoma cells when diluted ×62 and for Lewis lung carcinoma cells when diluted ×46.

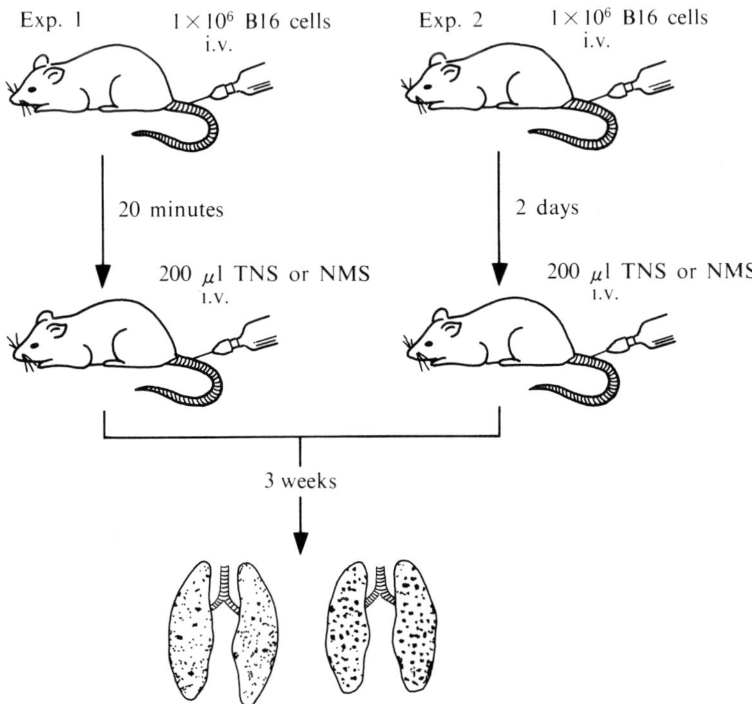

Fig. 1 Protocol of experiment on artificial metastasis by B-16 melanoma cells.

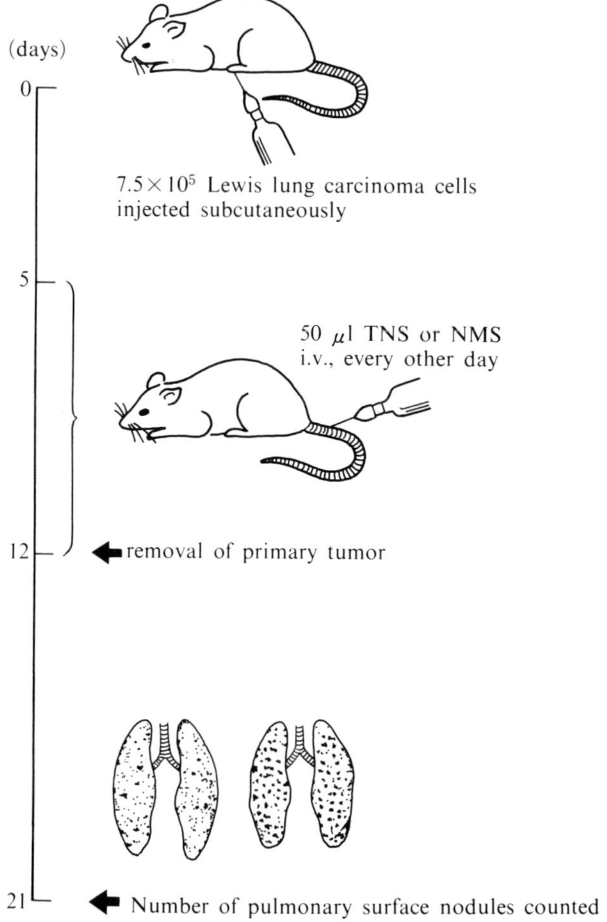

Fig. 2 Protocol of experiment on spontaneous metastasis by Lewis lung carcinoma cells.

Table 1 Cytotoxicity of TNF against B-16 melanoma and Lewis lung carcinoma cells

	Dilution of TNS for 50% cytotoxicity (mean ± SD)
B-16 melanoma cell	$\times 62 \pm 7$
Lewis lung carcinoma cell	$\times 46 \pm 4$

Clearance of TNF from blood

After intravenous injection of TNF, the half life was approximately 33 minutes. At least 80% of the injected TNF remained in the blood for 20

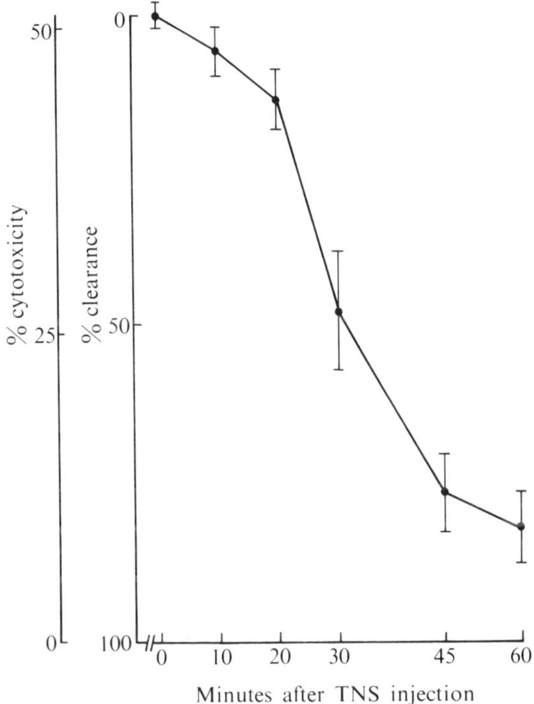

Fig. 3 Clearance of TNF in C57BL/6 mouse.

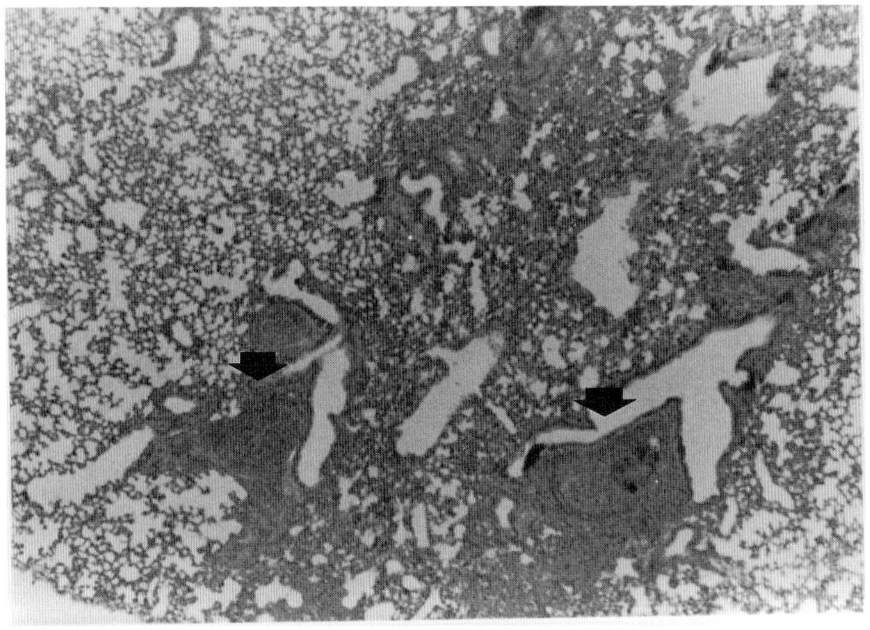

Fig. 4 Histology of lung 2 days after intravenous injection of B-16 melanoma cells showing micrometastasis (arrow). HE × 100

minutes after the injection (Fig. 3).

Induction of micrometastasis after intravenous injection of B-16 melanoma cells

The lung was resected on the lst, 2 nd and 3rd days after the intravenous injection of B-16 melanoma cells. Resected lung was examined by means of an optical microscope after HE staining. It was found that the formation of micrometastases had already begun 2 days after the injection of tumor cells (Fig. 4).

Anti-metastatic effect of TNF on artificial metastasis

TNS was administered at two points after the induction of artificial metastasis: in Exp. 1, it was administered immediately (20 minutes) after the implantation of tumor cells; in Exp. 2, it was administered when micrometastases had formed, i.e., 2 days after the injection of B-16 melanoma cells.

In Exp. 1, the number of metastatic foci was 88.4 ± 77.5 (mean ± SD) in the control group, and 0.8 ± 0.8 in the TNF-treated group, showing a dramatic suppressive effect of TNF on metastasis. In 2 out of 6 TNS-treated mice, no pulmonary metastatic focus was found (Table 2).

In Exp. 2, the number of metastatic foci was 80.5 ± 77.8 in the NMS-administered group, and 0.3 ± 0.5 in the TNS group, showing complete suppression of metastasis. In 4 out of 6 TNS-treated mice, no pulmonary metastatic focus was seen (Table 2).

Histological pictures of lung obtained in this experiment are shown in Fig. 5.

Table 2 Inhibitory effect of TNF on pulmonary metastasis after intravenous injection of B-16 melanoma cells

	Period of TNF challenge	No. of pulmonary surface nodules (mean±SD)	Incidence of pulmonary metastasis
Exp. 1			
Normal mouse serum	20 min after	88.4±77.5	6/6
Tumor necrosis serum	〃	0.8±0.8	4/6
Exp. 2			
Normal mouse serum	2 days after	80.5±77.8	6/6
Tumor necrosis serum	〃	0.3±0.5	2/6

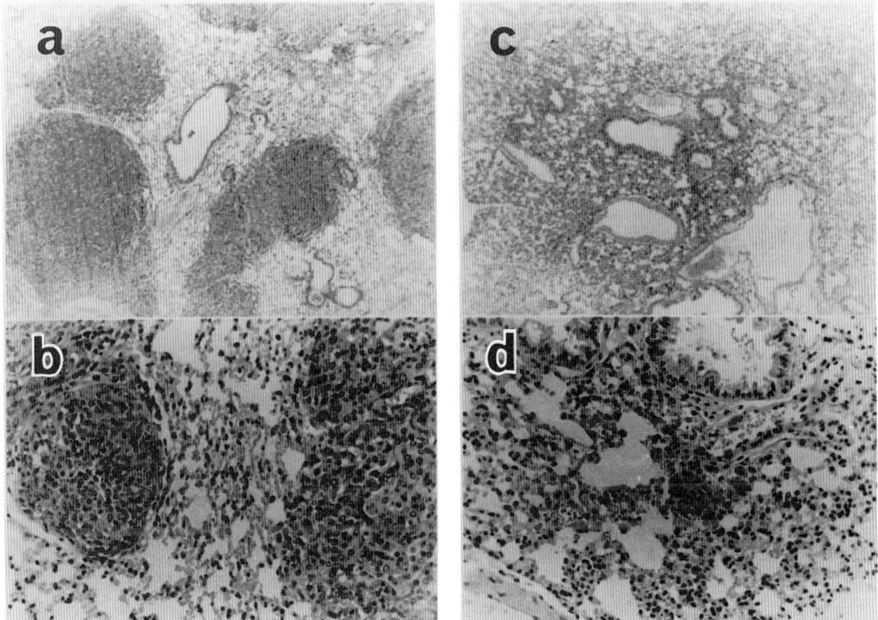

Fig. 5 Histology of mouse lung treated with NMS (a, b) and TNS (c, d) 3 weeks after intravenous injection of B-16 melanoma cells. HE. (a) (c) ×100, (b) (d) ×200

Typical metastatic foci are shown side by side in the NMS-administered control group, but only one metastatic focus is shown at the center in the TNS-administered group. No necrotic features or inflammatory cell infiltration are observed in the lung tissue.

Effect of TNF on hepatic tissue

In order to examine the effect of TNF on normal tissues, the hepatic tissue of the mice in the above-mentioned artificial metastasis experiment was examined histologically (Fig. 6).

No hepatic necrosis or infiltration of inflammatory cells was seen in the TNS-administered group.

Anti-metastatic effect of TNF on spontaneous metastasis

In the spontaneous metastatic experiment using Lewis lung carcinoma cells, there were 35.7 ± 12.9 metastatic foci in the NMS-administered control group, against 14.5 ± 8.9 in the TNS-administered group, revealing approximately 60% suppression of metastasis by TNS (Table 3).

The primary tumor of the resected forelimb was 3.1 g on average in the control group, and 1.2 g in the TNS-administered group, demonstrating 60% regression.

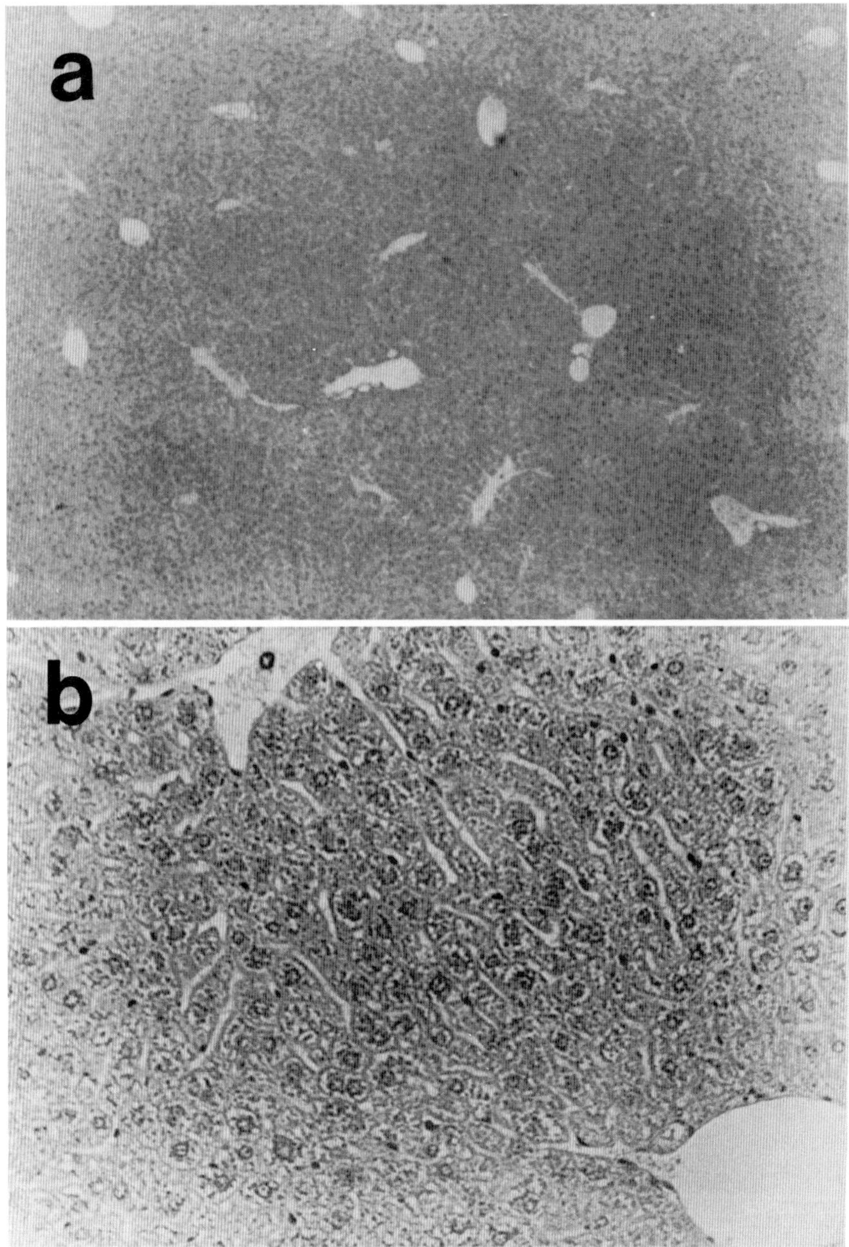

Fig. 6 Histology of liver of mouse treated with TNS. HE. (a) ×40, (b) ×200

Table 3 Inhibitory effect of TNF on pulmonary metastasis in mice bearing Lewis lung carcinoma cells

	No. of pulmonary surface nodules (mean ± SD)	Incidence of pulmonary metastasis	Tumor weight (mean, g)
Normal mouse serum	35.7 ± 12.9	10/10	3.06
Tumor necrosis serum	14.5 ± 8.9	7/9	1.21

DISCUSSION

The following methods for determining TNF activity *in vitro* have been used previously: morphological microassay using L cells as the target cell,[6] ^{51}Cr cytotoxic release assay,[6] and *in vivo* examination of the degree of necrosis of transplanted tumors[1] and of regression of tumors.[5]

However, the *in vivo* methods used so far all use the naked eye to judge the degree of necrosis. These methods lack objective quantitative evaluation, and are also unable to determine accurately whether or not the necrosis is caused by the direct cytotoxic effect of TNF on the tumor cells. Since TNF causes central necrosis, some additional action involving blood vessels may be suggested. In the present study, artificial metastasis and spontaneous metastasis were used for the investigation of the anti-metastatic effect of TNF.

In the artificial metastatic system, two experimental systems were used; that is, TNS was administered at two points: at the 20th minute and on the 2nd day after the administration of tumor cells. Marked suppression of pulmonary metastasis of tumors was observed after only a single administration of TNS. According to Fidler et al.,[7] approximately 90% of intravenously administered B-16 melanoma cells implant in the lung within 20 to 60 minutes of injection, while approximately 3% of the cells remain in the blood.

Since the half life of TNF clearance from blood was approximately 33 minutes, TNF administered 20 minutes after the injection of B-16 melanoma cells might be expected to be more effective on the lung-implanted tumor cells as well as on the residual tumor cells in the circulation.

Micrometastasis formation was already demonstrated 2 days after the administration of tumor cells; TNF administered at this stage showed a marked inhibitory effect on pulmonary metastasis, suggesting a prophylactic effect by TNF as well as a suppressive one. TNS was particularly effective against established micrometastases; therefore the mechanism of TNF activity may involve not only a direct effect by TNF but also some defense function of the host.

On the other hand, in the spontaneous metastatic system using Lewis lung carcinoma cells, regression of the primary tumor was seen in addition to suppression of pulmonary metastasis. The effect was slightly weaker (approximately 40% less) than that in the artificial metastasis. The reason may be that the tumor cells were administered intravenously into the caudal vein in the artificial metastatic system, whereas tumor cells may be liberated continuously from the primary foci in the spontaneous metastatic system. The sensitivity of Lewis lung carcinoma cells to TNF *in vitro* was lower than that of B-16 melanoma cells. In addition, the dose of TNS was lower in the spontaneous metastatic system.

The results obtained from both experimental systems confirmed that TNF exerted some cytotoxic effect on all the processes of tumor cell development including metastasis. Histopathologically, no cytotoxic effect of TNF was demonstrated other than its anti-metastatic action. However, these results apply only to the sensitive cell line used in the present experiment; needless to say, the result cannot be generalized to other tumor cell systems. Further studies will be needed to determine the efficacy of TNF against other types of tumor.

REFERENCES

1. Carswell, E.A., Old, L.J., Kassel, R.L., Green, S., Fiore, N. and Williamson, B. (1975): An endotoxin-induced serum factor that causes necrosis of tumors. *Proc. Acad. Sci. U.S.A.*, *72*, 3666.
2. Helson, L., Green, S., Carswell, E. and Old, L.J. (1975): Effect of tumor necrosis factor on cultured human melanoma cells. *Nature*, *258*, 731.
3. Old, L.J. (1976): Tumor necrosis factor. *Clin. Bull.*, *6*, 118.
4. Matthews, N. and Watkins, J.F. (1979): Tumor-necrosis factor from the rabbit. I. *Br. J. Cancer*, *38*, 302.
5. Helson, L., Holson, C. and Green, S. (1979): Effects of murine tumor necrosis factor on heterotransplanted human tumors. *Exp. Cell. Biol.*, *47*, 53.
6. Ruff, M.R. and Gifford, G.E. (1981): Rabbit tumor necrosis factor: Mechanism of action. *Infect. Immun.*, *31*, 380.
7. Fidler, I.J. (1970): Metastasis: Quantitative analysis of distribution and fate of tumor emboli labeled with ^{125}I-5-Iodo-2′-deoxyuridine. *J. Natl. Cancer Inst.*, *45*, 773.

Enhancement of experimental pulmonary metastasis of B16 melanoma in mice with granulocytosis

Makoto Ishikawa, Yutaka Koga, Masuo Hosokawa and Hiroshi Kobayashi

SUMMARY

The effect of granulocytosis on pulmonary metastasis of malignant melanoma in mice was investigated. When a methylcholanthrene-induced fibrosarcoma (BMT-11) was transplanted subcutaneously into syngeneic C57BL/6 mice, a progressive increase in the number of polymorphonuclear leukocytes (PMN) (more than $10^5/mm^3$) was observed as the tumors grew. The PMN from these tumor-bearing mice showed the same degree of cytostatic activity against B16 melanoma cells as those from normal mice. However, the number of pulmonary colonies of B16 melanoma and the lung retention of intravenously-injected radiolabeled melanoma cells were greater in mice bearing BMT-11, i.e., with granulocytosis, than those in normal mice. On the other hand, neither in BMT-11-bearing mice treated with the antileukemic drug, busulfan, which reduces the number of white blood cells, nor in mice bearing another fibrosarcoma which did not induce granulocytosis, was there a significant difference in the number of B16 cells retained compared with normal mice. These results suggest that increased numbers of PMN in the peripheral circulation cause enhancement of metastasis, although these PMN exhibit tumoricidal activity *in vitro*.

INTRODUCTION

Many reports have been published that focus on the antitumor activity of T-lymphocytes, natural killer cells or macrophages, yet relatively little attention has been directed toward polymorphonuclear leukocytes (PMN). There is increasing evidence, however, suggesting that PMN play

Table 1 Granulocytosis and splenomegaly in C57BL/6 mice bearing transplanted BMT-11 tumor or its clones

Clone[a]	White blood cell count[b] (No./mm^3)[c]	Spleen weight[b] (g)[c]
BMT-11		
parent line	179,300±26,000	0.73±0.10
clone 1	202,900±24,900	0.74±0.06
clone 3	186,600±25,900	0.76±0.13
clone 4	166,000±13,600	0.72±0.07
clone 5	140,000±14,600	0.49±0.03
clone 7	140,300±14,000	0.67±0.05
clone 9	307,200±18,000	0.74±0.05
clone 10	125,000±17,700	0.49±0.05
Normal[d]	9,300± 700	0.07±0.01

[a] Culture cells of the BMT-11 parent line or its clones (2×10^5 cells) were transplanted subcutaneously.
[b] White blood cell count and spleen weight were measured when tumors were more than 20 mm in diameter.
[c] Mean±SE.
[d] Value obtained from ten C57BL/6 mice.

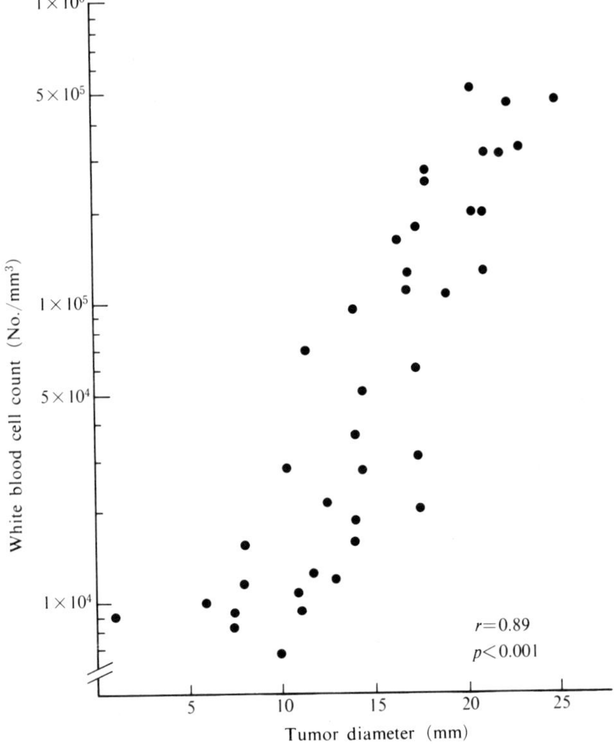

Fig. 1 Correlation between white blood cell count and tumor diameter in C57BL/6 mice bearing BMT-11 cl-9 fibrosarcoma. n=5.

a role in the host's natural mechanisms of resistance against neoplastic cells, such as a direct tumor cytotoxicity,[1,2] antibody- or lectin-dependent cellular cytotoxicity,[3,4] and the cytotoxicity induced by some BRMs.[5–7]

Recently, we found a marked degree of granulocytosis in C57BL/6 mice bearing transplantable fibrosarcoma, and this finding prompted us to investigate the function of PMN. This paper reports that these abnormally increased PMN may enhance pulmonary metastasis, even if the activity of the PMN *in vitro* is tumoricidal.

METHODS AND RESULTS

Granulocytosis in mice bearing BMT-11 fibrosarcoma

As is shown in Table 1, the inoculation of culture cells of the BMT-11 parent line and all its seven clones into C57BL/6 mice was accompanied by leukocytosis and splenomegaly; of them, clone 9 (BMT-11 cl-9) induced the most marked increase in the peripheral white blood cell (WBC) count. A linear relationship between the WBC count and tumor size was found (Fig. 1), and the differential counts revealed that PMN accounted almost completely for the increase in WBC (Fig. 2). This granulocytosis in tumor-bearing mice is similar to that reported in previous studies.[8–12]

Cytostatic activity of PMN

The cytostatic activity against B16 melanoma cells of PMN obtained from BMT-11 cl-9 tumor-bearing mice with granulocytosis, or from normal mice, is shown in Table 2. The PMN isolated from four sources (either peripheral blood or proteose-peptone-stimulated peritoneal exudate cells) exhibited cytostatic activity, and there were no large differences in the degree of the reactivity shown by the groups. In this growth inhibition assay system, thymocytes obtained from normal mice did not show any cytostatic activity.

Experimental metastasis of B16 melanoma in BMT-11 cl-9 tumor-bearing mice

In experimental systems where tumor cells are reinoculated into tumor-bearing animals, most reports, with one exception,[13] have shown that subsequent metastatic tumor growth is less in tumor-bearing animals than in normal hosts; this resistance against metastasis is called concomitant immunity (see review by Gorelik[14]). To exclude the effect of concomitant

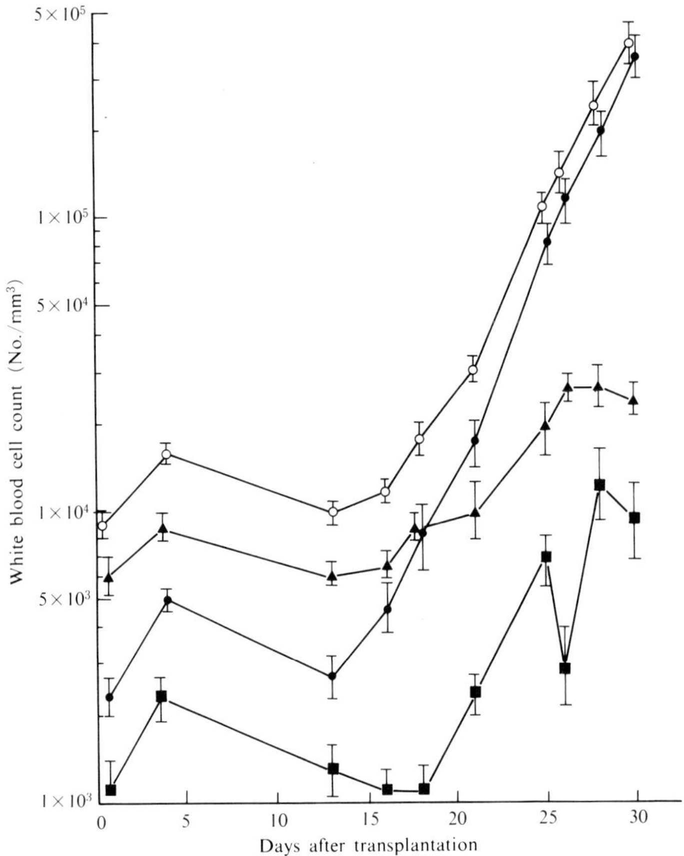

Fig. 2 Changes in the white blood cell and differential counts in C57BL/6 mice after transplantation with 2×15^5 BMT-11 cl-9 cells on Day 0. Total white blood cells (○); PMN (●); lymphocytes (▲); monocytes (■). n=5. Means±SEM.

immunity, antigenically different B16 melanoma cells were used for the intravenous challenge into BMT-11 cl-9 tumor-bearing mice. Intact mice were transplanted subcutaneously with 2×10^5 BMT-11 cl-9 tumor cells; 24 days later, these mice were challenged intravenously with 3.3×10^4 B16 melanoma cells. The mice bearing BMT-11 cl-9 tumor (mean WBC count: 153,100 at B16 injection, 474,700 at sacrifice), developed significantly more lung colonies than untreated controls (mean WBC count: 8,900 at B16 injection, 9,400 at sacrifice, Table 3). No extrapulmonary metastasis of B16 melanoma occurred in this experiment.

Table 2 Cytostatic activities of polymorphonuclear leukocytes (PMN) obtained from C57BL/6 mice against B16 melanoma cells

Effectors[a]	Donor of effectors	% growth inhibition[b] at E:T ratio[c]				
		50:1	25:1	12:1	6:1	3:1
Peripheral PMN	BMT-11 cl-9 bearing	94	75	67	42	9
Peritoneal PMN[d]	〃	93	83	57	16	9
Peripheral PMN	Normal	90	40	30	11	2
Peritoneal PMN[d]	〃	98	92	69	29	8
Thymocytes	Normal	16	0	-18	-28	-24

[a] Percentage decrease in [^{3}H]TdR uptake in a 24-hour assay.
[b] Purified PMN suspensions were obtained by the use of a Ficoll-Hypaque gradient (specific gravity: 1.077).
[c] E:T, effector:target
[d] Peritoneal PMN were isolated from proteose-peptone-stimulated peritoneal exudate cells.

Table 3 Experimental metastasis of intravenously injected B16 melanoma cells in C57BL/6 mice bearing BMT-11 cl-9 fibrosarcoma

Mice	No. of mice	WBC count (No./mm^3)[c] at B16 injection[b] (on Day 24)	WBC count (No./mm^3)[c] at sacrifice (on Day 37)	No. of pulmonary colonies per mouse	(mean ± SD)	Extrapulmonary metastases
BMT-11 cl-9 -bearing[a]	7	153,100±47,400	474,700±42,700	21[d], 21, 34, 38, 57, 58, 72	(43±20[e])	0/7
Normal	9	8,900±600	9,400±800	0, 1, 2, 4, 6, 6, 7, 10, 30	(7±9[e])	0/9

[a] BMT-11 cl-9 tumor cells (2×10^5) were transplanted s.c. on Day 0.
[b] 3.3×10^4 cells injected i.v.
[c] Mean±SE.
[d] Spontaneous metastatic nodules of BMT-11 cl-9 fibrosarcoma were found in this mouse only.
[e] Statistically significant ($p<0.005$).

Retention of radiolabeled B16 melanoma cells

The lung retention of ^{125}IUdR-labeled B16 cells was also determined 24 hours after intravenous injection (Fig. 3). Retention of B16 cells 20 days after BMT-11 cl-9 inoculation was three times greater than that in non-tumor-bearing control mice while 30 days after inoculation it was seven times greater ($p<0.001$). Treatment with the antileukemic drug, busulfan (BU), however, abrogated this enhancement of B16 retention (Fig. 3, Exp. I). From our preliminary experiment, BU administration had been found not to affect the growth of BMT-11 tumors but to decrease the WBC count, which reaches a minimal level approximately 5 days after drug administration. It seems unlikely that the decrease in the number of

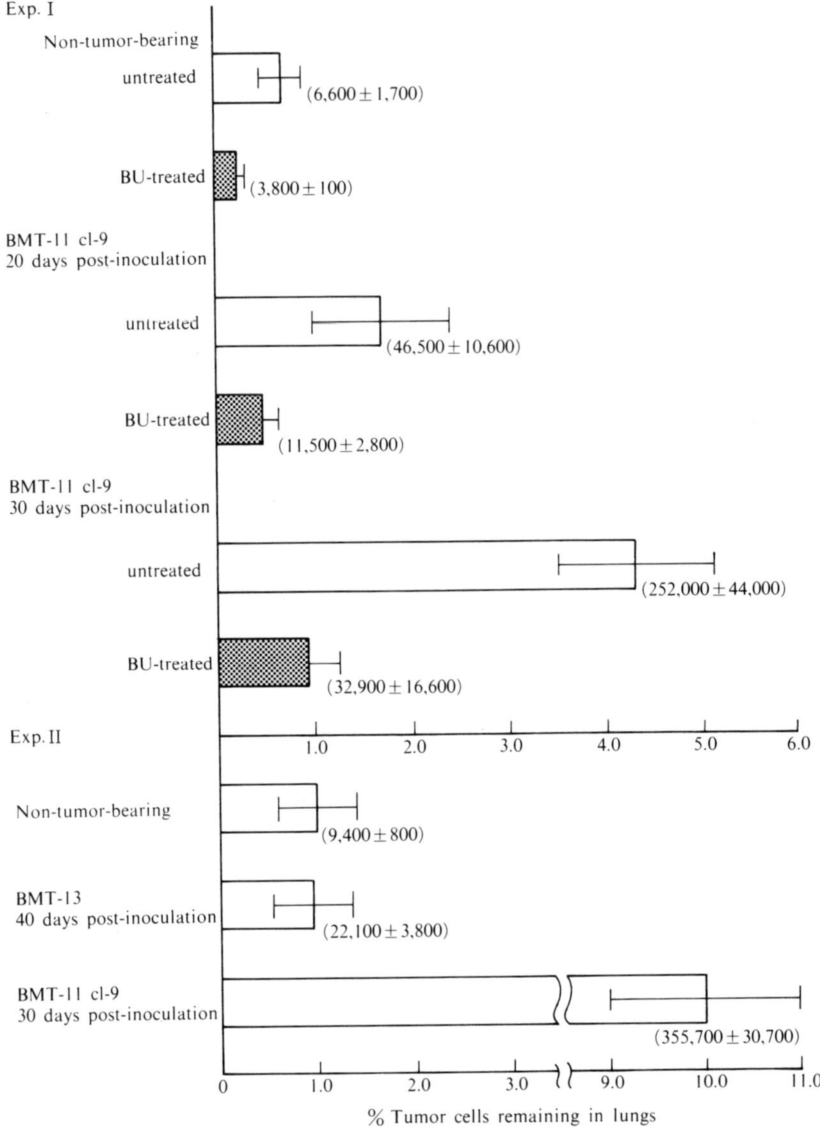

Fig. 3 Percentage of radioactivity retained in the lungs 24 hours after i.v. injection of 10^5 ^{125}IUdR-labeled B16 cells. Bars indicate standard errors of means. Busulfan (BU, 50 mg/kg, i.g.) was administered 5 days before the B16 cells. Figures in brackets indicate WBC counts (mean ± SE). n = 5 to 10 in each group.

tumor cells retained in BMT-11 cl-9 tumor-bearing mice produced by BU treatment was due to its therapeutic effect against B16 melanoma, since BU treatment did not show any inhibitory effect on B16 lung colonization (data not shown). When radiolabeled B16 cells were injected into mice inoculated 40 days previously with another fibrosarcoma, BMT-13, which did not induce granulocytosis, the retention of B16 cells was no different from that in control mice (Fig. 3, Exp. II).

DISCUSSION

This study demonstrated that tumor-bearing mice with granulocytosis developed more experimental pulmonary metastases than normal mice, although increased PMN in tumor-bearing mice showed tumoricidal activity (cytostasis) *in vitro*. This enhancement of metastasis was also identified by a decrease in the clearance from the lung of intravenously injected radiolabeled tumor cells, which is a system known to correlate with subsequent outgrowth of pulmonary tumor nodules.[15] These results suggest that the increased numbers of circulating PMN could be responsible for the enhancement of metastasis, and this phenomenon might be effected at an early stage of metastasis formation such as the attachment of cells to vascular endothelium and intravascular survival of tumor cells rather than at extravasation or subsequent tumor growth. Although the mechanism of this enhancement is still unclear, there are some possible explanations: 1) granulocytosis might influence the surface area of vascular endothelium available for adhesive interactions, or rheological factors such as the blood viscosity and the number of cells in circulation; 2) the high level of PMN might tend to form emboli with tumor cells which are similar to the emboli which form with lymphocytes and tumor cells,[16,17] these embolized tumor cells being arrested and surviving better to yield subsequent metastasis.

In addition, this experimental system may serve as a useful new tool for research into hematopoiesis, into the production of the colony-stimulating-factor by tumors and into the interaction between PMN and cancer cells, since the C57BL/6 mouse strain is widely used in experimental studies.

REFERENCES

1. Fisher, B. and Saffer, F.A. (1978): Tumor cell cytotoxicity by granulocytes from peripheral blood of tumor-bearing mice. *J. Natl. Cancer Inst.*, *60*, 687.
2. Korec, S., Herberman, R.B., Dean, J.H. and Cannon, G.B. (1980): Cytostasis of tumor cell lines by human granulocytes. *Cell. Immunol.*, *53*, 104.

3. Clark, R. and Klebanoff, S.J. (1977): Studies on the mechanism of antibody-dependent polymorphonuclear leukocyte-mediated cytotoxicity. *J. Immunol.*, *119*, 1413.
4. Tsunawaki, S., Oshima, H., Mizuno, D. and Yamazaki, M. (1983): Induction of polymorphonuclear leukocyte-mediated cytolysis by wheat germ agglutinin and antitumor antibody. *Gann*, *74*, 258.
5. Glaves, D. (1983): Role of polymorphonuclear leukocytes in the pulmonary clearance of arrested cancer cells. *Invasion Metastasis*, *3*, 160.
6. Inoue, T. and Sendo, F. (1983): *In vitro* induction of cytotoxic polymorphonuclear leukocytes by supernatant from a concanavalin A-stimulated spleen cell culture. *J. Immunol.*, *131*, 3508.
7. Watabe, S., Sendo. F., Kimura, S. and Arai, S. (1984): Activation of cytotoxic polymorphonuclear leukocytes by *in vivo* administration of a streptococcal preparation, OK-432. *J. Natl. Cancer Inst.*, *72*, 1365.
8. Bateman, L.C. (1951): Leukemoid reaction to transplanted mouse tumors. *J. Natl. Cancer Inst.*, *11*, 671.
9. Delmonte, L., Liebelt, A.G. and Liebelt, R.A. (1966): Granulopoiesis and thrombopoiesis in mice bearing transplanted mammary cancer. *Cancer Res.*, *26*, 149.
10. Kodama, T., Sendo, F. and Kobayashi, H. (1974): Leukemoid reaction in BALB/c mice bearing transplanted tumors. *Cancer Res.*, *34*, 176.
11. Lan, S., Rettura, G., Levenson, S.M. and Seifter, E. (1981): Granulopoiesis associated with the C3HBA tumor in mice. *J. Natl. Cancer Inst.*, *67*, 1135.
12. Bessho, M., Hirashima, K., Ando, K., Nara, N. and Momoi, H. (1984): Hemopoietic stem cell kinetics in mice bearing CSF-producing fibrosarcoma. *Acta Haematol. Jpn.*, *47*, 21.
13. Ando, K., Hunter, N. and Peters, L.J. (1979): Immunologically nonspecific enhancement of artificial lung metastasis in tumor-bearing mice. *Cancer Immunol. Immunother.*, *6*, 151.
14. Gorelik, E. (1983): Concomitant tumor immunity and the resistance to a second tumor challenge. *Adv. Cancer Res.*, *21*, 391.
15. Procter, J.W., Yamamura, Y., Diluzio, N.R., Mansell, P.W.A. and Harnaha, J. (1981): Development of bioassay for the antitumor activity of biological response modifiers of the reticuloendothelial stimulant class. *Cancer Immunol. Immunother.*, *10*, 197.
16. Fidler, I.J. (1974): Immune stimulation-inhibition of experimental cancer metastasis. *Cancer Res.*, *34*, 491.
17. Glaves, D. (1983): Correlation between circulating cancer cells and incidence of metastasis. *Br. J. Cancer*, *48*, 665.

The role of macrophages in the therapeutic effect of bleomycin on a rat fibrosarcoma

Kiyoshi Morikawa, Masuo Hosokawa, Jun-ichi Hamada, Michio Sugawara and Hiroshi Kobayashi

SUMMARY

The role of macrophages in bleomycin (BLM)-treatment of a fibrosarcoma, KMT-17, in syngeneic WKA rats was investigated. The therapeutic effects of BLM were demonstrated by significant prolongation of the mean survival time (MST) of rats bearing the ascitic tumor and reduction of deaths from subcutaneously inoculated tumors in the rats. It was also found that the therapeutic effects of BLM were significantly inhibited by the concomitant use of an anti-macrophage agent, carrageenan. It was found that the cytotoxic activity of spleen cells or peritoneal exudate cells (PEC) against KMT-17 cells, detected by the Winn test or the *in vitro* ^{125}IUdR release test, was augmented in BLM-treated tumor-bearing rats compared with that in untreated tumor-bearing and normal rats. The activity was not specific to KMT-17 cells and was cytotoxic against antigenically different tumor cells. The concurrent use of carrageenan inhibited the cytotoxic activity of effector cells. These results indicate that BLM activates macrophage antitumor activity and that the therapeutic effect of BLM may depend on the action of BLM-activated macrophages.

INTRODUCTION

The antitumor antibiotic, bleomycin (BLM), which was discovered by Prof. Umezawa and his colleagues,[1] is one of the most effective and widely used drugs in cancer treatment. The efficacy of the drug is believed to be due to its strong and direct action against tumor cells. The authors have observed, however, that the therapeutic effect of BLM depends not only on its direct action against tumor cells but also on antitumor immune responses in the host. We have already reported that BLM,[2,3] as well as cyclophosphamide[4] and busulfan,[5] augments antitumor immune responses through selective elimination of suppressor activity. Recently, it was found that the therapeutic effect of BLM against experimental tumors in rats was reduced by the concomitant administration of carrageenan, which is selectively toxic to macrophages. Thus a significant macrophage-mediated antitumor action was suspected to occur in BLM-treated tumor-bearing rats. This paper discusses the activation of macrophages by BLM.

METHODS AND RESULTS

Inhibition of the therapeutic effects of BLM on a syngeneic rat fibrosarcoma, KMT-17, by combined administration of carrageenan

The effects of the anti-macrophage agent, carrageenan, on the therapeutic effect of BLM against a syngeneic tumor, KMT-17, inoculated intraperitoneally into WKA rats (Fig. 1, Table 1) were investigated. Treatment

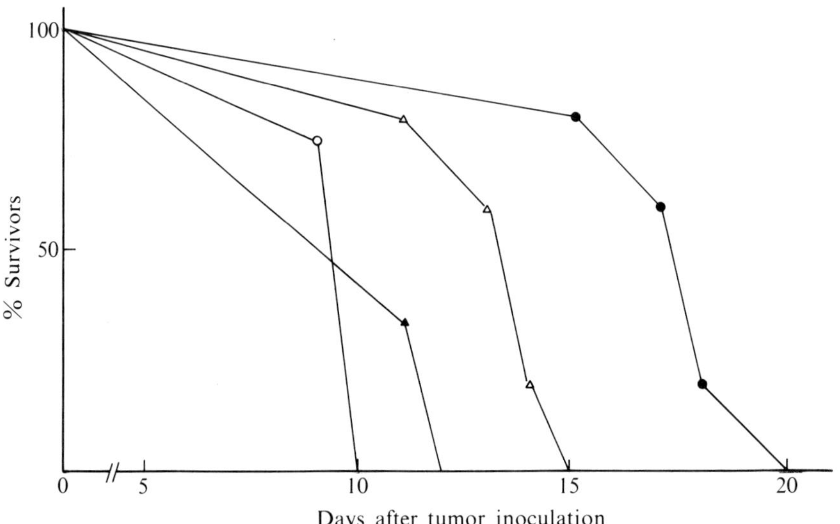

Fig. 1 Inhibition by carrageenan of therapeutic effects of BLM on KMT-17 inoculated i.p. into rats. KMT-17 cells (1×10^3) were implanted i.p. into WKA rats on Day 0 and BLM, 20 mg/kg/day i.p., was administered on Days 1 and 7. Carrageenan, 7 mg/rat i.p., was administered on Days 1 and 6. Untreated (n=12): —▲—. BLM-treated (n=5): —●—. BLM and carrageenan-treated (n=5): —△—. Carrageenan-treated (n=4): —○—.

Table 1 Inhibition of therapeutic effect of bleomycin (BLM) on KMT-17 by antimacrophage agent carrageenan

	KMT-17[a]	BLM[b] (on Day)	Carrageenan[c] (on Day)	Died/Used(%)	MST±SD (days)	ILS(%)
Exp. 1	i.p. (10^3)	No	No	12/12 (100)	11.3±0.5	—
	〃	Yes (1,7)	No	5/5 (100)	17.6±1.8**[d]	55.8
	〃	Yes (1,7)	Yes (-1,6)	5/5 (100)	13.4±1.5*[e]	18.6
	〃	No	Yes (-1,6)	4/4 (100)	9.8±0.5**	-13.3
Exp. 2	s.c. (10^5)	No	No	19/19 (100)	21.3±3.6	—
	〃	Yes (8∼12)	No	6/12** (50)	44.3±13.6**[f]	108.0
	〃	Yes (8∼12)	Yes (8,10)	10/15** (67)	29.8±5.8**[g]	39.9
	〃	No	Yes (8,10)	16/16 (100)	25.3±8.0	18.8

[a] WKA rats were implanted with KMT-17 (Exp. 1: 10^3 i.p., Exp. 2: 10^5 s.c.) on Day 0.
[b] BLM was administered 20 mg/kg i.p. ×2 (Exp. 1) or 5 mg/kg i.p. ×5 (Exp. 2) on indicated days.
[c] Carrageenan, 7 mg, was administered i.p. on indicated days.
[d] vs. [e] $p<0.01$.
[f] vs. [g] $p<0.05$.
Significant compared with untreated group: *$p<0.05$, **$p<0.01$.

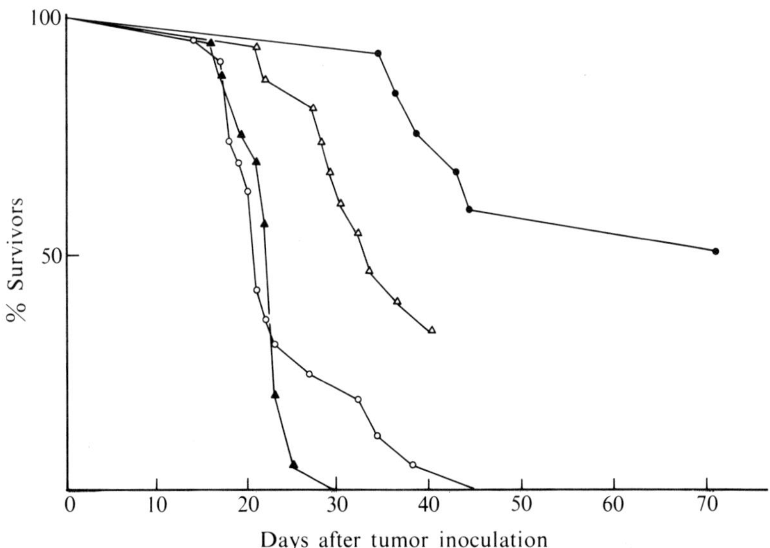

Fig. 2 Inhibition by carrageenan of therapeutic effects of BLM on KMT-17 inoculated s.c. into rats. KMT-17 cells (1×10^5) were implanted s.c. into WKA rats on Day 0 and BLM, 5 mg/kg/day i.p., was administered for 5 days from Day 8. Carrageenan, 7 mg/rat i.p., was administered on Days 8 and 10. Untreated (n=19): —▲—. BLM-treated (n=12): —●—. BLM and carrageenan-treated (n=15): —△—. Carrageenan-treated (n=16): —○—.

with BLM increased the survival time of rats significantly; the increase of life span (ILS) value was 55.8%. Concurrent treatment with carrageenan markedly inhibited the antitumor activity of BLM, as is shown by the significant decrease in survival time (ILS 18.6%) compared with the BLM-treated rats.

Similarly, in subcutaneous-tumor-bearing rats, inhibition of the therapeutic effects of BLM by carrageenan was observed (Fig. 2, Table 1). BLM treatment produced cures in 50% of animals with an ILS of 108%. The therapeutic effects of BLM were significantly reduced by carrageenan, as is shown by the significant decrease in the proportion of long-term survivors in the group subjected to this combined treatment (33% cured, ILS 39.9%), compared with the group of rats given BLM alone. In rats given combined treatment with carrageenan and BLM, the growth of

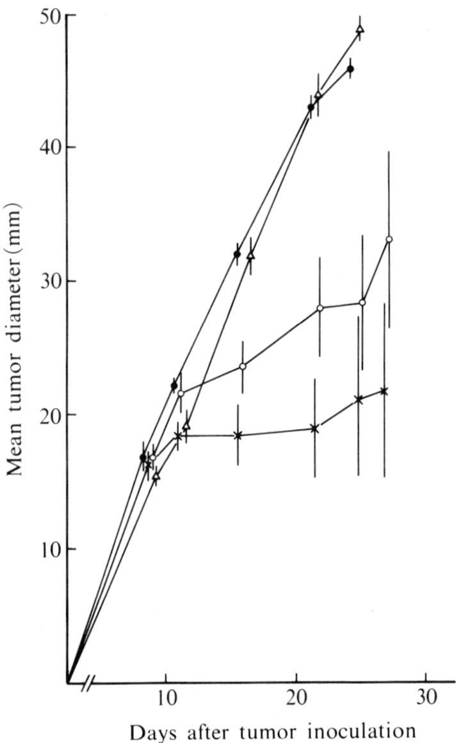

Fig. 3 Growth curves of KMT-17 tumor in rats treated with BLM and carrageenan. KMT-17 cells (1×10^5) were implanted s.c. into rats on Day 0 and BLM, 5 mg/kg/day i.p., was administered for 5 days from Day 8. Carrageenan, 7 mg/rat i. p., was administered on Days 8 and 10. Each value represents the mean diameter$\pm$SE (mm) of 12 to 19 tumors in each group. Untreated: —●—. BLM-treated: —×—. BLM and carrageenan-treated: —○—. Carrageenan-treated: —△—.

tumors was markedly enhanced compared with that in the BLM-treated rats (Fig. 3). On the other hand, when carrageenan alone was given, no significant change in the number of days of survival or in tumor growth could be seen compared with the untreated group (0% cured, ILS 18.8%).

These results suggest that the therapeutic effect of BLM depends not only on its direct tumoricidal activity but also on the activity of macrophages in both intraperitoneal and subcutaneous tumor-bearing rats.

Augmentation by BLM therapy of tumor-neutralizing activity of spleen cells and PEC in tumor-bearing rats

To ascertain whether host immune responses did in fact play a role in the therapeutic action of BLM, Winn's assay was used to examine the tumor-neutralizing activity of spleen cells and peritoneal exudate cells (PEC) obtained from tumor-bearing rats treated with BLM. The tumor-neutralizing activity of these cells was found to be significantly augmented compared with spleen cells and PEC from untreated rats (Table 2). This suggests that BLM-augmented tumor-neutralizing activity may play an important role in the regulation of tumor growth.

Table 2 Augmentation of tumor-neutralizing activity of spleen cells and peritoneal exudate cells (PEC) from KMT-17-bearing rats by administration of bleomycin (BLM)

	Effector[a] cells	Donor[b] of effector cells	Tumor-neutralizing activity	
			Tumor weight (g)±SD[c]	(%)Inhibition
Exp. 1	Spleen cells	BLM-treated TB[d] rats	0	(100)
	〃	Untreated TB rats	1.16±0.39[e]	(54.3)
	〃	Normal rats	1.59±0.09	(37.2)
	None	—	2.53±0.22	(0)
Exp. 2	PEC	BLM-treated TB rats	0.91±0.18[e]	(79.3)
	〃	Untreated TB rats	2.07±0.44[e]	(52.9)
	〃	Normal rats	1.50±0.34	(65.9)
	None	—	4.40±0.77	(0)

[a] Effector cells were harvested on Day 13.
[b] WKA rats were inoculated s.c. with KMT-17 cells (1×10^5) on Day 0 and BLM, 5 mg/kg/day i.p., was administered for 5 days from Day 8.
[c] Mean weight±SD of 5 tumars from recipient rats 11 days (Exp. 1) or 13 days (Exp. 2) after the inoculation of mixture of KMT-17 cells (1×10^5) and effector cells (1×10^7 spleen cells or 1×10^6 PEC).
[d] TB: tumor-bearing.
[e] $p<0.01$ compared with BLM-treated TB rats.

Table 3 Tumor-neutralizing activity of adherent and non-adherent spleen cells from KMT-17-bearing rats treated with bleomycin (BLM).

Group	Donor of spleen cells[a]	Spleen cells[b]		Tumor neutralizing activity	
		Fraction	Treated[c] with	Tumor weight (g)±SD[d] (% Inhibition) Exp. 1	Exp. 2
1	Tumor bearing rats treated with BLM	Unfractionated	Nil	1.4±0.9* (78)	ND[f]
2	〃	〃	anti+T+C'	1.4±0.7* (77)	ND
3	〃	〃	C' only	0.4±0.7**(93)	ND
4	〃	Adherent	Nil	1.2±0.5**(81)	0.7±0.5** (79)
5	〃	Non-adherent	Nil	0.8±0.7**(88)	0.3±0.3**[e](92)
6	〃	〃	anti+T+C'	ND	1.6±0.7[e] (54)
7	〃	〃	C' only	ND	0.5±0.6** (84)
8	Normal rats	Unfractionated	Nil	3.3±1.1 (37)	2.2±0.4 (35)
9	None (KMT-17 only)	—	—	5.2±1.5 (0)	3.4±1.2 (0)

[a] WKA rats were inoculated s.c. with KMT-17 cells (1×10^5) on Day 0 and administered BLM, (5 mg/kg/day) i.p., for 5 days from Day 8.

[b] Spleen cells were harvested on Day 13.

[c] Spleen cells were treated with anti-T lymphocyte serum (anti-T) and complement (C') for 1 hour at 37°C.

[d] Mean weight±SD of 5 tumors from recipient rats 13 days (Exp. 1) or 11 days (Exp. 2) after inoculation of mixture of KMT-17 cells (1×10^5) and spleen cells (unfractionated cells, non-adherent cells: 1×10^7; adherent cells: 1×10^6).

[e] $p<0.01$

[f] ND: not determined.

Significantly different from Group 8: $*p<0.05$, $**p<0.01$.

BLM-augmented tumor-neutralizing activity of spleen cells is a property of both glass non-adherent and adherent cells

To determine what cell populations of spleen cells in rats treated with BLM possess the tumor-neutralizing activity, this activity was examined by Winn's assay using spleen cells which were separated on the basis of glass adherence (Table 3). Activity was observed not only in the adherent cells but also in the non-adherent cell preparation. Treatment with anti-T cell serum and complement did not decrease the activity of unfractionated spleen cells, but significantly decreased the activity of non-adherent spleen cells. Morphologically, over 90% of the adherent cells were monocytes-macrophages. From these facts, it seemed that the BLM-augmented neutralizing activity of spleen cells depended on both T-cells and macrophages.

Augmentation by BLM therapy of cytolytic activity of peritoneal macrophages in tumor-bearing rats

To investigate further the role of macrophages in the anti-tumor activity

Table 4 Augmentation of cytolytic activity of peritoneal exudate cells (PEC) from KMT-17-bearing rats by administration of bleomycin (BLM)

PEC		Percent specific cytolysis at E: T ratio[c]		
Donor[a]	Fraction[b]	20:1	10:1	5:1
BLM treated TB rats[d]	Unfractionated	18.6	8.6	8.8
〃	Non-adherent	2.1	-4.1	NT[e]
〃	Adherent	28.9	21.1	18.1
Non-treated TB rats	Unfractionated	-4.5	0.5	3.4
〃	Non-adherent	-4.9	-7.7	NT[e]
〃	Adherent	12.1	6.1	4.7
Normal rats	Unfractionated	-6.3	-4.4	1.4
〃	Adherent	10.6	5.9	1.4

[a] Each group contained five rats. Rats were inoculated s.c. with KMT-17 cells (1×10^5) on Day 0 and BLM, 5 mg/kg/day i.p., was administered for 5 days from Day 8. Spleen cells were harvested on Day 13.

[b] PEC were fractionated by adhesion to glass.

[c] Percentage of specific ^{125}I released after 24 hours incubation using KMT-17 target cells. E/T ratio: ratio of effector to target cells.

[d] TB: tumor-bearing.

[e] Not tested.

of BLM, the cytolytic activity of PEC collected from BLM-treated tumor-bearing rats was assessed. By means of ^{125}IUdR release assay after 24 hours of incubation, PEC from BLM-treated rats showed significant cytotoxicity against KMT-17 cells, while PEC from untreated rats showed no cytotoxicity (Table 4). The enhanced PEC cytotoxicity was recovered in the adherent cell preparation, little activity being found in the non-adherent cells.

This PEC-mediated cytolytic activity after 24 hours of incubation was not tumor-specific, as PEC from BLM-treated rats also showed cytotoxicity against the antigenically different syngeneic tumors, KST-20 and WFT-2N, and against human leukemia cells, K562 (Table 5). It is noteworthy, however, that no cytotoxicity against K562 cells was detected after 6 hours of incubation. Therefore, these PEC, which have non-specific cytotoxic activity, have little natural killer cell activity against K562.

In vitro carrageenan treatment significantly reduced the cytotoxic effects of PEC from BLM-treated rats (Table 6). As mentioned previously, the concurrent use of carrageenan significantly reduced the therapeutic effects of BLM. Moreover, *in vivo* this combined treatment significantly reduced the cytotoxic activity of PEC compared with that of PEC from the group given BLM alone.

In summary, these data suggest that the augmented cytotoxicity of PEC in tumor-bearing rats treated with BLM may be mediated by

Table 5 Effect of administration of bleomycin (BLM) on cytolytic activity of peritoneal exudate cells (PEC) from KMT-17-bearing rats

Donor of PEC[a]	Incubation[b] time (h)	Percent specific cytolysis[c] E: T ratio, 20 : 1			
		KMT-17	K 562	KST-20	WFT-2N
BLM treated TB rats[d]	24	36.5	22.1	22.5	21.6
〃	6	0	0.9	NT[e]	NT[e]
Untreated TB rats	24	11.3	9.1	16.9	-4.4
〃	6	-0.9	-0.7	NT	NT[e]

[a] Rats were inoculated s.c. with KMT-17 cells (1×10^5) on Day 0 and BLM, 5 mg/kg/day i.p., was administered for 5 days from Day 8. PEC were harvested on Day 13.
[b] Incubation time for ^{125}IUdR release assay.
[c] Percentage of specific ^{125}I released.
[d] TB: tumor-bearing.
[e] NT: not tested.

Table 6 Inhibition of cytolytic activity of BLM-induced adherent PEC by *in vivo* and *in vitro* carrageenan treatment

Donor[a] treated with (*in vivo*)	PEC treated with (*in vitro*)	Percent specific cytolysis[e] at E: T ratio		
		40:1	20:1	10:1
BLM[b]	—	71.8	28.9	23.7
BLM	Carr.[c]	14.0	13.8	15.5
BLM+Carr.[d]	—	19.8	12.5	15.5
Nil	—	19.9	3.2	0.3

[a] Each group contained five rats. Rats were inoculated with KMT-17 (1×10^5) on Day 0. PEC were harvested on Day 13.
[b] BLM, 5 mg/kg/day i.p., was administered for 5 days from Day 8.
[c] PEC were treated with carrageenan (250 μg/ml) at 37°C for 2 hours.
[d] Carrageenan (7 mg/rat) was administered i.p. on Days 8 and 10.
[e] Percentage of specific ^{125}I released after 24 hours of incubation using KMT-17 target cells.

activated antitumor macrophages. BLM may contribute to the regulation of tumor growth by stimulating tumoricidal macrophage production as well as by acting directly on the tumors.

DISCUSSION

It has been found that BLM renders macrophages cytotoxic in tumor-bearing rats and that the macrophages may play a role in the therapeutic effects of BLM. The authors reported previously that when BLM is administered to KMT-17-tumor-bearing rats at a late stage after tumor inoculation, more marked therapeutic effects are observed than when the drug is administered earlier.[3] The results presented here provide more direct evidence suggesting host-mediated therapeutic effects of BLM.

Many investigators have reported that, following BLM treatment of cancer in man, a large number of giant macrophages appear in the region of the tumor.[6] Similarly, in the present ascitic tumor system, a large number of macrophages were observed to appear in the peritoneal cavity of rats and to become attached to tumor cells (data not shown). Because macrophages in tumor-bearing hosts may act as suppressor cells and inhibit antitumor immune responses,[7] the macrophage content of tumor tissue may require careful consideration. However, from the facts that the anti-macrophage agent, carrageenan, inhibits the therapeutic effects of BLM (Fig. 1, Table 1), and that BLM therapy does not suppress T cell-mediated antitumor activity (Table 3), the macrophages appearing in the tumor tissue during BLM therapy are thought to act as antitumor effector cells.

Moreover, it is speculated that these host-mediated therapeutic effects of BLM may complement the direct tumoricidal activity of the drug. Two possibilities for the mechanism of this therapeutic complementerity may be offered: 1) Tumor cells may be rendered more immunogenic by the drug,[8] thereby resulting in an enhancement of antitumor immune responses. It is possible that activation of macrophages may be a consequence of specific antitumor responses in tumor-bearing hosts treated with the drug. 2) The activated macrophages may preferentially destroy drug-damaged tumor cells. These possibilities are currently under further investigation.

The precise mechanisms of the activation of macrophages following BLM therapy are not presently known. It has been reported by other investigators that other antitumor chemotherapeutic drugs such as adriamycin,[9,10] cyclophosphamide[9,11] and mitomycin[12] also augment macrophage cytotoxicity. Direct action of drug on macrophages is possible in the augmentation of macrophage-mediated cytotoxicity, since Haskill has shown that adriamycin may be entrapped in macrophages.[10] It is possible that macrophages may merely transport the drug into the culture medium and thereby manifest the direct cytotoxic action of the drug against tumor cells. However, this mechanism appears unlikely in the present experimental system, because conditioned media from BLM-treated macrophages did not show cytotoxic activity against KMT-17 (data not shown). Therefore, it is speculated that the effects of BLM on macrophages seem to be related to the mechanisms of differentiation or activation of macrophages.

CONCLUSION

The host-mediated effects on experimental tumors in rats in BLM treatment were observed. The host-mediated therapeutic effects of BLM may complement the direct tumoricidal activity of the drug. To ensure more effective treatment of cancer, it is important that studies be made of promising regimens of chemotherapy in which antitumor drugs are able to exhibit host-mediated therapeutic effects as well as direct tumoricidal effects.

REFERENCES

1. Umezawa, H., Maeda, K., Takeuchi, T. and Okami, Y. (1966): New antibiotics bleomycin A & B. *J. Antibiot., 19A*, 210.
2. Hosokawa, M., Suzuki, Y., Takimoto, M., Morikawa, K., Mizushima, Y. and Kobayashi, H. (1985): Elimination of suppressor cells by bleomycin for augmentation of antitumor resistance in WKA rats immunized with irradiated tumor cells. *Cancer Res.*, (In press).
3. Morikawa, K., Hosokawa, M., Hamada, J., Sugawara, M. and Kobayashi, H. (1985): Host-mediated therapeutic effects produced by appropriately timed administration of bleomycin on a rat fibrosarcoma. *Cancer Res.*, (In press).
4. Terashima, M., Takeichi, N., Suzuki, K., Itaya, T., Gotohda, E. and Kobayashi, H. (1980): Enhanced immunogenicity of xenogenized tumor cells in rats pretreated with cyclophosphamide. *Tohoku J. Exp. Med., 132*, 355.
5. Mizushima, Y., Sendo, F., Takeichi, N., Hosokawa, M. and Kobayashi, H. (1981): Enhancement of antitumor transplantation resistance in rats by appropriately timed administration of Busulfan. *Cancer Res., 41*, 2917.
6. Burkhardt, A., Bommer, G., Gebbers, J.O. and Hötje, W.J. (1976): Reisenzellbildung bei bleomycintherapie oraler Plattenepithelcarcinome. *Virchow Arch. A. Path. Anath. und Histol., 369*, 197.
7. Mokyr, M.B., Hengst, J.C.D., Przepiorka, D. and Dray, S. (1979): Augmentation antitumor cytotoxicity of MOPC-315 tumor bearer spleen cells by depletion of DNP-adherent cells prior to *in vitro* immunization. *Cancer Res., 39*, 3928.
8. Fuji, H., Mihich, E. and Pressman, D. (1979): Differential tumor immunogenicity of DBA/2 mouse lymphoma L1210 and its sublines. *J. Natl. Cancer Inst., 62*, 1503.
9. Stoychkov, J.N., Schultz, R.M., Chiligos, M.A., Pavlidis, N.A. and Goldin, A. (1979): Effects of adriamycin and cyclophosphamide treatment on induction of macrophage cytotoxic function in mice. *Cancer Res., 39*, 3014.
10. Haskill, J.S. (1981): Adriamycin-activated macrophages as tumor growth inhibitors. *Cancer Res., 41*, 3852.
11. Schultz, R.M., Pavlidis, N.A., Chiligos, M.A. and Weiss, J.F. (1978): Effects of whole body X-irradiation and cyclophosphamide treatment on induction of macrophage tumoricidal function in mice. *Cell. Immunol., 38*, 302.

12 . Ogura, T., Shindo, H., Shinzato, O., Namba, M., Masuco, T., Inoue, T., Kishimoto, S. and Yamamura, Y. (1982): *In vitro* tumor cell killing by peritoneal macrophages from mitomycin C-treated rats. *Cancer Immunol. Immunother., 13*, 112.

Therapeutic implications of activation of human monocyte-macrophages to the tumoricidal state by liposomes containing biological response modifiers

Saburo Sone, Seiji Mutsuura, Mitsumasa Ogawara, Teruhiro Utsugi and Eiro Tsubura

SUMMARY

Human alveolar macrophages and peripheral blood monocytes can be activated to the tumoricidal state *in vitro* by incubation with liposomes containing muramyl dipeptide (MDP) or its lipophilic derivative, muramyl tripeptide-phosphatidylethanolamine (MTP-PE). Macrophages activated by this procedure destroy allogeneic tumor cells but leave non-tumorigenic cells unharmed. Negatively-charged liposomes are preferentially incorporated into monocyte-macrophages by phagocytosis. Liposome-encapsulated MDP and MTP-PE not only cause activation of human monocyte-macrophages at lower concentrations than free MDP but also maintain activation for a longer period than free MDP. These results indicate that systemic administration of liposomes containing MDP or MTP-PE should be useful for *in situ* activation of macrophages responsible for eradication of cancer metastases.

INTRODUCTION

The increasing evidence that activated macrophages are important in the host defense against primary and/or metastatic tumors has resulted in the discovery of new biological response modifiers (BRMs) that can enhance macrophage-mediated tumor cell killing. For example, muramyl dipeptide (MDP), which is synthesized in large quantities by *Mycobacterium*, is the main component of the preparation from this organism responsible for the immunopotentiating activity of Freund's complete adjuvant.[1] Soluble MDP is known to affect macrophage functions *in vitro*.[1] The authors demonstrated previously that encapsulation of MDP within the aqueous space of phospholipid vesicles (liposomes) greatly enhances its effect in rendering murine macrophages tumoricidal *in vitro*[2,3] *and in vivo*.[4,5] Moreover, systemic administration of liposome-entrapped MDP to tumor-bearing mice inhibits or eradicates disseminated metastatic disease.[6] We tried to apply these findings from animal studies to human systems. Recent studies in our laboratory have shown that free or liposome-encapsulated MDP potentiates the tumoricidal activity of human monocyte-macrophages *in vitro*.[7–9] The results also showed that a lipophilic derivative of MDP, muramyl tripeptidephosphatidylethanolamine (MTP-PE), encapsulated in the bilayer membrane of multilamellar (MLV) liposomes activated human monocytes to the tumoricidal state.[10] This paper provides a brief review of our *in vitro* studies, which provide a rationale for the clinical use of biological response modifiers (BRMs) encapsulated in liposomes for potentiating the host defense against primary and/or metastatic tumors.

MATERIALS AND METHODS

The origin, properties and cultivation of tumorigenic (A375 melanoma and KB epidermoid cell carcinoma) and non-tumorigenic (Flow-7000 foreskin fibroblast) target cell lines have been described previously.[7–10] Recognized methods were used for: the isolation of human alveolar macrophages[7,8] and peripheral blood monocytes from normal volunteers by adherence and then treatment with EDTA[10] or by the percoll gradient centrifugation method[11]; for the preparation of large MLV liposomes composed of phosphatidylserine (PS) and phosphatidylcholine (PC) in a molar ratio of 3:7 or 5:5[7–10]; for the activation of monocyte-macrophages by free or liposome-entrapped MDP or MTP-PE (Ciba-Geigy);[7–10] and for the quantitative assay of the cytotoxicity of treated and control monocyte-macrophages against ^{125}I-IUdR-labeled target cells.[7–10]

RESULTS AND DISCUSSION

The authors demonstrated previously that in animal models, *in situ* activation of the tumoricidal properties of alveolar macrophages (AM) by MDP in liposomes is closely associated with eradication of pulmonary metastases.[6] These findings prompted examination of whether liposomes containing BRMs could activate human alveolar macrophages to the tumoricidal state. Human alveolar macrophages incubated for 24 hours

Table 1 Cytotoxicity of human alveolar macrophages treated with free or liposome-entrapped MDP[7]

Treatment of alveolar macrophages	Cytotoxicity[b] against: Tumorigenic target cells		Normal target cells
	A375 melanoma	KB	Flow-7000
MDP (0.2 μg)	35%[c]	15%[c]	0%
Liposome-MDP[a]			
10 nmol	47%[c]	37%[c]	0%
50 nmol	42%[c]	31%[c]	0%
LPS[d] (0.1 μg)	59%[c]	38%[c]	0%

[a] 10 μg/ml of MDP was encapsulated in the aqueous space of MLV liposomes (10 μmol). Human macrophages were treated for 24 hours with the indicated agent before addition of labeled target cells. Assays were terminated after 72 hours.

[b] Percent increase in cytotoxicity over that of untreated macrophages.

[c] $p<0.05$ compared with untreated macrophages.

[d] Lipopolysaccharide.

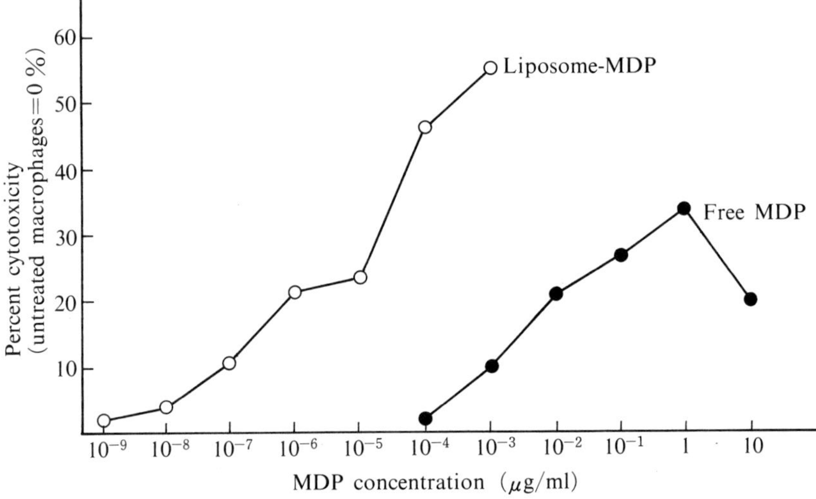

Fig. 1 *In vitro* tumoricidal activity of human alveolar macrophages treated with free MDP or liposomes containing different doses of MDP. AM were incubated in medium with the indicated agents for 24 hours before addition of labeled tumor cells. Assays were terminated after 72 hours.[7]

with free MDP or MDP in liposomes became cytotoxic to allogeneic tumor cells but did not kill non-tumorigenic cells (Table 1). Human alveolar macrophages exposed to liposomes containing MDP had higher cytotoxicity than those incubated with free MDP, even though the amount of MDP encapsulated in liposomes was much less than the amount of free MDP used (Fig. 1). These results confirm and extend the results of previous studies on mouse cells.[2,6]

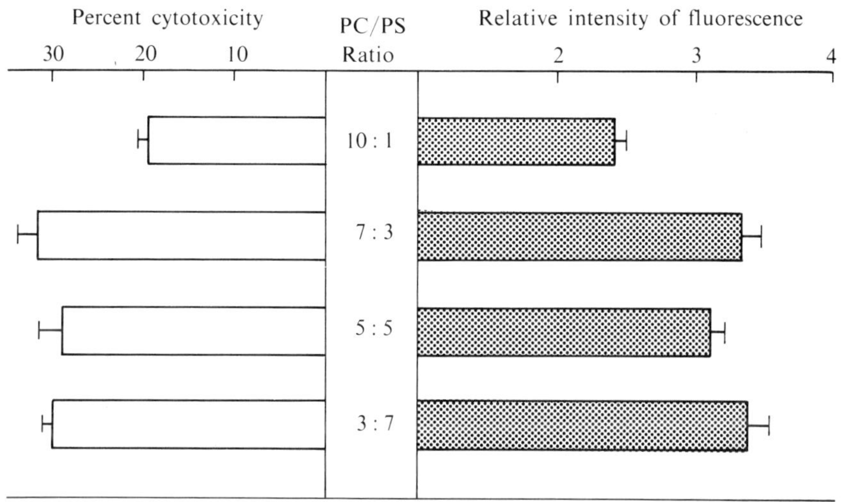

Fig. 2 Effect of molar ratio of lipids in liposomes on their phagocytosis by human alveolar macrophages and subsequent cytotoxicity of the macrophages.[8]

Phagocytic uptake of liposomes by macrophages is influenced by the liposome composition, and murine macrophages are known to phagocytize negatively-charged liposomes composed of PS and PC more rapidly than neutral liposomes.[12] Therefore, the effect of the liposome composition on the phagocytic and tumoricidal activities of human alveolar macrophages was examined. Human macrophages were incubated for 4 hours with liposome-encapsulated MDP composed of PS and/or PC in various molar ratios before cytotoxicity assay. The addition of PS to PC liposomes resulted in significant potentiation of their phagocytosis, measured fluorimetrically as the ability of human alveolar macrophages to phagocytize liposome-entrapped quinacrine (Fig. 2). Thus, human macrophages also phagocytized negatively-charged liposomes (PS/PC) at a significantly faster rate than neutral liposomes (PC alone).

Potentiation of the tumoricidal activity of human peripheral blood monocytes by liposomes containing the lipophilic MDP analog MTP-PE in the bilayer membrane is interesting for several reasons. First, lipophilic MTP-PE can be inserted directly into the lipid bilayer of MLV liposomes, whereas water-soluble MDP leaks out of the liposomes and is then excreted from the body. In fact, the authors demonstrated previously that MTP-PE encapsulated in liposomes is more effective than MDP in liposomes for activation of murine macrophages *in vitro* and *in vivo*.[5] Second, for significant activation of murine alveolar macrophages, MTP-PE in liposomes was found to be effective at a much lower concentration than free/soluble MDP.[5]

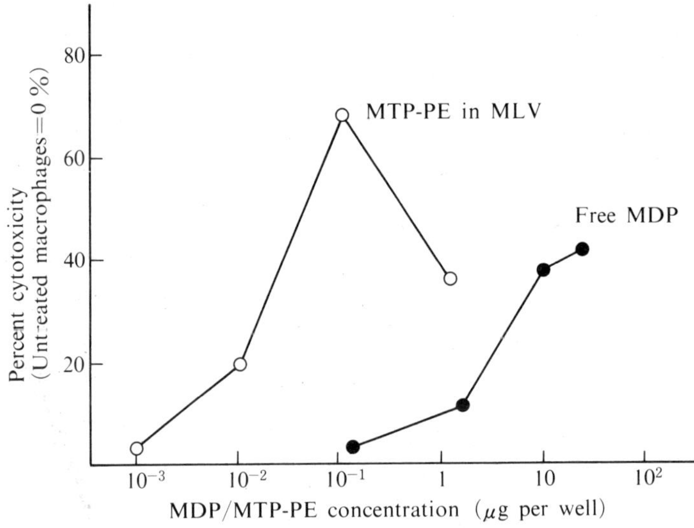

Fig. 3 *In vitro* tumoricidal activity of human monocyte-derived macrophages treated with free MDP or with liposomes containing different amounts of MTP-PE. Monocyte-derived macrophages (cultured in medium for 4 days) were treated with MDP or liposome-entrapped MTP-PE at the indicated doses for 24 hours before cytotoxicity assay.

The finding that systemic administration of liposomes containing MDP or its lipophilic analog, MTP-PE, resulted in eradication of established spontaneous pulmonary metastases[6,13] suggests that the direct interaction of circulating peripheral blood monocytes with MLV liposomes administered intravenously may be the first step in the *in situ* activation of tissue macrophages, such as alveolar macrophages or macrophages infiltrating tumors. The authors reported previously that noncytotoxic human blood monocytes (named monocyte-derived macrophages) that had been incubated for 4 days in medium were activated and rendered tumoricidal by liposome-entrapped MTP-PE at much lower concentrations than the effective concentration of free MDP (Fig. 3). Here, we examined whether monocytes that had been freshly isolated from peripheral blood on a percoll gradient could be activated and rendered tumoricidal by treatment *in vitro* with liposomes containing MTP-PE. Monocytes isolated by this procedure were not spontaneously cytotoxic but they too were activated to kill allogeneic tumor cells by liposome-MTP-PE in a dose of more than 10 nmol/well (5 μg/μmol) (Fig. 4). Freshly isolated monocytes also phagocytized negatively-charged MLV liposomes (Fig. 5). These results strongly suggest that monocytes circulating in the blood could be activated by liposome-entrapped MTP-PE administered intravenously.

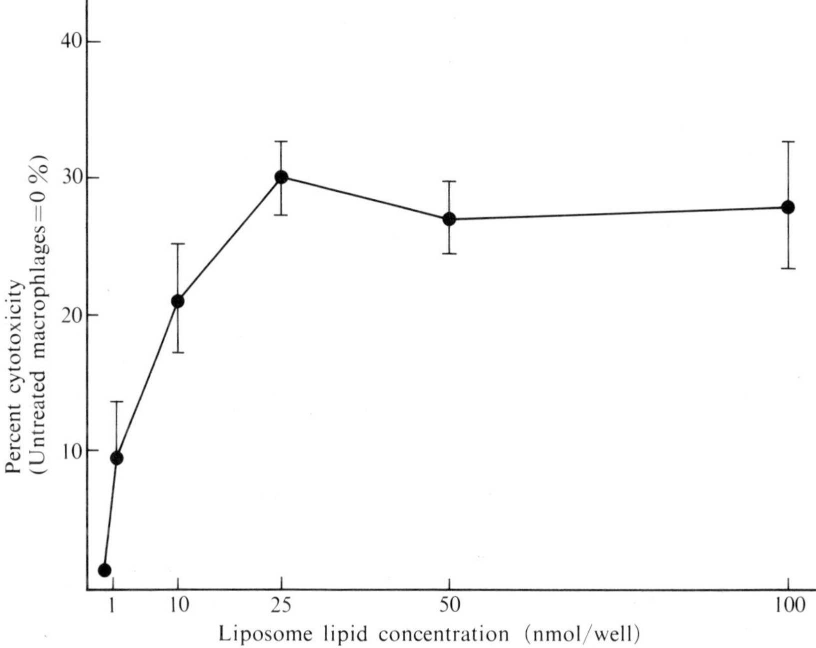

Fig. 4 Effect of the concentration of MLV liposomes containing MTP-PE on activation of monocytes freshly isolated by percoll gradient centrifugation and treated with different amounts of liposome lipid (5 μg of MTP-PE per μmol of lipid) for 24 hours before cytotoxicity assay.

In addition to MDP and its derivatives, some other factors or agents encapsulated in liposomes have been reported to potentiate host defenses. For example, liposomes containing bioproducts such as lymphokines containing macrophage-activating factor (MAF) and C-reactive protein (CRP) have also been demonstrated to be effective in the treatment of cancer metastasis in murine models.[14,15] Moreover, two different activators (MAF and MDP) encapsulated in liposomes have been reported to have synergistic effects on macrophage activation and eradication of cancer metastasis.[4,16] On the other hand, the authors found recently that a synthetic acyltripeptide and its derivatives, which are structurally very similar to *Streptomyces* cell-wall peptidoglycan peptides, are potent activators of rat alveolar macrophages *in vitro*, and that encapsulation of these compounds in MLV liposomes resulted in increased macrophage-mediated tumor cell killing *in vitro*.[17] Thus, further attempts to find new BRMs with macrophage-activating capability, such as bioproducts or synthetic substances, are required in order to develop more effective combinations for use in liposomes.

It will be very interesting to see whether liposomes containing MDP

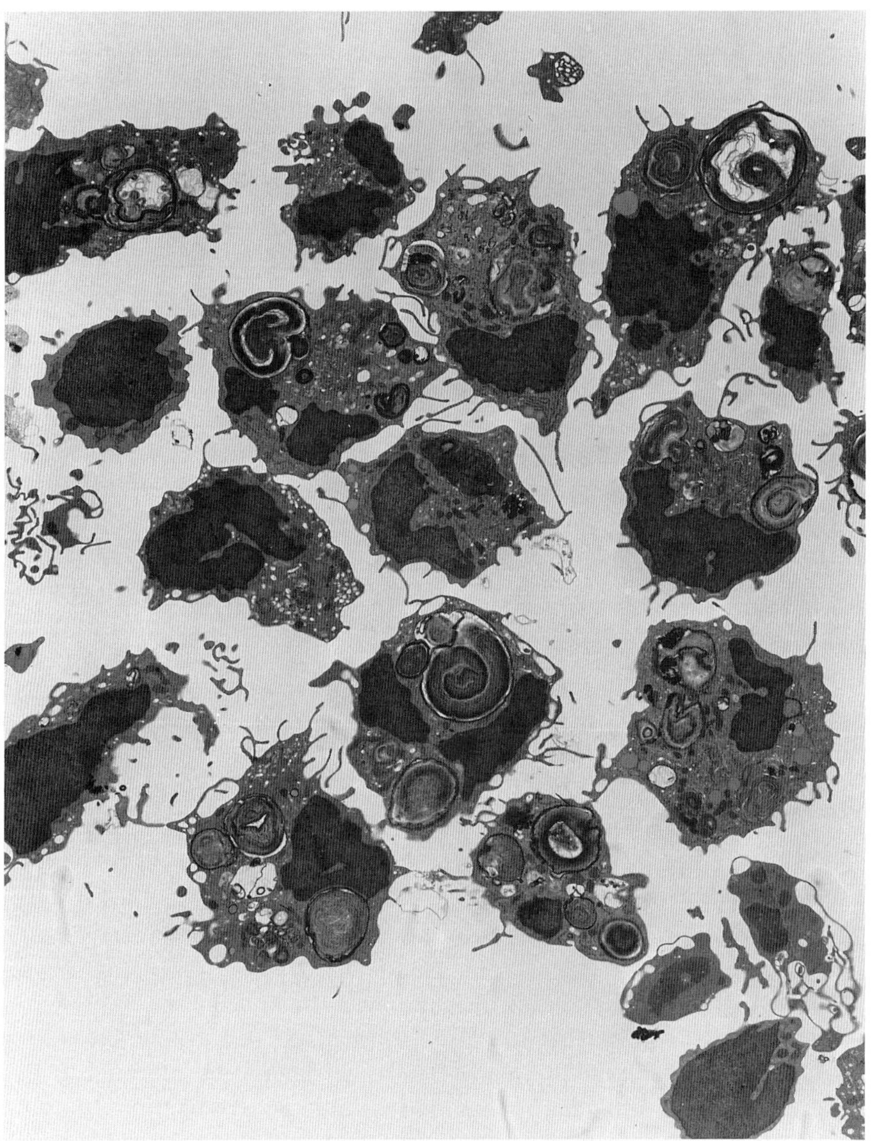

Fig. 5 Human blood monocytes containing phagocytized MLV liposomes.

or MTP-PE are effective for the treatment of disseminated diseases in cancer patients. There is promising evidence on their clinical use. Recently, Lopez-Berestein et al.[18] studied the pharmacokinetics and organ distribution of negatively charged ^{99m}Tc-labeled MLV liposomes in cancer patients, and found that 24 hours after intravenous injection of the MLV liposomes, they were localized in organs rich in reticuloendothelial cells, i.e., the liver, spleen, lungs and bone marrow, in that order. These findings suggest that appropriate agents encapsulated in liposomes should be effective macrophage activators. Moreover, it is noteworthy that systemic administration of MLV liposomes is safe and results in no adverse side effects.[18] These observations, together with the authors' findings that liposome-entrapped MDP or MTP-PE can activate human monocyte-macrophages to the tumoricidal state, and results on the therapeutic effect of these liposomes on murine cancer metastasis, indicate that administration of MLV liposomes should be useful for the treatment of disseminated metastatic diseases in humans.

ACKNOWLEDGEMENT

This research was supported by a Grant-in-Aid for Cancer Research and a Grant-in-Aid for Scientific Research from the Ministry of Education, Science and Culture of Japan. We wish to thank Dr. Cora Bucana for providing the photograph shown in Fig. 5.

REFERENCES

1. Adam, A. and Lederer, E. (1984): Muramyl dipeptides: Immunomodulators, sleep factors, and vitamins. *Med. Res. Rev.*, *4*, 111.
2. Sone, S. and Fidler, I.J. (1981): *In vitro* activation of tumoricidal properties in rat alveolar macrophages by synthetic muramyl dipeptide encapsulated in liposomes. *Cell. Immunol.*, *57*, 42.
3. Sone, S. and Fidler, I.J. (1981): Activation of rat alveolar macrophages to the tumoricidal state in the presence of progressively growing pulmonary metastases. *Cancer Res.*, *41*, 2401.
4. Sone, S. and Fidler, I.J. (1980): Synergistic activation by lymphokines and muramyl dipeptide of tumoricidal properties in rat alveolar macrophages. *J. Immunol.*, *125*, 2454.
5. Fidler, I.J., Sone, S., Fogler, W.E., Smith, D., Braun, D.G., Tarcsay, V., Gisler, R.H. and Schroit, A.J. (1982): Efficacy of liposomes containing a lipophilic muramyl dipeptide derivative for activating the tumoricidal properties of alveolar macrophages *in vivo*. *J. Biol. Res. Modif.*, *1*, 43.
6. Fidler, I.J., Sone, S., Fogler, W.E. and Barnes, Z.L. (1981): Eradication of spontaneous metastases and activation of alveolar macrophages by intravenous injection of liposomes containing muramyl dipeptide. *Proc. Natl. Acad. Sci. U.S.A.*, *78*, 1680.
7. Sone, S. and Tsubura, E. (1982): Human alveolar macrophages: Potentiation of their tumoricidal activity by liposome-encapsulated muramyl dipeptide. *J. Immunol.*, *129*, 1313.
8. Sone, S., Tachibana, K., Shono, M., Ogushi, M. and Tsubura, E. (1984): Potential value of liposomes containing muramyl dipeptide for augmenting the tumoricidal activity of human alveolar macrophages. *J. Biol. Res. Modif.*, *3*, 185.
9. Sone, S., Tachibana, K. and Tsubura, E. (1983): Therapeutic implications of tumor cell destruction *in vitro* by human alveolar macrophages activated with muramyl dipeptide entrapped in liposomes. *Recent Advances in RES Res.*, *22*, 187.

10. Sone, S., Mutsuura, S., Ogawara, M. and Tsubura, E. (1984): Potentiating effect of muramyl dipeptide and its lipophilic analog encapsulated in liposomes on tumor cell killing by human monocytes. *J. Immunol.*, *132*, 2105.
11. Utsugi, T., Sone, S., Mutsuura, S., Ogawara, M., Shirahama, T., Ishii, K. and Tsubura, E. (1985): Generation *in vitro* of human monocyte tumoricidal potential by interferon alpha and beta. In: *Rationale of Biological Response Modifiers in Cancer Treatment.* p. 74. Excerpta Medica. Tokyo.
12. Raz, A., Bucana, C., Fogler, W.E., Poste, G. and Fidler, I.J. (1981): Biochemical, morphological and ultrastructural studies on the uptake of liposomes by murine macrophages. *Cancer Res.*, *41*, 187.
13. Schroit, A.J. and Fidler, I.J. (1982): Effects of liposome structure and lipid composition on the activation of the tumoricidal properties of macrophages by liposomes containing muramyl dipeptide. *Cancer Res.*, *42*, 161.
14. Kleinerman, E.S., Schroit, A.J., Fogler, W.E. and Fidler, I.J. (1983): Tumoricidal activity of human monocytes activated *in vitro* by free and liposome-encapsulated human lymphokines. *J. Clin. Invest.*, *72*, 304.
15. Deodhar, S.D., James, K., Chiang, T., Edinger, M. and Barna, B.P. (1982): Inhibition of lung metastases in mice bearing a malignant fibrosarcoma by treatment with liposomes containing human C-reactive protein. *Cancer Res.*, *42*, 5084.
16. Fidler, I.J. and Schroit, A.J. (1984): Synergism between lymphokines and muramyl dipeptide encapsulated in liposomes: *in situ* activation of macrophages and therapy of spontaneous cancer metastases. *J. Immunol.*, *133*, 515.
17. Sone, S., Mutsuura, S., Ogawara, M., Utsugi, T. and Tsubura, E. (1984): Activation by a new synthetic acyltripeptide and its analogues entrapped in liposomes of rat alveolar macrophages to the tumor cytotoxic state. *Cancer Immunol. Immunother.*, (In press).
18. Lopez-Berestein, G., Kasi, L. and Rosenblum, M.G. (1984): Clinical pharmacology of ^{99m}Tc-labeled liposomes in patients with cancer. *Cancer Res.*, *44*, 375.

Macrophage activating factor for cytotoxicity produced by human T cell hybridomas

Toshiaki Osawa and Masahiro Higuchi

SUMMARY

Human macrophage activating factor for cytotoxicity (MAF-C)-producing hybridomas, H2-E3-5 and H3-E9-6, were prepared by somatic cell fusion of phytohemagglutinin (PHA)-activated human peripheral blood lymphocytes with emetine-actinomycin D-treated cloned human acute lymphatic leukemia cells (CEM). It was revealed that there are at least two human MAF-Cs, differing in the maturational stages of the cells they affect. MAF-C from H2-E3-5 culture supernatants activated differentiated macrophages but not monocytes, while MAF-C from H3-E9-6 culture supernatants could activate both macrophages and monocytes.

INTRODUCTION

Cytotoxic macrophages play a crucial role as effector cells in host defense mechanisms against tumor cells. The lymphokine which stimulates and increases the metabolic, secretory and cytotoxic activities of macrophages is known as macrophage activating factor (MAF). However, it was an important unanswered question whether or not most of these phenomena were exerted by one molecule. Since activated lymphocytes produce MAF in very tiny amounts, the authors constructed MAF-producing human T cell hybridomas and showed that at least three different molecules, MAF-G (for glucose consumption), MAF-O (for O_2^- formation) and MAF-C (for cytotoxicity), are involved in the activation of macrophages.[1,2]

This paper describes two kinds of MAF-C produced by human T cell hybridomas. One of them activated differentiated macrophages but not monocytes [MAF-C (macrophage)], while the other activated monocytes [MAF-C (monocyte)] as well as differentiated macrophages. These results may suggest that even MAF-C is heterogeneous with respect to target cells.

MATERIALS AND METHODS

Stimulation of human peripheral blood lymphocytes with a T cell mitogen

Human peripheral blood lymphocytes (PBL) were isolated from a healthy donor by Ficoll-Urografin density gradient centrifugation.[3] Contaminating red cells were lysed in 0.87% Tris-buffered NH_4Cl. The lymphocytes (10^6 cells/ml) were cultured for 40 hours at 37°C in RPMI 1640 containing 60 mg/l of kanamycin, 2 mM glutamine, 5×10^{-5} M 2-mercaptoethanol, 10% fetal calf serum (enriched medium) and 5 μg/ml of phytohemagglutinin-P (PHA-P; Difco, Detroit).

Treatment of a clone of CEM (CEM 11) with emetine and actinomycin D

Emetine and actinomycin D-treated cloned human acute lymphatic leukemia cells (CEM) were prepared essentially by the method described previously.[4] Briefly, a clone of CEM (CEM 11) was suspended at a cell density of 2×10^6/ml in RPMI 1640 containing 20 mM HEPES (pH 7.2) and then treated with 5×10^{-5} M emetine hydrochloride (Nakarai Chemicals Ltd., Kyoto, Japan) and 0.25 μg/ml of actinomycin D (Makor Chemicals Ltd., Jerusalem) at 37°C for 2 hours. These concentrations of emetine hydrochloride and actinomycin D completely inhibited proliferation of CEM 11 cells. The cells were washed four times with 10 mM sodium phosphate buffer (pH 7.2) containing 0.15 M NaCl (PBS) in order to remove free emetine and actinomycin D.

Hybridization

PHA-P-activated PBL were centrifuged and incubated with 0.1 M N-acetyl-D-galactosamine at 37°C for 20 minutes to remove cell-bound PHA-P. These PBL were fused with emetine-actinomycin D-treated CEM 11 cells, as described previously.[4] Mitomycin C-treated CEM 11 cells were added to the fused cells. The mixture was subcultured in 96×0.2 ml culture wells (Falcon microplate No. 3042). Every day during the first week, 100 μl of the medium in each well was replaced by 100 μl of fresh enriched medium. The hybrid cell lines showed good growth in all of the wells within 2 weeks of fusion. However, in the control wells to which emetine-actinomycin D-pretreated CEM 11 cells or mitomycin C-pretreated CEM 11 cells had been added, no cell growth was observed.

Preparation of supernatants of PHA-P-activated PBL

PBL were cultured at a density of 10^6 cells/ml in enriched medium containing 5 μg/ml of PHA-P at 37°C for 48 hours. After centrifugation, the supernatants (sup) were stored at −20°C. PHA-P itself does not show MAF-C activity.

Preparation of 0-80% ammonium sulfate precipitate fraction of the culture supernatant of H2-E3-5

Ammonium sulfate was added to the H2-E3-5 culture supernatant to a saturation of 80%. After centrifugation, the precipitates formed at 0-80% saturation were dissolved in PBS and dialyzed against PBS to remove ammonium sulfate. By this procedure, 300 ml of the culture supernatant was concentrated to 25 ml.

Assay for tumor cytotoxicity of human monocyte-derived macrophages [MAF-C (macrophage)]

MAF-C activity was evaluated as the cytotoxicity toward tumor cells of monocyte-derived macrophages, using a modification of the method of Cameron et al.[5] Briefly, PBL freshly isolated from human blood were suspended at a concentration of 2.5×10^6 cells/ml in minimal essential medium with 10% human blood group type AB serum. Two-hundred microliter aliquots of the cell suspension were added to Falcon microtiter plate wells (No. 3042, Oxnard, Calif.). After incubation for 1 hour at 37° C, the nonadherent cells were removed by gently washing twice with warm (37°C) RPMI 1640. Two hundred microliters of RPMI 1640 containing 10% human blood group type AB serum was added to each well and the monocyte preparations were allowed to develop into macrophages by incubation for 5 to 6 days at 37°C. After this incubation period, the medium was removed and the macrophages incubated for an additional 24 hours with test samples. Then the number of macrophages adhering to the wells were counted and washed. ^{3}H-TdR-prelabeled K562 cells were added to each well (effector:target cell ratio=10:1). After 48 hours of incubation, release of incorporated ^{3}H-TdR from K562 was determined by counting radioactivity. MAF-C activity was expressed as the percentage of tumor cytotoxicity where:

$$\% \text{ Tumor cytotoxicity} = \frac{\text{release in test sample} - \text{spontaneous release}}{\text{total count} - \text{spontaneous release}} - \frac{\text{release in control sample} - \text{spontaneous release}}{\text{total count} - \text{spontaneous release}} \times 100$$

To quantify MAF-C activity, 100 units of MAF-C was defined as the amount of MAF-C in 1 ml of the ammonium sulfate precipitate fraction of the H2-E3-5 culture supernatant. To determine the amount of MAF-C activity, serial dilutions were assayed.

Assay for tumor cytotoxicity of human monocytes [MAF-C (monocyte)]

Instead of monocyte-derived macrophages, plastic-adherent monocytes were used for the MAF-C assay. Other details were as above.

Assay for tumor cytotoxicity of mouse macrophages

Peritoneal exudate macrophages were isolated from DBA/2 female mice (6-8 weeks old) 4 days after intraperitoneal injection of 2 ml of proteose peptone. Cells were cultured at a concentration of 2×10^5 cells/well on a 96-well plate (Falcon Plastics, Oxnard, Calif.) in RPMI 1640 medium supplemented with 10% fetal calf serum. After 120 minutes at 37°C, the cultures were washed twice to remove nonadherent cells. More than 95% of the adherent cells were macrophages, as judged by their ability to take up latex beads and by morphological observation. The macrophages thus obtained were incubated for 24 hours with test samples and the cytotoxicity was tested using ^{3}H-TdR-prelabeled P815 cells as target cells. Other details were the same as in the case of human monocyte-derived macrophages.

Assay for interferon

Interferon (IFN) activity was determined by a cytopathic-effect-inhibition assay with vesicular stomatitis virus in WISH (HeLa) cells.

RESULTS

Establishment of hybridomas

PHA-P-activated PBL were successfully fused with emetine- and actinomycin D-treated CEM 11 cells, a clone of CEM cells, as described under Materials and Methods. Within 2 weeks of fusion, good growth of hybridomas was observed in all wells, while both emetine- and actinomycin D-treated CEM 11 cells and mitomycin C-treated CEM 11 cells in control cultures completely lost their proliferating activity within a week, suggesting that all of the growing cells were hybrid cells.

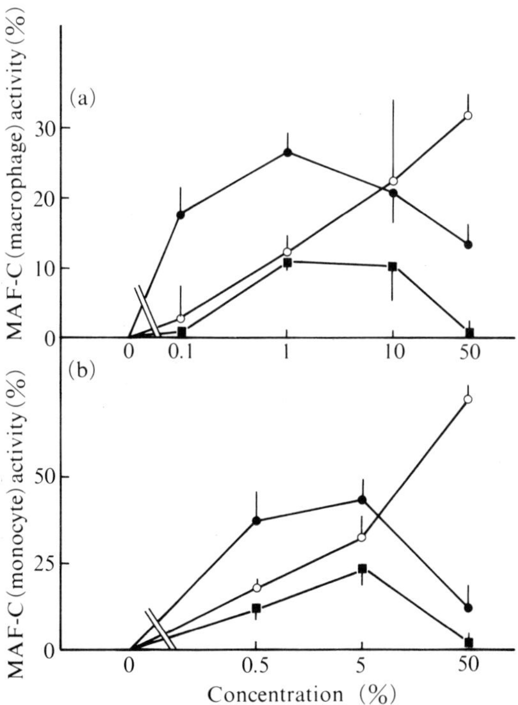

Fig. 1 (a) Dose-response curves of MAF-C (macrophage) activity of PHA sup (○), H2-E3-5 sup (●) and CEM 11 sup (■). (b) Dose-response curves of MAF-C (monocyte) activity of PHA sup (○), H3-E9-6 sup (●) and CEM 11 sup (■).

MAF-C production by H2-E3-5 and H3-E9-6

In order to obtain MAF-C-producing hybridoma cells, we assayed MAF-C activity in the culture supernatant of all hybrid cell lines using human monocytes and monocyte-derived macrophages as target cells, and obtained an MAF-C (macrophage)-producing hybrid cell line, H2-E3, and an MAF-C (monocyte)-producing hybrid cell line, H3-E9. The cloning of H2-E3 and H3-E9 was carried out by limited dilution (0.5 cells/well) using mitomycin C-treated CEM 11 cells as feeder cells. Thus, a high MAF-C (macrophage)-producing hybrid clone, H2-E3-5, and a high MAF-C (monocyte)-producing hybrid clone, H3-E9-6, were obtained. Next comparison was made of the MAF-C activity of PHA-P-activated PBL culture supernatant (PHA sup), CEM 11 culture supernatant (CEM 11 sup), and H2-E3-5 and H3-E9-6 culture supernatants. Both H2-E3-5 and H3-E9-6 produced more MAF-C than PHA-P-activated PBL, whereas CEM 11 produced much weaker MAF-C activity (Fig. 1). At high concentrations of the hybridoma culture supernatants (10-50%), an inhibitory effect was observed.

Effect of H2-E3-5 concentrated supernatant on human monocyte-derived macrophages and human monocytes

In order to clarify which stage of differentiation of macrophages is stimulated by MAF-C from H2-E3-5, not only monocyte-derived macrophages but also monocytes were used as effector cells. Table 1 shows the tumoricidal activities of these effector cells activated with PHA sup, H2-E3-5 concentrated supernatant (H2-E3-5 conc. sup) or lipopolysaccharide (LPS). PHA sup activated both monocyte-derived macrophages and monocytes, whereas H2-E3-5 conc. sup and LPS activated monocyte-

Table 1 Tumor cytotoxicity by activated monocytes and monocyte-derived macrophages

	Activity(%)			
	Sample (final concentration in culture medium)			
Effector cells	PHA sup (50%)	PHA sup (10%)	H2-E3-5 conc. sup(10%)	LPS (10 μg/ml)
Monocytes				
Exp. 1	17.8±1.3	10.2±0.4	2.7±0.7	–
Exp. 2	8.7±1.2	–	–	1.0±0.9
Monocyte-derived-macrophages				
Exp. 1	36.2±1.9	26.2±1.9	29.0±2.8	–
Exp. 2	15.0±1.9	–	–	40.5±2.3

Table 2 MAF-C activity in H3-E9-6 culture supernatant

Sample (final concentration in culture medium)	Activity (%)		
	MAF-C (monocytes)	MAF-C (monocyte-derived macrophages)	MAF-C (mouse macrophages)*[1]
H3-E9-6 sup (0.5%)	37.2±8.7	–	–
(1%)	–	27.8±1.2	–
(5%)	43.0±6.0	–	–
(10%)	–	–	10.9
PHA sup (0.5%)	18.6±1.3	–	–
(10%)	–	61.7±13.7	–
Mouse PHA sup (50%)	–	–	-2.5
LPS (10 ng/ml)	–	–	3.4
Mouse PHA sup (50%) +LPS (10 ng/ml)	–	–	73.3
Mouse PHA sup (50%) +H3-E9-6 sup (10%)	–	–	52.5
LPS (10 mg/ml) +H3-E9-6 sup (10%)	–	–	10.5

*[1] Average values for duplicate determinations.

derived macrophages but not monocytes. These results suggest that different molecules are concerned in the activation of macrophages and monocytes to kill tumor cells.

Effect of H3-E9-6 supernatant on human monocyte-derived macrophages, human monocytes and mouse macrophages

The MAF-C in the H3-E9-6 culture supernatant can activate human monocytes, human monocyte-derived macrophages and even proteose peptone-elicited mouse peritoneal exudate cells (Table 2). Furthermore, it was found that the activation of the cytotoxicity of mouse macrophages by the H3-E9-6 sup was markedly enhanced by the addition of culture supernatants of PHA-activated mouse spleen cells while the addition of LPS had no effect.

DISCUSSION

The data presented in this paper demonstrate that there are at least two human MAF-Cs, differing in the maturational stages of the cells they affect. One of them, derived from H2-E3-5 and LPS, was found to activate tumor cell killing by differentiated macrophages only, while the other, derived from H3-E9-6 and PHA sup, could activate both monocytes and monocyte-derived macrophages. However, it is not certain whether or not a single molecular species in the H3-E9-6 sup or the PHA sup is responsible for activity toward the two kinds of cells.

The current investigation has revealed that two signals are required to generate tumoricidal activity in mouse macrophages; mouse MAF is generally considered to be the first signal which primes the macrophages for triggering by a second signal.[6–10] Hammerstrøm[7] reported that LPS activation of tumoricidal activity of human monocytes occurred at a very low rate but gradually increased during an *in vitro* culture; he suggested that the *in vitro* culture acts as a priming signal and LPS as a triggering signal. Our results suggest that human MAF-C derived from H2-E3-5 may function as a triggering signal. Moreover, the fact that the tumoricidal activation of mouse macrophages by the H3-E9-6 sup was remarkably enhanced by the addition of culture supernatants of PHA-activated mouse spleen cells, but not by the addition of LPS, suggests that the MAF-C in the H3-E9-6 sup is also a triggering signal, at least toward mouse macrophages, and that the PHA sup contains certain priming signals.

We could not detect any antiviral activity in the H2-E3-5 and H3-E9-6 culture supernatants. These results seem to suggest at least that MAF-Cs produced by our human T cell hybridomas are distinct from IFN-γ. However, Svedersky et al.[11] have reported recently that a tiny amount of murine recombinant IFN-γ, too little to be detectable in antiviral assays, can exert potent macrophage activation activity if a second signal (LPS) is present. Since the MAF-C obtained from either H2-E3-5 or H3-E9-6 acts as a triggering signal in the tumoricidal activation of macrophages, the possibility that these MAF-Cs and IFN-γ are the same molecular species is remote. However, to verify this assumption further, a neutralization test with an antibody raised against the purified preparation of human IFN-γ may be necessary.

REFERENCES

1. Higuchi, M., Asada, M., Kobayashi, Y. and Osawa, T. (1983): Human T cell hybridomas producing migration inhibitory factor and macrophage activating factors, *Cell. Immunol., 78*, 236.
2. Higuchi, M., Nakamura, N., Tsuchiya, S., Kobayashi, Y. and Osawa, T. (1984): Macrophage activating factor for cytotoxicity produced by a human T cell hybridoma. *Cell. Immunol., 87,* 626.
3. Kawaguchi, T., Matsumoto, I. and Osawa, T. (1974): Studies on hemagglutinins from *Maackia amurensis* seeds. *J. Biol. Chem., 249*, 2786.
4. Kobayashi, Y., Asada, M., Higuchi, M. and Osawa, T. (1982): Human T cell hybridomas producing lymphokines. I. Establishment and characterization of human T-cell hybridomas producing lymphotoxin and migration inhibitory factor. *J. Immunol., 128*, 2714.
5. Cameron, D.J. and Churchill, W.H. (1980): Cytotoxicity of human macrophages for tumor cells: Enhancement by bacterial lipopolysaccharides (LPS). *J. Im-*

munol., 124, 708.

6. Weinberg, J.B., Chapman, H.A., Jr. and Hibbs, J.B., Jr. (1978): Characterization of the effects of endotoxin on macrophage tumor cell killing. *J. Immunol., 121*, 72.
7. Hammerstrøm, J. (1979): In vitro influence of endotoxin on human mononuclear phagocyte structure and function. 2. Enhancement of the expression of cytostatic and cytolytic activity of normal and lymphokine-activated monocytes. *Acta Path. Microbiol. Immunol. Scand., Sect. C., 87*, 391.
8. Meltzer, M.S. (1981): Tumor cytotoxicity by lymphokine-activated macrophages: Development of macrophage tumoricidal activity requires a sequence of reactions. *Lymphokines, 3*, 319.
9. Ratliff, T.L., Thomasson, D.L., McCool, R.E. and Catalona, W.J. (1982): Production of macrophage activation factor by a T-cell hybridoma. *Cell. Immunol., 68*, 311.
10. Schreiber, R.D., Altman, A. and Katz, D.H. (1982): Identification of a T cell hybridoma that produces large quantities of macrophage activating factor. *J. Exp. Med., 156*, 677.
11. Svedersky, L.P., Benton, C.V., Berger, W.H., Rinderknecht, E., Harkins, R.N. and Palladino, M.A. (1984): Biological and antigenic similarities of murine interferon-γ and macrophage-activating factor. *J. Exp. Med., 159*, 812.

In vitro activation of human pleural macrophages with *Nocardia rubra* cell wall skeleton (N-CWS)

Mitsunori Sakatani, Tomiya Masuno, Ichiro Kawase, Takeshi Ogura, Susumu Kishimoto and Yuichi Yamamura

SUMMARY

Nocardia rubra cell wall skeleton (N-CWS) augmented *in vitro* cytostatic activity of human pleural macrophages for human lung cancer cells. Macrophage activity was increased following direct interaction of macrophages with N-CWS or following incubation of macrophages with supernatant culture fluids from pleural lymphocytes with N-CWS. Maximal augmentation was observed after 24 hours of incubation of macrophages with 10 μg/ml N-CWS in the presence of lymphocytes. The culture fluids of pleural lymphocytes with N-CWS contained macrophage activation factor (MAF)-like substance other than interferon (IFN)-γ.

INTRODUCTION

In a previous report, the authors showed the clinical effectiveness of local adjuvant immunotherapy with *Nocardia rubra* cell wall skeleton (N-CWS) for malignant pleural effusion.[1] In an animal model, intraperitoneal adjuvant immunotherapy with N-CWS resulted in marked increases not only in peritoneal exudate cell number but also in the tumoricidal activity of peritoneal exudate macrophages.[2,3] These results indicate an important role of macrophages in developing an immunotherapeutic effect in nonspecific immunotherapy.

The purpose of the work reported in the present paper was to examine the ability of N-CWS to augment *in vitro* cytotoxic activity of human pleural macrophages and to investigate in more detail the role of N-CWS in macrophage activation.

MATERIALS AND METHODS

Patients

Specimens of pleural effusions (usually 100 to 200 ml) were harvested from 18 patients into heparinized glass bottles by thoracentesis. Histological diagnosis of the primary tumors revealed that all 18 patients had adenocarcinoma of the lung. The 11 male and 7 female patients, ranging in age from 42 to 78 years, had not received any anticancer chemotherapy before the time of thoracentesis.

Pleural washings were obtained from another 30 patients with lung cancer during surgery. Most of them were patients in the Department of Chest Surgery, Osaka Medical Center for Adult Diseases. The pleural cavity was washed with 500 ml of warmed sterile saline solution and washings were collected in heparinized glass bottles. Sixteen patients had squamous cell carcinoma and 14 had adenocarcinoma. Twenty of the patients were male and 10 were female; their ages ranged from 34 to 73 years.

Pleural mononuclear cells

Pleural effusions and pleural washings harvested in heparinized glass bottles were immediately centrifuged at 400 g for 5 minutes. The cells were washed twice with Eagle's minimum essential medium (MEM) and suspended in 20 ml of complete medium (RPMI 1640 medium supplemented with 100 μU/ml of penicillin, 100 μg/ml of streptomycin, 2 mM glutamine and 10% heat-inactivated fetal calf serum). Mononuclear cells (MNC) were isolated by Ficoll-Hypaque (Ficoll-Paque; Pharmacia Fine Chemical, Uppsala, Sweden) density gradient centrifugation, washed twice and resuspended in complete medium.

Preparation of macrophage monolayers

After determination of viability using the trypan blue dye exclusion test, 1×10^5 MNC suspended in 0.2 ml complete medium were dispensed into the flat-bottomed wells of 96-well culture plates (#25860; Corning Glass Works, Corning, NY). After incubation at 37°C for 2 hours, nonadherent cells were removed by repeated washings with MEM, producing monolayers of adherent cells which consisted of esterase staining-positive cells and showed the typical morphology of macrophages by Giemsa staining. In some experiments, before MNC dispensation, T-lymphocytes were removed by centrifugation of the rosetting cells with sheep red blood cells (E-rosetting cells).

Reagents

Nocardia rubra cell wall skeleton (N-CWS) was supplied as a lyophilized preparation containing 2 mg of N-CWS, 4 mg of squalene, 1 mg of polysorbate-80 and 28.2 mg of mannitol (Fujisawa Pharmaceutical Co., Ltd., Osaka, Japan). Prior to use, it was redispersed with 0.85% NaCl solution at a concentration of 0.1 mg/ml.

Cell culture and preparation of culture supernatants

Pleural MNC (1×10^5), adherent macrophages or nonadherent cells (5×10^4) were incubated with or without N-CWS (10 μg/ml) at 37°C in a 5% CO_2-air humidified atmosphere. After 24 hours of incubation, the supernatants were centrifuged, passed through a 0.45 μm cellulose nitrate filter (Sartorius GbH, Göttingen, FRG) and frozen at −20°C until tested. The adherent macrophages that remained in the culture plates were washed twice with fresh medium and were used for cytostasis assay.

Assay for macrophage-mediated tumor cytostasis

In vitro tumor cytostasis was assayed using human lung adenocarcinoma PC-9 cells, which had been kindly supplied by Dr. Hayata of Tokyo Medical College. The assay was based on the method of Evans and Alexander.[4] Briefly, 1×10^4 tumor cells were added to culture wells containing macrophages. The culture plates were incubated at 37°C in a 5% CO_2-air humidified atmosphere for 24 hours. Cells in each well were pulsed with 0.5 μCi (^{3}H)-TdR for the last 6 hours and harvested with a cell harvester. Cellular DNA was precipitated on glass fiber filters and the radioactivity of the (^{3}H)-TdR incorporated was determined in a liquid scintillation counter. The mean cpm were obtained from triplicated cultures, and results were presented as percentage cytostasis which was calculated by the following formula:

$$\%\ \text{cytostasis} = \frac{(A-B)}{A}\times 100$$

where A is the cpm of the culture containing tumor cells alone, and B is the cpm of the culture containing experimental macrophages. The significance of the difference between the percentage cytostasis of the control and that of experimental macrophages was determined by Student's *t*-test.

Macrophage activating factor

Macrophage activating factor (MAF) activities in the culture supernatants mentioned above were determined by measuring their ability to induce cytostatic activity toward PC-9 cells in human pleural macrophages. The fresh macrophage monolayers in 96-well culture plates were incubated in 200 μl of complete medium and 100 μl of culture supernatants. After 24 hours of incubation, macrophage monolayers were washed twice with MEM and 1×10^4 PC-9 cells were added to each well for the assay of macrophage-mediated tumor cytostasis.

Interferon assay

Interferon (IFN) in the culture supernatants was quantitated by a virus plaque reduction assay with the use of human amnion FL-WISH cells and vesicular stomatitis virus (VSV). IFN activity was expressed in National Institutes of Health (NIH) reference units with recombinant human leukocyte IFN-α (La Roche Co., Ltd., Basel, Switzerland).

Interleukin-1 assay

Interleukin-1 (IL-1) activities in the culture supernatants were determined by measuring the proliferative effects on mouse thymocytes.[5] Thymocytes (5×10^5/well) from 6- to 8-week old C3H/HeJ mice were cultured in 0.1 ml of complete medium containing 0.1% phytohemagglutinin (PHA) in flat bottomed 96-well culture plates, to which 0.1 ml of supernatant was added and cultured for 3 days at 37°C; for the last 20 hours of incubation, 0.5 μCi of (^{3}H)-TdR was added. The cultures were harvested on glass fiber filters and the radioactivity of the filters was measured with a liquid scintillation counter.

Assay for glucose consumption

The glucose consumption in macrophages[6] was determined by measuring the incorporation of (^{3}H)-2-deoxy-D-glucose. Macrophage monolayers in 96-well culture plates were incubated with phosphate buffer solution (PBS) containing 8.2×10^{-2} mg/ml 2-deoxy-D-glucose (2-DG) for 10 minutes. After incubation, the wells were pulsed with 0.2 μCi (^{3}H)-2-DG (New England Nuclear, Boston, Mass) for 40 minutes. The wells were washed twice with cold (4°C) PBS containing 2-DG. The cells were then harvested with a cell harvester and precipitated on glass fiber filters. The (^{3}H)-2-DG radioactivity incorporated was determined with a liquid

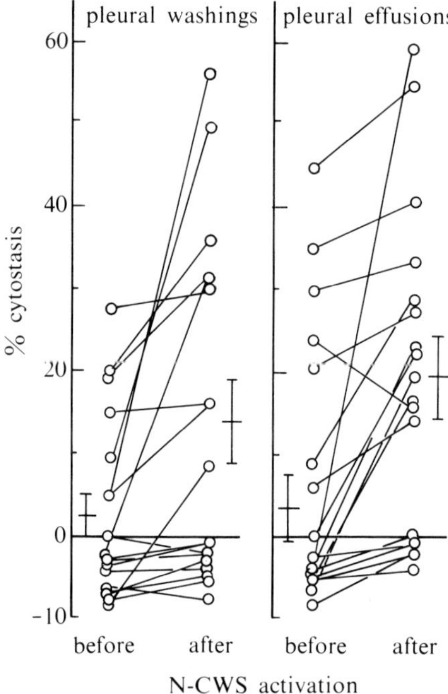

Fig. 1 Human pleural macrophage cytostatic activity and effect of N-CWS. Bars indicate means$\pm$SE.

scintillation counter.

Heat and acid stability studies

Samples of culture supernatants were incubated at 56°C in a constant-temperature bath with a circulator. After 30 minutes, sample tubes were removed, rapidly cooled in an ice bath, and then assayed for residual MAF and IFN activities. Samples of culture supernatants were dialysed against 0.1 M glycine-HCl-0.15 M NaCl buffer (pH 2.0) for 24 hours at 4°C, followed by a further 24 hours dialysis against RPMI-1640 medium, and then assay for residual IFN activity.

RESULTS

Cellular composition of pleural effusions and washings

In 12 of 18 effusions, no malignant cells were found on routine cytological examination. The yields of MNC ranged from 1×10^6 to $10\times$

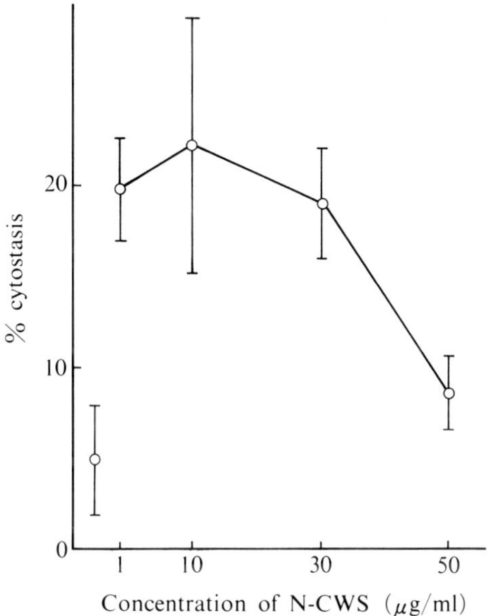

Fig. 2 Relation of N-CWS concentration to macrophage activation. Results are means ± SE of triplicate cultures at each concentration.

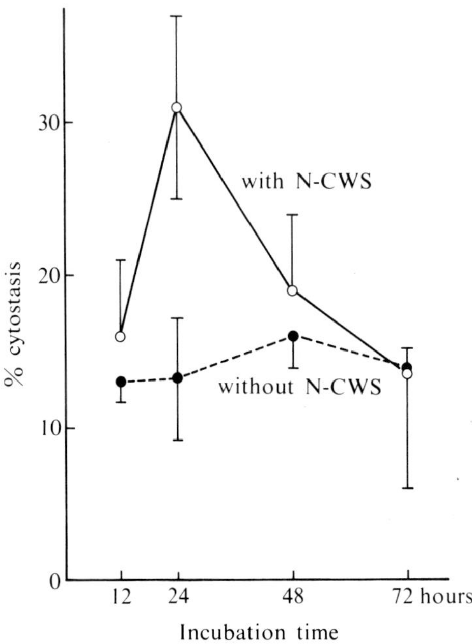

Fig. 3 Kinetics of macrophage activation with N-CWS. Results are means ± SE of triplicate cultures.

10^6 cells. The percentage of adherent macrophages varied among the 18 effusions, ranging from 15% to 40% of the initial cells dispensed. Evaluated on a morphological basis, almost all of the nonadherent cells consisted of lymphoid cells. The percentage of tumor cells varied considerably among the six effusions in which they were found.

In the 30 washings, yields of MNC ranged from 0.8×10^6 to 1.6×10^6 cells, Approximately 40% to 60% of MNC dispensed were adherent macrophages and almost all nonadherent cells were lymphoid cells. Eighteen washings were used for cytostasis assay, and the other 12 washings for analysis of macrophage activation mechanisms.

Effect of N-CWS on macrophage cytostatic activity

The overall results from 36 patients (18 patients with pleural effusions and 18 surgically operated patients) are shown in Fig. 1. Pleural macrophages were incubated in the presence of nonadherent cells for assay of macrophage-mediated cytostasis. Increased cytostasis was observed in 7 (38.9%) of 18 effusions without N-CWS treatment and mean cytostasis ($\pm$ SE) was $24.5 \pm 5.2\%$. After N-CWS treatment, 12 (66.7%) effusions showed increased cytostatic activity, ranging from 14.0% to 59.8%. The mean activity in these 12 effusions was $29.7 \pm 4.4\%$. Increased cytostasis was observed in seven washings without N-CWS treatment and nine washings with N-CWS treatment. The mean cytostasis values were $14.3 \pm 3.2\%$ and $30.6 \pm 5.2\%$ respectively. In a total of 36 cases tested, the cytostatic activity of N-CWS-treated macrophages was significantly higher than that of nontreated macrophages ($p < 0.05$). The difference between the mean activities of the effusions and the washings was not statistically significant. Regarding the dose response and kinetics of activation by N-CWS, cytostatic activity was increased after 12 hours of incubation and maximal activation required 24 hours of incubation at an N-CWS concentration of 10 μg/ml (Figs. 2 and 3).

Table 1 *In vitro* augmentation of macrophage activity by N-CWS

	cytostatic activity[a]		2-DG uptake[b]		IL-1 activity[c]	
	N-CWS		N-CWS		N-CWS	
case No.	(−)	(+)	(−)	(+)	(−)	(+)
37	-6.9	19.6	1709	2307	523	2776
38	-4.3	16.5	2447	3593	5787	11844
39	-2.8	0.3	366	699	220	303
40	-2.1	59.8	1890	3959	504	4944

[a] percent cytostasis against PC-9 cells.
[b] (^{3}H)-2-DG uptake (dpm) by 1×10^5 macrophages in 40 minutes.
[c] (^{3}H)-TdR uptake (dpm) by mouse thymocytes incubated with supernatant tested.

Other characteristics of N-CWS-activated macrophages

Staining for nonspecific esterase was clearly positive in N-CWS-treated macrophages. Glucose metabolism, measured by 2-DG-incorporation, was increased in N-CWS-treated macrophages. IL-1 activities were significantly higher in supernatants from MNC cultures with N-CWS (Table 1).

Role of T-lymphocytes in macrophage activation with N-CWS

To examine the interaction between macrophages and co-existing lymphocytes, whole MNC and adherent macrophages depleted of T-lymphocytes with E-rosetting cells were incubated separately with N-CWS. The removal of T-lymphocytes produced partial reduction of cytostatic activity (Fig. 4). To elucidate the underlying mechanism, culture supernatants from whole MNC, adherent macrophages or nonadherent cells were assayed for their ability to increase cytostatic activity of allogeneic pleural macrophages. MAF activity was detected in the culture supernatants of whole MNC and nonadherent cells but not of adherent macrophages alone (Fig. 5). Six out of eight supernatants of MNC cultures with N-CWS showed increased MAF activity (Table 2).

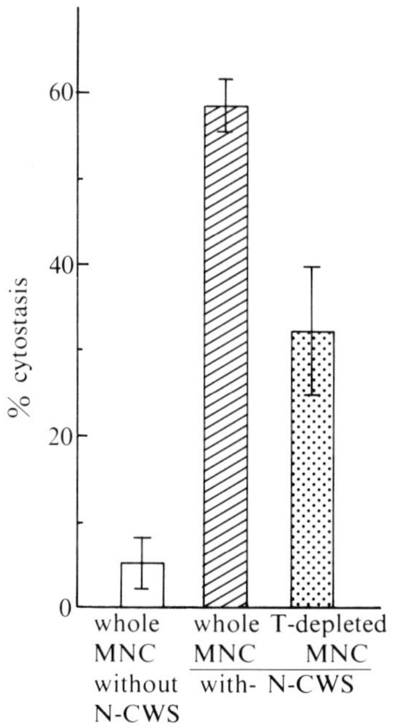

Fig. 4 Effect of presence of T-lymphocytes on macrophage activation with N-CWS. Results are means±SE of triplicate cultures.

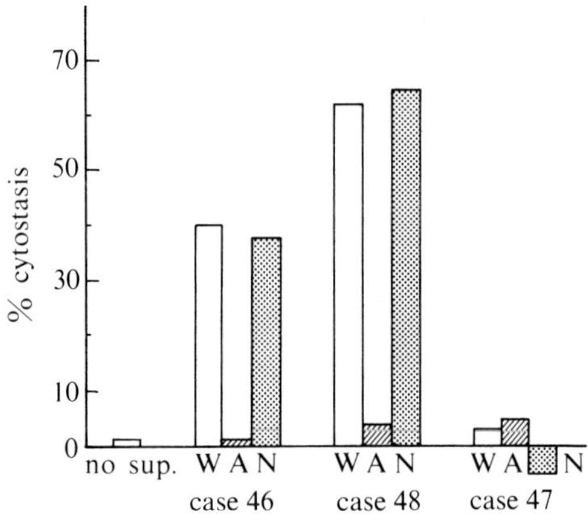

Fig. 5 MAF activity in supernatants (sup) from cultures of whole MNC (W), adherent cells (A) or nonadherent cells (N) with N-CWS. Results are means of duplicate cultures.

Table 2 MAF and IFN activities in supernatants of MNC cultures with N-CWS

	Treatment at 56°C for 30 minutes				Dialysis against pH 2 buffer
	Pretreatment		Post-treatment		
case No.	MAF[a]	IFN[b]	MAF[a]	IFN[b]	IFN[b]
41	31.3	<4	28.9	<4	<4
42	20.6	64	22.6	<4	<4
43	20.5	256	2.8	<4	<4
44	3.1	<4	NT	<4	<4
45	26.7	512	39.4	<4	<4
46	40.1	<4	NT	<4	<4
47	3.2	<4	NT	<4	<4
48	61.6	<4	NT	<4	<4

[a] cytostatic activities of macrophages incubated with supernatants tested (%).
[b] units/ml.
NT: not tested.

IFN activity in culture supernatants

As Table 2 shows, IFN activity was detected only in three of six supernatants showing MAF activity, ranging from 64 to 512 units/ml. Two supernatants without MAF activity showed no significant IFN activity. Heat and acid stability study revealed that the IFN activity detected in the three supernatants was not stable. In contrast, in three of four samples studied, increased MAF activities were not affected after incubation at 56° C for 30 minutes.

DISCUSSION

There is considerable evidence from animal studies that macrophages can be activated to nonspecific tumor cytotoxicity by a variety of treatments.[2,7–15] In a few papers, *in vitro* exposure to lymphokine supernatants,[15] IFN,[16,17] endotoxin[18,19] or muramyl dipeptide[20,21] has been reported to enhance the tumoricidal activity of human monocytes and macrophages obtained from peripheral blood,[16–18,21] bronchial washings[19,20] or malignant ascitic fluid.[16]

The present results demonstrated that *in vitro* treatment of human pleural macrophages with N-CWS augmented glucose consumption and IL-1 release as well as the cytotoxic potential of macrophages. The cytostatic activity of macrophages was maximally increased after 24 hours of incubation with 10 μg/ml N-CWS in the presence of pleural lymphocytes. Activity was detectable but decreased in the absence of lymphocytes. Macrophages were also stimulated by culture supernatants of pleural lymphocytes incubated with N-CWS, indicating direct and indirect activation of macrophages by N-CWS. Regarding direct activation, Sone et al.[22] reported that rat alveolar macrophages were rendered tumoricidal following direct interaction with N-CWS. Masuno[23] found that culture supernatants of spleen cells with N-CWS could make mouse peritoneal macrophages tumoricidal. The present results seem to be consistent with these earlier observations on rodent macrophages.

IFN activity was detected in three of six supernatants strongly activating macrophages for tumor cytostasis. The heat-stability study, in which IFN activity in the culture supernatants was lost while MAF activity was not affected, indicated that these culture supernatants contained an MAF-like substance other than IFN-γ. Our results are in agreement with the findings of Mantovani et al.[16] that in lymphokine supernatants IFN plays an important role for macrophage activation and that lymphocyte mediators other than IFN can also augment macrophage activity.

Further studies for the definition of the mechanism(s) by which IFN and MAF are released by N-CWS may provide new approaches for more successful local immunotherapy of malignant pleural effusions.

REFERENCES

1. Yamamura, Y., Ogura, T., Sakatani, M., Hirao, F., Kishimoto, S., Fukuoka, M., Takada, M., Kawahara, M., Furuse, K., Kuwahara, O., Ikegami, H. and Ogawa,

N. (1983): Randomized controlled study of adjuvant immunotherapy with *Nocardia rubra* cell wall skeleton for inoperable lung cancer. *Cancer Res., 43*, 5575.

2. Ogura, T., Namba, M., Hirao, F., Yamamura, Y. and Azuma, I. (1979): Association of macrophage activation with antitumor effect on rat syngeneic fibrosarcoma by *Nocardia rubra* cell wall skeleton. *Cancer Res., 39*, 4706.
3. Ogura, T., Shinzato, O., Sakatani, M., Shindo, H., Namba, M., Kishimoto, S. and Yamamura, Y. (1982): Analysis of therapeutic effect in experimental chemoimmunotherapy for rat ascitic tumor. *Cancer Immunol. Immunother., 14*, 67.
4. Evans, R. and Alexander, P. (1970): Cooperation of immune lymphoid cells with macrophages in tumor immunity. *Nature (London), 228*, 620.
5. Pollack, S., Micall, A., Kinne, D.W., Enker, W.E., Gellen, N., Oettigen, H.F. and Hoffman, M.K. (1983): Endotoxin-induced *in vitro* release of Interleukin-1 by cancer patients' monocytes. *Int. J. Cancer, 32*, 733.
6. Sober, A.J., Haynie, M. and David, J. (1979): Enhanced uptake of ^{3}H-glucosamine by macrophages stimulated by macrophage-activating factor. *J. Immunol., 122*, 1731.
7. Zwilling, B.S. and Campolito, L.B. (1977): Destruction of tumor cells by BCG-activated alveolar macrophages. *J. Immunol., 119*, 838.
8. Olivotto, M. and Bomford, R. (1974): *In vitro* inhibition of tumor cell growth and DNA synthesis by peritoneal and lung macrophages from mice injected with *Corynebacterium pavum. Int. J. Cancer, 13*, 478.
9. Weinberg, J.B., Chapman, H.A. and Hibbs, J.B., Jr. (1978): Characterization of the effects of endotoxin on macrophage tumor cell killing. *J. Immunol., 121*, 72.
10. Alexander, P. and Evans, R. (1971): Endotoxin and double-stranded RNA render macrophage cytotoxic. *Nature New Biology, 232*, 76.
11. Stoychkov, J.N., Schultz, R.M., Chirigos, M.A., Pavlidis, N.A. and Goldin, A. (1979): Effect of adriamycin and cyclophosphamide treatment on induction of macrophage cytotoxicity function in mice. *Cancer Res., 39*, 3014.
12. Ogura, T., Shindo, H., Shinzato, O., Namba, M., Masuno, T., Inoue, T., Kishimoto, S. and Yamamura, Y. (1982): *In vitro* tumor cell killing by peritoneal macrophages from mitomycin-C-treated rats. *Cancer Immunol. Immunother., 13*, 112.
13. Wang, B.S., Lumanglas, A.L., Ruszala-Mallon, V.M. and Durr, F.E. (1984): Activation of tumor-cytostatic macrophages with the antitumor agent 9,10-Anthracene di-carboxaldehyde Bis [(4,5-dihydro-1 H-imidazole-2-yl) hydrazone] Dihydrochloride (Bisantrene). *Cancer Res., 44*, 2363.
14. Meltzer, M.S., Benjamin, W.R. and Farrar, J.J. (1982): Macrophage activation for tumoricidal activity by lymphokines from EL-4, a continuous T cell line. *J. Immunol., 129*, 2802.
15. Sone, S., Poste, G. and Fidler, I.J. (1980): Rat alveolar macrophages are susceptible to activation by free and liposome-encapsulated lymphokines. *J. Immunol., 124*, 2197.
16. Mantovani, A., Dean, J.H., Jerrells, T.R. and Herberman, R.B. (1980): Augmentation of tumoricidal activity of human monocytes and macrophages by lymphokines. *Int. J. Cancer, 25*, 691.
17. Le, J., Prensky, W., Yip, Y.K., Chang, Z., Hoffman, T., Stevenson, H.C., Blazs, I., Sadlik, J.R. and Vilĉek, J. (1983): Activation of human monocyte cytotoxicity by natural and recombinant immune interferon. *J. Immunol., 131*, 2821.
18. Cameron, D.J. and Churchill, W.H. (1980): Cytotoxicity of human macrophages for tumor cells: Enhancement by bacterial lipopolysaccharides (LPS). *J. Im-*

munol., 124, 708.
19. Sone, S., Moriguchi, S., Shimizu, E., Ogushi, F. and Tsubura, E. (1982): *In vitro* generation of tumoricidal properties in human alveolar macrophages following interaction with endotoxin. *Cancer Res., 42*, 2227.
20. Sone, S. and Tsubura, E. (1982): Human alveolar macrophages: Potentiation of their tumoricidal activity by liposome-encapsulated muramyl dipeptide. *J. Immunol., 129*, 1313.
21. Lopez-Berestein, G., Mehta, K., Mehta, R., Juliano, R. and Hersh, E.M. (1983): The activation of human monocytes by liposome-encapsulated muramyl dipeptide analogues. *J. Immunol., 130*, 1500.
22. Sone, S., Pollack, V.A. and Fidler, I.J. (1980): Direct activation of tumoricidal properties in rat alveolar macrophages by *Nocardia rubra* cell wall skeleton. *Cancer Immunol. Immunother., 9*, 227.
23. Masuno, T. (1980): Activation of mouse peritoneal macrophages by *Nocardia rubra* cell wall skeleton. *Osaka Univ. Med. J., 32*, 81. (In Japanese).

Generation *in vitro* of human monocyte tumoricidal potential by interferon alpha and beta

Teruhiro Utsugi, Saburo Sone, Seiji Mutsuura, Mitsumasa Ogawara, Toyohiro Shirahama, Kiyoshi Ishii and Eiro Tsubura

SUMMARY

Human blood monocytes separated by a continuous percoll gradient method were plated for 1 hour and then washed at least three times. The resultant monocyte-rich adherent monolayers contained up to 2.0% natural killer (NK) cells as assessed with a monoclonal antibody marker (Leu-7). The monocytes were not cytotoxic to allogeneic melanoma (A375) cells, but were activated to become tumoricidal by incubation for 24 hours with interferon (IFN)-α or IFN-β at concentrations of more than 1000 IU/ml. Maximal activation of the monocytes was achieved by incubating them with 50,000 IU/ml of IFN-α or IFN-β for 24 hours. Monocyte density was closely correlated with the development of monocyte-mediated cytotoxicity. Pretreatment of isolated monocyte preparations with anti-NK cell monoclonal antibodies (Leu-7 and Leu-11b) to deplete them of NK cell activity did not inhibit the monocyte-mediated cytotoxicity. Pre-exposure of tumor target cells to IFN-α resulted in increased sensitivity to cytotoxicity mediated by IFN-α-activated monocytes. These results indicate that IFN-α and IFN-β directly activate human monocytes to the tumoricidal state, although more than 1000 IU/ml of IFN-α or IFN-β is required for maximal expression of monocyte activation.

INTRODUCTION

Human monocytes and macrophages can be activated to destroy tumorigenic cells *in vitro* by treatment with bacterial preparations and various lymphokine preparations.[1–5] These *in vitro* findings suggest that the resultant tumoricidal macrophages may be important in the host defense against primary and/or metastatic cancers. Indeed, there is increasing evidence from animal models that *in situ* activation of the tumoricidal property of macrophages is closely associated with eradication of cancer metastasis.[6–8] Recently, interferon alpha (IFN-α) and interferon beta (IFN-β) have been shown to activate murine and human macrophages to destroy tumorigenic cells.[9–13] Several investigations have suggested that a variable but detectable proportion of lymphoid cells with natural killer (NK) activity contaminating adherent monocyte preparations may contribute to most, if not all, of the cytotoxicity mediated by IFN-treated monocytes, since IFN is a potentiator of NK cells. The authors, therefore, examined the nature of the effector cells involved in killing of tumor cells by monocyte-rich preparations using monoclonal antibodies against NK cells. The kinetics of monocyte activation by IFN-α and IFN-β were also studied.

MATERIALS AND METHODS

Cell cultures

Cell line A375, derived from a human melanoma,[3–5] was maintained on plastic in RPMI 1640 medium supplemented with 10% heat-inactivated fetal bovine serum and gentamicin (named CRPMI 1640) at 37°C in a humidified atmosphere of 5% CO_2 in air.

Reagents

RPMI 1640 medium and fetal bovine serum (FBS) were purchased from M. A. Bioproducts, Walkersville, Md. Human IFN-α and IFN-β were kindly supplied by Otsuka Pharmaceutical Co., Tokushima, Japan, and Toray Industries, Inc., Tokyo. Anti-NK cell antibodies (Leu-7 and Leu-11)[14,15] were purchased from Becton Dickinson Monoclonal Center, Inc., Mountain View, Calif.

Isolation and culture of human peripheral blood monocytes

Mononuclear cells were obtained from healthy donors, and separated by discontinuous gradient centrifugation on lymphocyte separation medium (LSM, Litton Bionetics, Kensington, Md). Monocytes were isolated from the mononuclear cell sample on a percoll gradient.[2] The resulting

Table 1 Cellular compositions of monocyte-rich preparations and adherent monocyte monolayers

Monocyte-rich preparations		Adherent monocyte monolayers	
% monocytes	% NK cells (mean±SD)	% monocytes	% NK cells (mean±SD)
≧76	9.3±9.4	≧97	1.1±0.9

monocyte-rich preparation contained≧76% monocytes (Table 1), as determined by nonspecific esterase staining and morphological examination, and the cells were≧97% viable, as judged by trypan blue dye exclusion.

Monocyte-mediated cytotoxicity

Cytotoxicity was assayed by measuring the release of radioactivity as described in detail previously.[5] ^{125}I-IUdR-labeled target cells (10^4) were plated into wells containing 10^5 monocytes. After 16 hours, the cells were washed to remove nonadherent and dead cells and re-fed with fresh CRPMI 1640. After a further 56 hours, the monocyte-target cell cultures were washed twice with phosphate buffered saline; adherent, presumably viable, cells were lysed with 0.1 ml of 0.1 N NaOH; and radioactivity was measured with a gamma counter.

The percentage of cytotoxicity mediated by activated human monocytes was calculated by the following formula:

$$\text{Percentage of specific cytotoxicity mediated by activated monocyte's} = \frac{A-B}{A} \times 100$$

where A represents the cpm in cultures of untreated monocytes and target cells, and B represents the cpm in cultures of test monocytes and target cells.

Statistical analysis

The statistical significance of differences between test groups was analyzed by Student's two-tailed *t*-test.

RESULTS

In vitro activation of human monocytes by IFN-α and IFN-β

The cellular compositions of monocyte-rich preparations and adherent

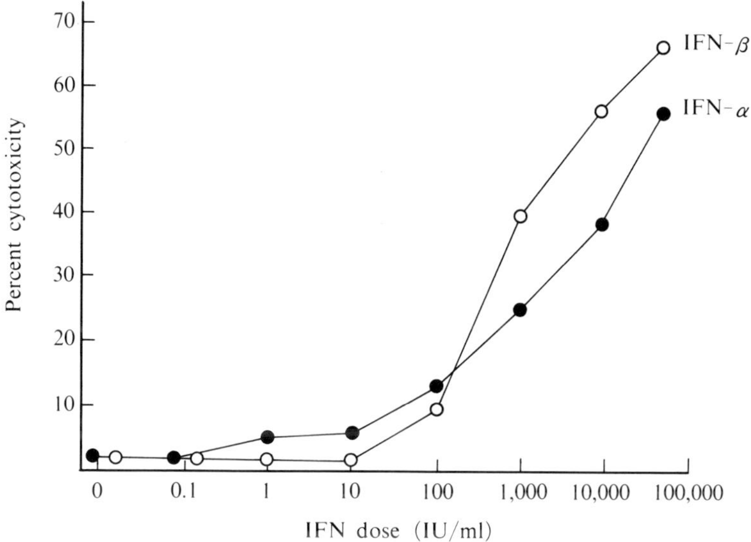

Fig. 1 Relation of activation of human monocytes to the tumoricidal state to dose of IFN-α or IFN-β. Cytotoxicity is shown as percent increase over that of untreated monocytes.

Table 2 Activation of monocytes in suspension by IFN-α and IFN-β

Monocyte density ($\times 10^5$/well)	% Cytotoxicity*1 of monocytes treated with				
	Medium	IFN-α*2		IFN-β*2	
2	2821±54	1953±98	(31)*3	2150±103	(24)*3
1.5	2825±39	2260±192	(20)*3	2274±108	(20)*3
1	2870±33	2406±162	(16)*3	2527±147	(12)*3
0.5	2988±71	2606±157	(13)	2598±210	(13)
0.25	2890±113	2753±90		2839±7	
0.1	2877±144	2752±245		2816±52	
0.05	2818±126	2796±52		2871±51	

*1 Mean cpm±SD for triplicate cultures. Representative results from three independent experiments.

*2 Figures in brackets are percent increase in cytotoxicity over that of untreated monocytes at the corresponding density.

*3 $p<0.05$.

monocyte monolayers were examined. Monocyte-rich preparations separated by continuous percoll gradient centrifugation were plated for 1 hour, washed three times with RPMI 1640, and stained with fluorescent anti-NK cell monoclonal antibody (Leu-7). Monocyte-rich preparations consisted of ≧76% monocytes; contaminating NK cells comprised 9% of cells (Table 1). When the cells had been plated for 1 hour and washed three times, contaminating NK cells comprised 0% to 2.0% of cells (mean±SD,

1.1±0.9) as assessed using anti-NK cell monoclonal antibodies (Leu-7 and Leu-11b).

For activation of monocytes by IFN, monocyte monolayers were incubated for 24 hours in medium with or without different doses of IFN-α or IFN-β, and the monolayers were washed thoroughly. ^{125}I-IUdR-labeled target A375 melanoma cells were then added to the wells. The untreated monocytes were not cytotoxic to allogeneic A375 melanoma cells, but significant and maximal activation of monocytes to the tumoricidal state was observed when monocytes were activated with more than 1,000 IU/ml of IFN-α or IFN-β for 24 hours (Fig. 1). Significant and reproducible monocyte-mediated cytotoxicity was obtained when monocytes were pretreated with 10,000 IU/ml of IFN-α or IFN-β.

In a parallel experiment, human monocytes in suspension were incubated for 24 hours in medium with 10,000 IU/ml of IFN-α. They were then plated for one hour and washed three times before the addition of labeled A375 melanoma cells. Assays were terminated 72 hours later. Results showed that suspended, but not plated, monocytes were activated to the tumoricidal state by interaction *in vitro* with IFN-α (or IFN-β) (Table 2).

Effect of monocyte density on activation of human monocytes by IFN-α or IFN-β

Human monocytes ranging in number from 0.05×10^5 to 2×10^5 cells/well (16 mm in diameter) were plated for 1 hour and thoroughly washed; the resulting monocyte monolayers were incubated for 24 hours with 10,000 IU/ml of IFN-α or IFN-β. Labeled A375 melanoma cells were then added. Assays were terminated 72 hours later. Results showed that, at densities of more than 5×10^4/well, monocytes were fully activated to destroy tumor cells in the presence of IFN-α or IFN-β (Table 3).

Table 3 Effect of monocyte density on activation of human monocytes by IFN-α and IFN-β

Monocyte density ($\times10^5$/well)	% Cytotoxicity against A375 cells*1 with:	
	IFN-α	IFN-β
0.01	9	12
0.05	11	22*2
0.1	10	20*2
0.5	64*2	61*2
1.0	61*2	62*2
2.0	53*2	56*2

*1 Percentage increase in cytotoxicity over that of untreated monocytes at the corresponding monocyte density.
*2 $p<0.05$.

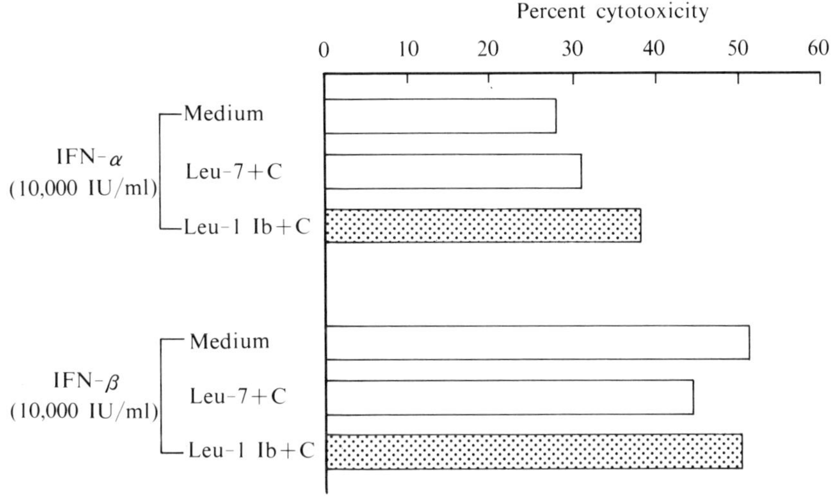

Fig. 2 Effect of NK cell depletion on monocyte activation by IFNs. Cytotoxicity is shown as percent increase over that of untreated monocytes.

Effect of NK cell depletion on monocyte activation by IFNs

To rule out the possibility that small populations of NK cells contaminating the monocyte monolayers were responsible for most, if not all, of the cytotoxicity mediated by IFN-treated monocytes, monocyte-rich monolayers were treated for 30 minutes with anti-NK cell antibodies (Leu-7 and Leu-11b), and then for 60 minutes with rabbit complement. The monocyte monolayers were then washed thoroughly and incubated with 10,000 IU/ml of IFN-α or IFN-β, and labeled A375 cells were added. These anti-NK cell monoclonal antibodies did not affect monocyte activation by IFN-α or IFN-β, indicating that both IFNs directly activate monocytes to kill human tumorigenic cells (Fig. 2).

Increased sensitivity of IFN-treated target cells to tumor cell killing by activated monocytes

Human A375 melanoma cells were exposed for 1 hour to different concentrations of IFN-α (1 to 100 IU/ml) before their addition to monocyte monolayers that had been incubated in medium with IFN-α for 24 hours. Pre-exposure of A375 melanoma cells to 100 IU/ml of IFN-α resulted in a significant increase in sensitivity to cytotoxicity mediated by monocytes treated with 1,000 or 10,000 IU/ml of IFN-α (Table 4).

Table 4 Effect of different doses of IFN-α on monocyte-mediated cytotoxicity against IFN-α-pretreated A375 melanoma cells

Treatment of target A375 melanoma cells		Cytotoxicity of monocytes*[1] treated with		
		Medium	IFN-α (1,000 IU)	IFN-α (10,000 IU)
Medium		2294±83	2102±96 (8)	1638±43 (29)*[2]
IFN-α	1 IU/ml	2289±45	2021±31 (12)*[2]	1671±54 (27)*[2]
	10 IU/ml	2324±22	2049±87 (11)*[2]	1639±25 (29)*[2]
	100 IU/ml	2216±67	1849±21 (19)*[2]	1490±53 (35)*[2]

*[1] Cpm±SD of triplicate cultures. Representative data from three independent experiments. Figures in brackets indicate percent increase in cytotoxicity over that of untreated monocytes.

*[2] $p<0.05$.

DISCUSSION

The present studies demonstrated that peripheral blood monocytes from healthy volunteers, separated on a percoll continuous gradient, were rendered tumoricidal by interaction *in vitro* with IFN-α or IFN-β, and that removal of NK cells with complement plus the newly-developed monoclonal antibodies that react specifically with NK cells[14,15] did not affect monocyte activation by IFN-α or IFN-β. The results also showed that activation of human monocytes by IFNs was closely correlated with the monocyte density, and that monocytes in suspension were also activated by IFNs to destroy tumor cells.

Little or no spontaneous cytotoxicity was observed with this assay in untreated blood monocytes isolated by continuous percoll gradient centrifugation. This is in contrast to our previous findings[5] and those of others[11,16] that monocytes isolated by adherence and then treated with a chelating agent such as EDTA were highly cytotoxic without activation stimuli. Thus these manipulations may affect the cell membrane, resulting in cell activation. Recently the small numbers of NK cells contaminating monocyte preparations were suggested to be responsible for some or all of the spontaneous cytotoxicity mediated by adherent monocyte populations. Monocyte preparations harvested by adherence only were found to contain 2% to 8% NK cells.[16,17] The present preparations of monocyte monolayers, isolated first by separation on a percoll gradient and then by adherence, contained much fewer NK cells (less than 2%) than preparations isolated by adherence alone. Moreover, the adherent monocyte monolayers were not tumoricidal without activation stimuli.

In the studies on the effects of IFN-α and IFN-β on monocyte activation, it was possible that some contaminating NK cells might have been activated, and perhaps more adherent, and thus have contributed to development of the observed cytotoxic activity. Therefore, the monocyte monolayers used in these experiments were incubated for 24 hours and washed before the monocyte-mediated cytotoxicity assay. This procedure should eliminate contaminating NK cells from the adherent monocytes, since adherent lymphoid cells with NK activity have been shown to become detached during the first 24 hours of culture. As conclusive evidence that NK cells were not responsible for the cytotoxicity, it was further shown that anti-NK cell monoclonal antibodies plus complement did not affect monocyte activation by IFN-α or IFN-β (Fig. 1). Thus the results clearly show that human monocytes respond directly to IFN-α and IFN-β, although relatively high doses of IFN (1,000 IU/ml) are required for significant monocyte activation.

Territo et al.[18] reported that monocytes from patients receiving intramuscular injections of 0.75 to 50×10^4 U of IFN-α for 7 days did not show any increase in tumoricidal potential. The present finding that significant activation of monocytes not only in monolayers but also in suspension requires interaction *in vitro* for 24 hours with 1,000 IU/ml of IFN may explain why the low blood levels of IFN-α produced by intramuscular injection did not activate peripheral monocytes in the experiments of Territo et al. Indeed, Yamazaki et al.[19] reported that the serum IFN-α level ranged from 30 to 60 IU/ml after intramuscular injection of 3×10^6 IU of IFN-α. In order to mimic *in vivo* conditions for monocyte-tumor cell interaction, target tumor cells were exposed to IFN-α at concentrations of 1 to 100 IU/ml for 2 hours. Pretreatment of tumor cells with 100 IU/ml of IFN-α increased their susceptibility to killing by IFN-α.

ACKNOWLEDGEMENTS

This work was supported by a Grant-in-Aid for Cancer Research from the Ministry of Education, Science and Culture of Japan, and a grant from the Japan Foundation for Clinical Pharmacology. We thank Ms. K. Kashihara for her excellent technical assistance.

REFERENCES

1. Cameron, D.J. and Churchill, W.H. (1979): Cytotoxicity of human macrophages for tumor cells: activation by lymphocyte mediators. *J. Clin. Invest., 63*, 977.
2. Kleinerman, E.G., Schroit, A.J., Fogler, W.E. and Fidler, I.J. (1983): Tumoricidal activity of human monocytes activated *in vitro* by free and liposome-encapsulated human lymphokines. *J. Clin. Invest., 72*, 304.
3. Sone, S., Moriguchi, S., Shimizu, E., Ohgushi, F. and Tsubura, E. (1982): *In vitro* generation of tumoricidal properties in human alveolar macrophages following

interaction with endotoxin. *Cancer Res., 42*, 2227.
4. Sone, S. and Tsubura, E. (1982): Human alveolar macrophages; potentiation of their tumoricidal activity by liposome-encapsulated muramyl dipeptide. *J. Immunol., 129*, 1313.
5. Sone, S., Mutsuura, S., Ogawara, M. and Tsubura, E. (1984): Potentiating effect of muramyl dipeptide and its lipophilic analog encapsulated in liposomes on tumor cell killing by human monocytes. *J. Immunol., 132*, 2105.
6. Hibbs, J.B., Jr. (1976): Role of activated macrophages in nonspecific resistance to neoplasia. *Res. J. Reticulothel. Soc., 20*, 223.
7. Fidler, I.J., Sone, S., Fogler, W.E. and Barnen, Z.L. (1981): Eradication of spontaneous metastases and activation of alveolar macrophages by intravenous injection of liposomes containing muramyl dipeptide. *Proc. Natl. Acad. Sci. USA, 78*, 1680.
8. Sone, S. and Fidler, I.J. (1982): *In situ* activation of tumoricidal properties in rat alveolar macrophages and rejection of experimental lung metastases by the intravenous injection of *Nocardia rubra* cell wall skeleton. *Cancer Immunol. Immunother., 12*, 203.
9. Stanwick, T.L., Campbell, D.E. and Nahima, R.J. (1980): Spontaneous cytotoxicity mediated by monocyte-macrophages against human fibroblasts infected with herpes simplex virus: augmentation by interferon. *Cell. Immunol., 53*, 413.
10. Jett, J.R., Mantovani, A. and Herberman, R.B. (1980): Augmentation of human monocyte-mediated cytolysis by interferon. *Cell. Immunol., 54*, 425.
11. Fischer, D.G., Golightly, M.G. and Koren, H.S. (1983): Potentiation of the cytolytic activity of peripheral blood monocytes by lymphokines and interferon. *J. Immunol., 130*, 1220.
12. Dean, R.T. and Virelizier, J.L. (1983): Interferon as a macrophage-activating factor. I. Enhancement of cytotoxicity by fresh and matured human monocytes in the absence of other soluble signals. *Clin. Exp. Immunol., 51*, 501.
13. Blasi, E., Herberman, R.B. and Varesio, L. (1984): Requirement for protein synthesis for induction of macrophage tumoricidal activity by IFN-α and IFN-β, but not by IFN-γ. *J. Immunol., 132*, 3226.
14. Abo, T., Cooper, M.D. and Balch, C.M. (1982): Postnatal expansion of the natural killer cell and killer cell population in humans identified by the monoclonal HNK-1 antibody. *J. Exp. Med., 155*, 321.
15. Lanier, L.L., Le, A.M., Phillips, J.H., Warner, N.L. and Barner, N.L. (1983): Subpopulations of human natural killer cells defined by expression of the Leu-7 (HNK-1) and Leu-11 (NK-15) antigens. *J. Immunol., 131*, 1789.
16. Horwitz, D.M., Bakka, A.C., Abo, W. and Nishiya, K. (1984): Monocyte and NK cell cytotoxic activity in human adherent cell preparation: Discriminating effects of interferon and lactoferin. *J. Immunol., 132*, 2370.
17. Freundlich, B., Trinchieri, G., Perusia, B. and Zurier, R.B. (1984): The cytotoxic effector cells in preparations of adherent mononuclear cells from human peripheral blood. *J. Immunol., 132*, 1255.
18. Territo, M., Sarma, G. and Figlin, R. (1983): Effect of *in vitro* administration of interferon on human monocyte function. *J. Biol. Res. Modif., 2*, 450.
19. Yamazaki, S. (1983): Current status of clinical interferon research in Japan. *Jpn. J. Med. Sci. Biol., 36*, 261.

Neutrophil activating factor (NAF) as a possible mediator in anticancer effector mechanisms

Fujiro Sendo

SUMMARY

The cytotoxicity of neutrophils was augmented by supernatants of cultures of lymphoid cells. The factor which renders neutrophils cytotoxic was tentatively named neutrophil activating factor (NAF). Human peripheral blood leukocytes and mouse and rat spleen cells produced NAF when stimulated with a streptococcal preparation, OK-432, or concanavalin A. Two culture cell lines also produced NAF. Regulation of neutrophil cytotoxicity by a serum factor is discussed.

INTRODUCTION

Neutrophils make up more than 50% of peripheral blood leukocytes and infiltrate to an inflammatory focus as the initial effector cells. The bacteriocidal activity of neutrophils has been studied by many researchers, and the biochemical mechanisms of the extra-cellular killing of bacteria and tumor cells have been well documented by Clark and Klebanoff.[1] Furthermore, it has been well established that neutrophils interact with humoral factors, mainly antibody and complement, in phagocytosis.

On the other hand, there has been relatively little interest in the possibility that neutrophils may work as initiators of a sequence of responses from inflammation to acquired specific immunity. In this area, the work of Yoshinaga et al.[2] indicating that polymorphonuclear leukocytes (PMN) produce factor(s) which stimulate lymphocyte proliferation, is worthy of attention. Furthermore, the interaction of PMN with macrophages and lymphocytes is poorly understood compared with that of macrophages with other lymphoid cells. Fewer cytokines are known to act on PMN; those that do are leukocyte migration inhibitory factor[3] and granulocyte chemotactic factor.[4] The differentiation of these factors is still inadequate, as purification of these factors has not been successful.

FACTOR(S) WHICH ACT ON NEUTROPHILS AND RENDER THEM CYTOTOXIC

Over the past few years, the author and his colleagues have been engaged in work on neutrophils cytotoxic to tumor cells. In the course of this study, it was found that culture supernatants of concanavalin A (Con A)-stimulated rat spleen cells showed activity that renders rat neutrophils cytotoxic.[5] The agent of this activity was tentatively named neutrophil activating factor (NAF). Subsequently, attempts were made to obtain NAF in various experimental systems. Table 1 summarizes the recent results of these attempts. Spleen cells from rat, mouse and human peripheral blood lymphocytes (PBL) were used as sources of NAF. These lymphoid cells were stimulated with Con A or a streptococcal preparation, OK-432. Two culture cell lines were also used as sources of NAF: Jurkat human lymphoma and a mouse natural killer (NK) line (a gift from Dr. Kumagai of Tohoku University). Target cells from various species were used. NAF was detected in various systems (Table 1).

The stability of NAF to physicochemical treatments was examined in a number of experimental systems, where it was revealed that NAF from different sources showed different stabilities. The preliminary results on purification of NAF from Con A-stimulated rat spleen cells show that

Table 1 Production of neutrophil activating factor (NAF) in various different systems

Species of NAF source	Origin of lymphoid cell	Stimulator	Species of responder PMN*	Stability at 60°C for 30 minutes
Rat	Spleen	Con A	Rat Mouse	Yes
Rat	Spleen	OK-432	Rat Mouse	NT**
Mouse	Spleen	Con A	Rat Mouse	NT
Mouse	Spleen	OK-432	Rat Mouse	No
Human	Peripheral Blood	Con A Sepharose	Human	NT
Human	Peripheral Blood	OK-432	Human	NT
Mouse	NK line	No	Rat	Yes
Human	Jurkat	No	Rat	Yes

* PMN from the described species at least can respond to NAF. In some systems, PMN from other species have not yet been tested.

** NT: not tested.

substances which had NAF activity were heterogeneous in terms of their molecular weight.

From these results it can be stated that the presence of factors which render neutrophils cytotoxic in certain supernatants of lymphoid cell cultures is not restricted to a single system; this phenomenon may be observed in various different species and in different experimental systems. At least two molecular species may have NAF activity.

REGULATION OF NEUTROPHIL CYTOTOXICITY

Two important questions to be clarified with reference to NAF are: 1) the *in vivo* role of NAF, and 2) the discrimination of NAF from other lymphokines which act on PMN.

Concerning the first point, preliminary experiments performed by the author and his colleagues produced interesting results: it was accidentally found that neutrophil cytotoxicity in fetal calf serum (FCS)-free Iscove's medium was significantly higher than that in the RPMI 1640 medium supplemented with 10% FCS which was routinely used in the neutrophil cytotoxicity studies. From this result, it was speculated that some factor(s) in FCS might inhibit neutrophil cytotoxicity. Experiments were carried out to test the validity of this hypothesis.

When FCS was added to Iscove's medium, neutrophil cytotoxicity was diminished. The inhibition of cytotoxicity by FCS affected not only neutrophils but also macrophages. However, cytotoxicity by natural killer cells and alloreactive cytotoxic T cells (CTL) was not affected by the addition of FCS to Iscove's medium.

These results suggest that the *in vivo* regulation of neutrophil cytotoxicity needs clarification before the *in vivo* role of NAF and NAF-activated cytotoxic neutrophils can be meaningfully discussed. The results also suggest that the four main effector cells in cell-mediated cytotoxicity, CTL, NK, macrophages and PMN, may be classified into two groups: CTL and NK versus macrophages and PMN. Inasmuch as the cytotoxicity of the former was not inhibited by FCS while that of the latter was, CTL and NK may work intravascularly, and macrophages and PMN extravascularly, mainly in inflammatory fields.

REFERENCES

1. Clark, R. and Klebanoff, S.J. (1975): Neutrophil-mediated tumor cell cytotoxicity: role of the peroxidase system. *J. Exp. Med.*, *141*, 1442.
2. Yoshinaga, M., Nakamura, S. and Hayashi, H. (1975): Interaction between lymphocytes and inflammatory exudate cells. I. Enhancement of thymocyte

response to PHA by product(s) of polymorphonuclear leukocytes and macrophages. *J. Immunol.*, *115*, 533.
3. Rocklin, R.E. (1974): Products of activated lymphocytes: leukocyte inhibitory factor (LIF) distinct from migration inhibitory factor (MIF). *J. Immunol.*, *112*, 1461.
4. Ward, P.A., Remold, H.G. and David, J.R. (1969): Leucotactic factor produced by sensitized lymphocytes. *Science*, *163*, 1079.
5. Inoue, T. and Sendo, F. (1983): *In vitro* induction of cytotoxic polymorphonuclear leukocytes by supernatant from a concanavalin A-stimulated spleen cell culture. *J. Immunol.*, *131*, 2508.

Recombinant human interleukin 2 functions as a differentiative signal in induction of T-lymphocyte cytotoxicity, but does not support long-term T cell growth

Seiko Yamasaki, Keiko Amikura, Shinsuke Taki, Ryota Yoshimoto and Junji Hamuro

SUMMARY

Not only interleukin 2 (IL2) purified by cell culture but also genetically homogeneous recombinant IL2 (G-IL2) induced secondary cytotoxic T-lymphocytes (2° CTL) from *in vitro* and *in vivo* alloantigen-primed T cells, by functioning as a differentiative signal more than as a proliferative signal. G-IL2 certainly augmented the induction of primary allo-CTL, and hapten-specific H-2 restricted CTL when added to culture. During prolonged culture, antigen-primed memory CTL tended to gradually lose their IL2 receptors, resulting in unresponsiveness to IL2. G-IL2 did not support the growth of concanavalin A (Con A)-activated T cell blasts, alloantigen-primed CTL or memory CTL in long-term culture, indicating the absence of a long-term T cell growth-supporting nature to IL2 itself. Crude conditioned medium derived from mitogen-stimulated human T cell leukemia exerted a stronger proliferative and differentiative impact on these activated T cells. G-IL2 augmented the induction of allo-CTL when splenocytes were used as responder cells, even in the absence of accessory cells, and when ultraviolet (UV)- or heat-inactivated stimulator cells were applied, but not when thymocytes were used as responder cells in the absence of accessory cells. A new lymphokine(s), T cell-growth-potentiating factor(s) (TCGPF), augmented the proliferative responses of thymocytes in synergy with IL2 in the absence of accessory cells. On the basis of G-IL2's augmentation of *in vivo* induction of CTL and NK activation, recombinant human IL2 may well be a candidate for use in immunotherapy of cancer.

INTRODUCTION

Interleukin 2 (IL2), first designated a T cell growth factor by Gallo,[1] is known to have diverse biological functions. However, the results of studies on the functions of IL2 in various immune systems using unpurified or partially purified IL2 preparations have been very controversial and ambiguous, probably due to contamination by other lymphokines which exert biological activities themselves or in synergy with IL2. Recombinant DNA technology has made it possible to obtain pure IL2 as a single gene product, thus enabling treatment with pure IL2 containing no other biologically active lymphokines.[2]

Aiming to clarify the functional roles of the IL2 molecule in T cell maturation and differentiation, the authors investigated whether IL2 acts as a differentiation factor as well as a proliferation factor. In this context, we investigated whether recombinant IL2 (G-IL2) plays a role as a differentiative signal in the induction of secondary cytotoxic T-lymphocytes (2° CTL) from antigen-primed memory T cells and in the activation of natural killer (NK) cells. It was concluded that G-IL2 does function qualitatively as a differentiation factor in the induction of both effector cells, because 2° CTL and NK cells were activated even in the absence of cell proliferation when a DNA synthesis blocker, mitomycin C (MMC), was present, although the activation required both RNA and protein synthesis. The absence of accessory cells such as macrophages ($M\phi$) did not alter the functional activities of G-IL2, although reductions in the degree of augmentation were observed.[3,4]

In this study, the role of the IL2 molecule as a differentiation factor rather than a growth factor in the induction of CTL is discussed further, to widen the range of possible applications of recombinant IL2 as an immunomodulator in cancer treatment.

MATERIAL AND METHODS

Animals and cell lines

Adult C3H/HeN, DBA/2 and C57BL/6 mice were purchased from Charles River (Atsugi, Kanagawa, Japan) and maintained in a specific pathogen-free environment. P815 tumor cells were grown in suspension culture *in vitro* and used as sensitizing alloantigens as well as target cells for cytotoxicity tests. A mouse cytotoxic T cell line (CTLL) was maintained according to the method described by Gillis and Smith[5] with a small modification.

Conditioned medium, IL2 and T cell-growth-potentiating factor

Con A-conditioned medium was produced by Con A stimulation (25 μg/ml) of human T cell leukemia cell line JPIII, cloned from Jurkat cells for 48 hours ; the contaminating Con A was removed by two filtrations on a Sephadex G50 column. Purified IL2 from this conditioned medium was obtained according to the procedures described in Table 1. T cell-growth-potentiating factor (TCGPF) was obtained as the culture supernatant of HUT 102 cells growing for 4 days at an initial cell density of 1×10^5 cells/ml in RPMI-1640 medium supplemented with 100 U/ml of penicillin, 100 μg/ml of streptomycin sulfate and 5% fetal bovine serum (FBS).

Preparation of memory cells

Memory cells were prepared by *in vitro* one-way mixed lymphocyte culture (MLC) as described by Wagner and Röllinghoff.[6] For the generation of memory CTL, cultivation was maintained for 12 to 15 days from the initial establishment of the MLC. The collected cells were fractionated by velocity sedimentation using Ficoll-Paque (Pharmacia, Uppsala, Sweden). *In vivo* induction of memory cells was carried out by sensitization of C57BL/6 mice by intraperitoneal injection of 5×10^5 P815 cells ; spleen cells were harvested 16 days after sensitization.

Functional assays

IL2 activity was measured according to the methods described by Gillis et al.[7] using an IL2-dependent murine CTLL. Primary CTL induction was performed in 24-well Nunc culture plates using 4×10^6 responder cells per well and X-irradiated (2000 R) stimulator cells which were cultured for 5 days. After culture, the harvested cells were tested for their cytotoxicity by a conventional 3-hour ^{51}Cr-release assay. For secondary CTL induction, only 1×10^6 responder cells per well were used and the culture was maintained for 3 days. The induction by IL2 of 2° CTL in the absence of antigen was carried out in 96-well multi-dish culture plates (Corning 25860, Corning, NY) in Click/RPMI-1640 medium. Various amounts of IL2 were cultured with the memory cells (usually 2×10^5) for 3 days, and generated cytotoxicity was determined against histocompatible target cells with primary stimulator cells. NK cell activation was performed according to the methods described previously[5] and cytotoxicity was measured in a 4-hour ^{51}Cr-release assay using YAC-1 cells as the target cell. Con A blast and primary CTL proliferation assays were performed in a similar way to the CTLL proliferation assay. Thymocyte proliferation assay was carried out in 96-well microplates using 5×10^5 thymocytes per well by culturing for 72 hours in Dulbecco's modified Eagle's medium (DMEM); the cultured cells were pulsed with 0.5 μCi of ^3H-TdR for the final 8 hours.

RESULTS AND DISCUSSION

IL2 purification

Recombinant human IL2 extracted from *E. coli* was purified to homogeneity using multi-step purification procedures including high performance liquid chromatography (HPLC) as the final step (Table 1). These purification procedures gave 12,500-fold purification and the IL2 obtained was calculated to have a specific activity of 5×10^7 units/mg protein as assessed by ^3H-TdR incorporation assay using an IL2-dependent murine CTLL. The IL2 activity recovered corresponded to 28% of the original activity in the *E. coli* extract. Thus one unit of IL2 corresponded to 20 pg of IL2 protein. Consequently 100 to 200 pg of IL2 protein was confirmed to be sufficient to manifest its immunological activities, such as NK cell activation, induction of 2° CTL from alloantigen-primed memory T cells, and proliferation of IL2-dependent T cell lines.

IL2 functions as both a differentiative and a proliferative signal

The authors have previously demonstrated using G-IL2 that IL2 alone is able to trigger the differentiation *in vitro* of alloantigen-primed memory CTL with no specific lytic activity into functionally activated lytic CTL.[3] To reconfirm the nature of IL2 as a differentiation factor in the induction of 2° CTL, splenocytes harvested 16 days after sensitization by intraperitoneal injection with 5×10^5 alloantigens were co-cultured with G-IL2 for 3 days in the absence or presence of the sensitized antigen. As expected, restimulation with the antigen *in vitro* gave rise to significant lytic activity in the absence of G-IL2, while the presence of G-IL2 together with antigen further augmented the lytic activity from 39.8% to 67.2% (Table 2). The observed synergistic augmentation may imply that IL2 is capable of augmenting 2° CTL induction under normal conditions. In contrast, primary CTL activity could not be detected even in the presence of G-IL2 under these culture conditions (a sub-optimum number of

Table 1 Purification of recombinant IL2

	Volume ml	Protein mg	IL 2 activity $\times 10^4$ units	Specific activity $\times 10^4$ U/mg	Degree of purification	Recovery %
Cell extract	106	1883	723	0.38	$\times$1	100
CPG* eluate	165	601	518	0.86	$\times$2.26	72
CM** eluate	58	50	329	6.85	$\times$17.3	46
Sephadex-G-75 eluate	18	3.4	957	281	$\times$739	132
Phenyl-Sepharose eluate	18	0.58	230	396	$\times$1042	32
HPLC	3.0	0.042	200	4726	$\times$12532	28

* Controlled pore glass ** Carboxymethyl

Table 2 Augmentation of *in vivo* generated allo-CTL activity by recombinant human IL2 during *in vitro* culture*

Antigen dose for sensitization (*in vivo*)	Restimulation *in vitro* (2.5×10^5/well)	IL2 added *in vitro* (200U/ml)	% specific lysis of P815 cells			
			E:T ratio (culture base)			
			30	7.5	1.8	0.47
0[a]	−	−	−0.3	−0.8	1.5	−0.9
		+	−0.4	−0.3	−1.4	−1.2
	+	−	3.0	0.6	2.9	1.1
		+	−0.1	−0.4	0.8	0.8
5×10^5[b]	−	−	5.8	1.1	1.0	−1.3
		+	33.1	−	7.1	0
	+	−	39.8	14.2	4.8	0.5
		+	67.2	43.1	17.7	6.1

* C57BL/6 ♀ ——16 days——
↑ P815 i.p. ↓ splenocytes ⟶ cultured for 3 days ⟶ ^{51}Cr release (3 hours)
+/−IL2, +/−stimulator

a,b CTL activities of day 16 splenocytes were 0% and 29.4% for a) and b) at E:T=50:1 respectively.

responder cells were used).

It is also noteworthy that 2° CTL could be induced in the absence of antigen when G-IL2 was added, in which case the induced lytic activity was equivalent to that induced by antigen restimulation. This induction of 2° CTL activity by G-IL2 in the absence of antigen reflects the probable function of IL2 as a differentiation factor in the induction of 2° CTL from *in vivo* alloantigen-primed memory T cells as well as from *in vitro* primed

T cells, as previously reported by Yoshimoto et al.[4] However, the possibility could not be excluded that primary CTL remaining 16 days after *in vivo* antigen sensitization were induced to proliferate by IL2 rather than memory CTL being stimulated to differentiate into functional 2° CTL. In the absence of antigen restimulation and IL2, lytic activity was only marginal (5.8%), whereas IL2 alone produced 33.1% activity. Thus the clonal expansion necessary to account for the increment observed would be more than 16 times higher during a 3-day culture. Therefore the observed increase in lytic activity induced by G-IL2 probably cannot be ascribed solely to the proliferation of primary CTL contaminating the 16-day memory CTL pool. Thus IL2 alone probably functions as a differentiation factor for *in vivo* alloantigen-primed memory CTL.

That the augmented 2° CTL activity induced by IL2 and antigen restimulation was higher than that induced by either of these alone suggests the possibility of the production during the course of antigen restimulation of other unknown proliferative and/or differentiative factor(s), which might function in synergy with IL2; or that the amount of IL2 produced *in situ* by antigen restimulation was insufficient for optimal 2° CTL induction.

G-IL2, functioning both as a differentiative and a proliferative factor, was confirmed to augment primary allo-CTL and Trinitrophenyl (TNP)-specific H-2-restricted CTL induction in a normal 5-day mixed lymphocyte culture (data not shown). About one tenth of the number of stimulator cells was sufficient to induce the same level of lytic activity elicited in the absence of G-IL2, provided exogenous G-IL2 was added during the 5-day culture. The same level of lytic activity was also observed at an effector to target cell ratio five to ten times smaller with effector cells induced in the presence of G-IL2. Thus exogenous IL2 further supplements the biological activities of IL2 produced *in situ* during primary antigen stimulation, which is consistent with the observation of 2° CTL induction in the presence of antigen restimulation and IL2. At present it is not clear which of the proliferative and differentiative signals manifested by IL2 contributes more to the augmentation of primary CTL induction.

IL2 was originally identified as a T cell-growth factor (TCGF), but it has not been clarified whether IL2 alone is responsible for the long-term T cell growth or whether IL2 contributes only to the proliferative response of activated T cells. To confirm whether IL2 contained in conditioned medium in which mitogen-stimulated human T cell leukemic cells had been grown showed quantitatively similar proliferative and/or differentiative functions as G-IL2, IL2 activities of pure IL2- and crude IL2-containing conditioned medium were arbitrarily calculated in different assay systems. Each of the three IL2 preparations tested showed the

Table 3 Proliferative responses induced by crude IL2, purified C-IL2 and G-IL2

Assay	Critical activity	Time (hours)	IL2 dilution manifesting critical activity*		
			G-IL2	C-IL2**	J-IL2†
CTLL proliferation (2×10^4/ml)	50% max ^{3}H-TdR uptake	4	1,000 (1)	1,000 (1)	1,000 (1)
NK augmentation (5×10^6/ml)	20% lysis	20	84 (1.50)	104 (1.80)	58 (1)
2° CTL activation (1×10^6/ml)	30% lysis	72	124 (0.24)	147 (0.28)	512 (1)
Con A blast growth (1×10^4/ml)	3-fold increase	96	50 (0.20)	111 (0.43)	256 (1)
Primary CTL growth (1×10^4/ml)	3-fold increase	96	175 (0.50)	119 (0.34)	350 (1)

* Figures in parentheses indicate value relative to J-IL2.
** C-IL2: purified Jurkat cell culture-derived IL2.
† J-IL2: culture supernatant of Jurkat cells stimulated by Con A.

same activity in a CTLL proliferation assay. Table 3 shows the dilutions of these preparations which manifested various critical biological activities. The relative activities of each preparation were compared with those of conditioned medium. As is evident from Table 3, purified IL2 showed relatively less biological activity than the crude conditioned medium obtained from mitogen-stimulated T cell leukemia cells, except for NK cell activation. Consequently, it can safely be said that the crude conditioned medium contained unknown factors which played roles in the differentiation and proliferation of activated T cells either in an additive or a synergistic manner, although IL2 itself acts as a proliferative and a differentiative signal.

Scope and limitations of the biological functions of IL2

In repeated trials, G-IL2 alone failed to support the long-term growth of activated T cells such as Con A-activated T cell blasts, primary CTL, and memory CTL. This may be accounted for by the gradual decline of IL2 receptors expressed on activated T cells during the course of long-term culture which was confirmed by ^{125}I-IL2 binding experiments (data not shown). Thus, in order to sustain the IL2 receptors expressed on activated T cells, further experiments will be necessary on the mechanism of the up or down regulation of IL2 receptors by IL2 and on the role of lymphokine(s) contributing to the maintenance or expression of IL2 receptors.

As mentioned above, IL2 was capable of augmenting primary CTL

Table 4 Effect of recombinant IL2 and T cell-growth-potentiating factor (TCGPF) on thymocyte proliferation

Thymocytes (5×10^5/well)	Additives*	^{3}H-TdR uptake ($\times 10^{-4}$ cpm)					
		Con A concentration (μg/ml)					
		0	0.075	0.15	0.31	0.63	1.25
Whole	(−)	0.0	0.0	0.1	0.4	2.4	10.2
	TCGPF	0.2	0.3	0.4	0.8	3.0	18.1
	IL2	0.3	0.4	0.7	2.3	10.2	21.1
	TCGPF+IL2	3.3	3.9	4.4	5.4	10.7	19.9
Nylon wool −passed	(−)	0.0	0.0	0.0	0.0	0.2	0.9
	TCGPF	0.2	0.4	0.3	0.6	0.9	8.0
	IL2	0.1	0.1	0,2	0.4	2.6	13.1
	TCGPF+IL2	4.8	5.5	6.4	6.3	8.3	17.3

* IL2: 50 U/ml, TCGPF: 25% (v/v)

induction in normal MLC when X-irradiated splenocytes were used as stimulator cells. On the other hand, no CTL activity was detected when stimulator cells were inactivated either by UV or heat treatment. However, addition of exogeneous G-IL2 induced a significant level of lytic activity. This result indicates that exogenous IL2 can compensate for the lack of IL2 produced *in situ* when intact stimulator cells stimulate IL2 producer cells. When splenocytes were used as responder cells, the absence of accessory cells in responder and/or stimulator cells did not alter the augmentation by G-IL2 of the induction of allo-CTL, even when inactivated stimulator cells were used. When thymocytes were used as responder cells, either deletion of accessory cells from responder cells or inactivation of stimulator cells completely abolished the generation of CTL activity even in the presence of G-IL2. These results suggest that there is a difference in the maturation of IL2-responding CTL precursor cells or in the capabilities of thymocytes and splenocytes to recognize an antigen.

Preliminary experiments show the presence of a new lymphokine, T cell-growth-potentiating factor (TCGPF), in the culture supernatant of human T cell leukemia cells. TCGPF triggered the proliferation of thymocytes synergistically with IL2 in the absence of accessory cells, whereas IL2 or TCGPF alone did not function as a mitogen to thymocytes even in the presence of accessory cells (Table 4). It is of interest that the synergistic proliferative effect of IL2 and IL2 receptor-inducing Con A requires the presence of at least some accessory cells, in contrast with the synergy observed between IL2 and TCGPF. Detailed analysis is now under way of the role of TCGPF in synergy with IL2 in the proliferation of T cells, in terms of the effect on IL2 receptor expression.

In conclusion, IL2 functions as a differentiation factor as well as a proliferation factor in the induction of CTL, as is the case for NK cell activation as previously reported by Amikura et al.[3] Furthermore, it augments primary and secondary CTL induction. At the same time, other unknown lymphokines may also participate in differentiation, maturation and proliferation of activated T cells and thymocytes. TCGPF may be one of these lymphokines. Rationalization of the appropriate application of recombinant IL2 in cancer treatment awaits further studies on the roles of the biological activities manifested by purified IL2.

REFERENCES

1. Morgan, D. A., Ruscetti, F. W. and Gallo, R. C. (1976): Selective *in vitro* growth of T-lymphocytes from normal human bone marrow. *Science, 193,* 1007.
2. Taniguchi, T., Matsui, H., Fujita, T., Takaoka, C., Kashima, N., Yoshimoto, R. and Hamuro, J. (1983): Structure and expression of a cloned cDNA for human interleukin 2. *Nature, 302*, 305.
3. Amikura, K., Ohno, K., Yoshimoto, R., Kashima, N., Hanzawa, Y. and Hamuro, J. (1984): Biological and immunological activities of human recombinant interleukin 2. In: *Manipulation of Host Defence Mechanisms*. p. 93. Editors: T. Aoki, E. Tsubura and I. Urushizaki. Excerpta Medica, Amsterdam.
4. Yoshimoto, R., Kashima, N., Ohno, K., Amikura, K. and Hamuro, J. (1984): Human interleukin 2, as a single gene product, differentiates memory killer-T cells into activated cytotoxic states. ibid., (In press).
5. Gillis, S. and Smith, K.A. (1977): Long term culture of tumor-specific cytotoxic T cells. *Nature, 268*, 154.
6. Wagner, H. and Röllinghoff, M. (1976): Secondary cytotoxic allograft responses *in vitro*. II. Differentiation of memory T cells into cytotoxic T lymphocytes in the absence of cell proliferation. *Eur. J. Immunol., 6*, 15.
7. Gillis, S., Ferm, M. M., Ou, W. and Smith, K.A. (1978): T cell growth factor: parameters of production and a quantitative microassay for activity. *J. Immunol., 120*, 2027.

Anti-Tac antibody does not necessarily recognize the same epitope as that which is defined by specific IL2 binding

Nobuo Kondoh, Michiyuki Maeda, Junji Yodoi and Junji Hamuro

SUMMARY

A monoclonal antibody generally called anti-Tac has been said to be probably able to recognize a certain epitope of a human interleukin 2 receptor (IL2-R) expressed on activated T cells, suggesting the presence of close molecular linkage between the IL2-R and the Tac antigen.

Aiming to define the molecular resemblance between these two molecules further, the binding sites of homogeneous recombinant IL2 on human malignant cell lines were compared numerically with those of anti-Tac. Three human T cell leukemia cell lines (HTL), ATL-2, MT-1 and HUT-102, were found to have the same concentrations of anti-Tac binding sites (20-40 $\times$ 10^4/cell), whereas the latter two cell lines were found to express no detectable IL2 binding sites, in contrast to the presence of 4. 3 $\times$ 10^4 IL2 binding sites on ATL-2. Furthermore, a natural killer cell line, YT, was found to express around ten times more binding sites for IL2 than for anti-Tac (5.4 $\times$ 10^4 versus 0.64 $\times$ 10^4 per cell), indicating molecular dissociation of the IL2-R from the Tac antigen. The probable molecular dissociation is additionally favored by the findings that IL2 was unable to inhibit the binding of anti-Tac to ATL-2, although the inverse competitive inhibition, of IL2 binding by anti-Tac, was clearly observed. Taking all of these results into censideration, it can be argued that anti-Tac does not necessarily recognize the epitope sharing a common structure with the functionally relevant IL2-R that is defined by specific IL2 binding.

INTRODUCTION

A monoclonal antibody, anti-Tac, originally established by Waldman and Uchiyama,[1] recognizes a putative antigen called Tac on activated T cells such as mitogens or antigen-stimulated T cells. Since then, much effort has been focused on elucidating the functional roles of the Tac antigen (Ag) in T cell-mediated immune responses but no distinct conclusion has yet been reached. Recent studies have revealed the presence of the Tac Ag on activated or EBV-transformed B cells.

Independent functional roles manifested by interleukin 2 (IL2) have been gradually clarified since cloned recombinant IL2 has become available. Consequently, it has been proven that IL2 functions both as a proliferation and a differentiation factor and the magnitudes of IL2-triggered T cell proliferation and differentiation are regulated by an IL2 ligand-IL2 receptor (IL2-R) interaction. Thus the IL2-R is currently considered to be a crucial molecule in IL2-driven immune responses.

Many controversial observations on the molecular linkage between the Tac Ag and the IL2-R have been reported[1,2]: some insist on the identity of the Tac Ag with the IL2-R while others claim dissociation of the functional roles of the Tac Ag from those of the IL2-R.

Additional interest in the relation of the Tac Ag to the IL2-R is based on the fact of constitutive expression of the Tac Ag on human T cell leukemia (HTL) and adult T cell leukemia (ATL) cells transformed by human T cell leukemia retrovirus (HTLV) in relation to the gene products controlling the autonomous growth of HTL.[3,4,5]

So far, the work on IL2-R has been done using anti-Tac in the absence of a definitive conclusion on the molecular identity between the Tac Ag and the IL2-R. In order to define more precisely the molecular correlation of these two molecules, the anthors analysed directly and numerically the binding sites of IL2 and anti-Tac expressed on humam malignant cell lines such as the HTL cell lines, ATL-2, MT-1, HUT 102 and, HUT 78, and a natural killer cell line YT, almost all of which are known to express Tac antigens constitutively. This paper describes results favoring the dissociation of the epitope recognized by anti-Tac from the fine structure of IL2 binding sites, and discusses the possible molecular structure of the functionally more relevant IL2 receptor(s) responsible for IL2-driven responses through ligand-receptor interactions.

MATERIALS AND METHODS

Cells

ATL-2, MT-1, HUT-102 and YT lines are Tac Ag-positive cells. HUT-78 line is a Tac Ag-negative line. CTLL-2, a murine IL2-dependent cell line, was used to ascertain the biological activity of ^{125}I-labelled IL2. All neoplastic cell lines were cultured *in vitro* in RPMI 1640 supplemented with 10% fetal calf serum (FCS).

Monoclonal antibody

A monoclonal anti-Tac antibody (mouse IgG2a) was kindly provided by Dr. Uchiyama of Kyoto University.

Iodination of human recombinant IL2

Human recombinant IL2, purified to homogeneity, was iodinated by a lactoperoxidase-glucose oxidase catalysed reaction. One hundred microliters of a solution of IL2 (360 μg/ml) in 0.25 M CH_3 COOH-NEt_3 (pH 4.0) containing 50% of n-propanol, was added to 0.4 ml of 0.4 M Tris-HC1 (pH 7.8, followed by the addition of 5 μl of a glucose oxidase solutios (1 mg/ml), 10 μl of 1 M glucose and 500 μCi of Na^{125}I (New England Nuclear). After incubation at room temperature for 60 minutes, 10 μl of 1 M sodium azide was added to the reaction mixture. The reaction mixture was applied to a Sephadex G-25 column (bed volume 10 ml), eqilibrated and eluted with PBS containing 1.0% of bovine serum albumin (BSA). Eluents in the void volume containing ^{125}I-labelled IL2 were pooled and dialyzed against PBS, and radiospecific actiity was determined. Radiospecific activity was found to be 2,200 cpm/ng of IL2 protein.

Binding experiment

Cultured cells were washed three times with RPMI-1640 medium and pelleted cells were then suspended in Dullbecco's Modified Eagle's Medium (DMEM) containing 1.0% of BSA. One milliliter of cell suspensions was placed in Falcon 1058 tubes and adjusted to a cell density of 2×10^6 cells/ml. To measure the total IL2 binding, labelled IL2 was added to one set of tubes, and the same concentration of labelled IL2 was

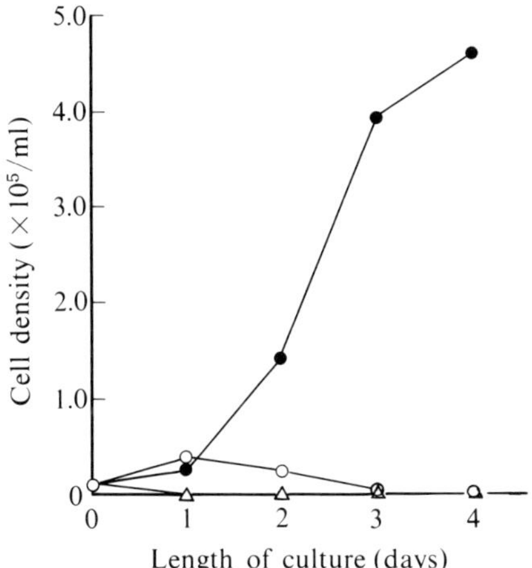

Fig. 1 Effect of the addition of ^{125}I-labelled IL2 on the proliferation of CTLL-2 cells. CTLL-2 cells were cultured in the presence of ^{125}I-labelled IL2. -●-: 20 ng/ml of ^{125}I-labelled IL2. -○-: 32 ng/ml of ^{125}I-labelled IL2. -△-: no ^{125}I-labelled IL2.

added to another set of tubes in the presence of a large excess amount of unlabelled IL2. After incubation, the tubes were centrifuged for 5 minutes at 2,000 rpm. The supernatants were removed and cell pellets were resuspended in cold DMEM and washed with the same medium. After a final washing, cell pellets were lysed with 0.1 M aqueous NaOH. Radioactivity in the cell lysate was determined using a γ-counter. Specific binding was calculated by subtracting the radioactivity of the nonspecific binding in the presence of cold IL2 from the total radioactivity bound. The nonspecific IL2 binding on CTLL-2 cells was less than 20% of the total IL2 binding.

RESULTS

Preparation of ^{125}I-labelled IL2

^{125}I-labelled IL2 was prepared in order to determine numerically the IL2 binding sites on human neoplastic cell lines. The addition of 20 ng/ml of ^{125}I-labelled IL2 (equivalent to 20,000 cpm/ml of radioactivity) induced sufficient proliferation of CTLL-2 (Fig. 1). The binding of ^{125}I-labelled IL2 to CTLL-2 followed the saturation curve shown in Fig. 2 and the binding was competitively inhibited by simultaneous addition of excess cold IL2 (data not shown, suggesting specific IL2 binding by ligand-

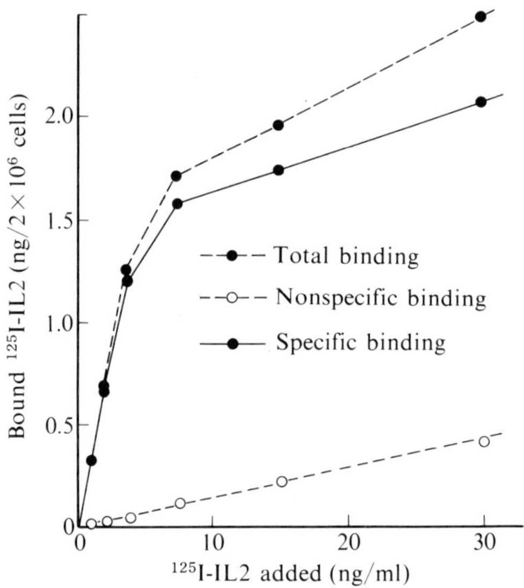

Fig. 2 Saturation of ^{125}I-labelled IL2 binding to CTLL-2 cells. CTLL-2 (2×10^6) cells were incubated with various concentrations of ^{125}I-labelled IL2 at 37°C for 40 minutes, and radioactivity bound on cells was measured. Specific binding was determined by subtracting the amount of nonspecifically bound radioactivity, i.e., the radioactivity bound in the presence of a large excess of unlabelled IL2, from total bound radioactivity, i.e., radioactivity bound in the absence of IL2.

receptor interaction.

Expressen of IL2 receptors and Tac antigens on human neoplastic cell lines

The number of anti-Tac and IL2 binding sites on the ATL-2, MT-1, HUT-102 and HUT-78 cell lines were estimated using radiolabelled IL2 and anti-Tac. All the HTL cell lines were found to have anti-Tac binding sites at the level of 20-40 $\times$ 10^4/cell (Fig. 3); the apparent affinity constants ranged from 0.5 to 1.0 $\times$ 10^{10}/M. In contrast, clear specific IL2 binding was observed only for ATL-2, while the other three cell lines showed no detectable IL2 binding under the same experimental conditions (Fig. 4). The number of IL2 binding sites on ATL-2 was found to be 3.9 $\times$ 10^3/cell and the affinity constant, calculated by Scatchard analysis, was 3.1 $\times$ 10^{10}/M. These observations clearly indicate the presence of a discrepancy between the molecular fine structures of the Tac Ag and IL2 binding sites (IL2 receptors).

A natural killer cell line, YT, was found to express around ten times more binding sites for IL2 than for anti-Tac (5.4 $\times$ 10^4 versus 0.64 $\times$ 10^4

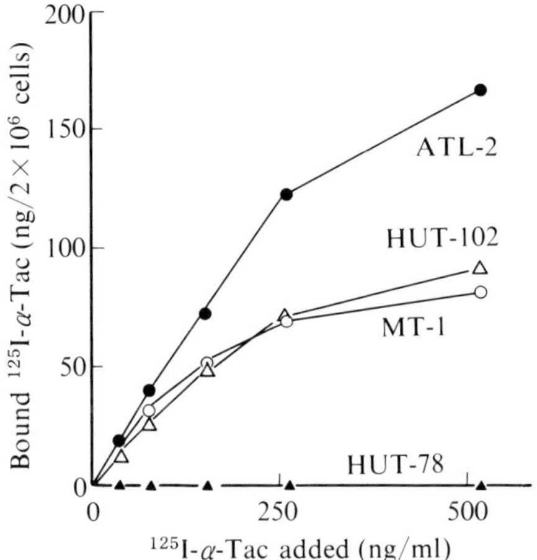

Fig. 3 ^{125}I-labelled anti-Tac binding to human neoplastic cell lines. Various concentrations of ^{125}I-labelled anti-Tac were incubated with ATL-2, MY-1, HUT-102 and HUT-78 cells, and radioactivity bound on cells was measured.

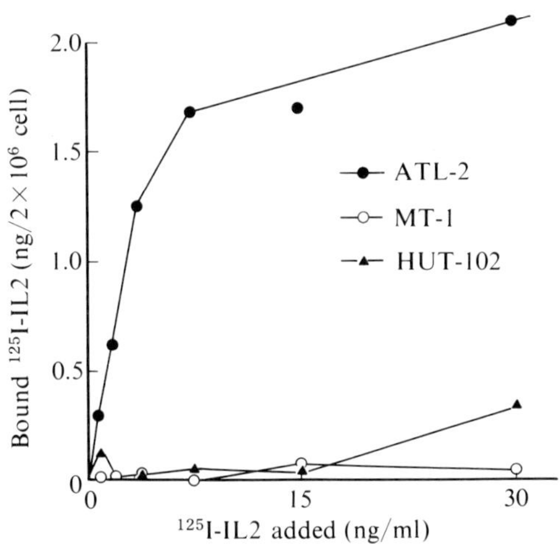

Fig. 4 ^{125}I-labelled IL2 binding to human neoplastic cell lines. Various concentrations of ^{125}I-labelled IL2 were incubated with ATL-2, MT-1 and HUT-102 cells, and radioactivity bound on cells was measured.

per cell), indicating again the presence of molecular dissociation of the IL2-R from the Tac Ag (Table 1).

Table 1 IL2 Receptor and Tac-Ag expression on human tumor cell lines

Cell line	IL2R (/cell)	Ka (M^{-1})	Tac-Ag (/cell)	Ka (M^{-1})	IL2-binding inhibition by α-Tac	α-Tac-binding inhibition by IL2
YT	5.4×10^4	0.77×10^{10}	0.64×10^4	1.8×10^{10}	partial	partial
ATL-2	4.3×10^4	3.1×10^{10}	38×10^4	2.9×10^{10}	Yes	No
MT-1	$<10^3$	—	22×10^4	0.96×10^{10}	—	No
HUT-102	$<10^3$	—	23×10^4	0.38×10^{10}	—	No
HUT-78	$<10^3$	—	ND	—	—	—

ND: not detectable

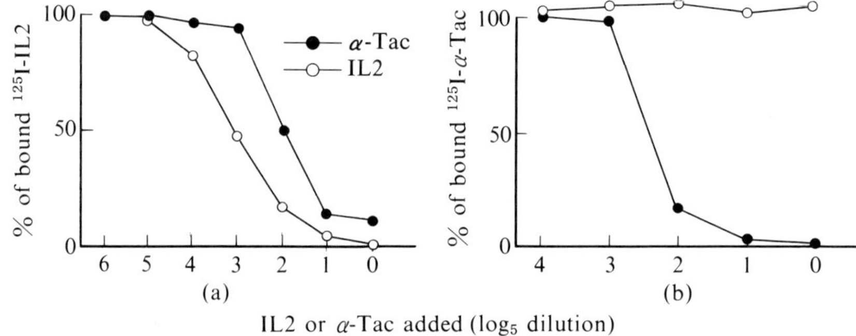

Fig. 5 Competitive binding inhibition by unlabelled IL2 and anti-Tac.
(a): Competitive inhibition of ^{125}I-labelled IL2 binding to ATL-2 cells by unlabelled IL2 and anti-Tac. ATL-2 cells were simultaneously incubated with varying concentrations of purified IL2, anti-Tac and ^{125}I-labelled IL2 (15 ng/ml) at 37°C for 40 minutes. Purified IL2 (13 μg/ml) and anti-Tac (100-fold diluted ascitic fluid) were diluted serially five times, and 0.1 ml of each diluted sample was added to the ATL-2 cells, followed by the ^{125}I-labelled IL2.
(b): Competitive inhibition of ^{125}I-labelled anti-Tac antibody binding by unlabelled IL2 and anti-Tac antibody. ATL-2 cells were simultaneously incubated with varying concentrations of purified IL2, anti-Tac antibody and ^{125}I-labelled anti-Tac antibody (250 ng/ml) at 37°C for 40 minutes, Purified IL2 (13 μg/ml) and anti-Tac antibody (100-fold diluted ascitic fluid) were diluted serially five times and 0.1 ml of each diluted sample was added to the ATL-2 cells, followed by the ^{125}I-labelled anti-Tac.

Competitive binding inhibition

An experiment on competitive inhibition of binding was carried out to define the molecular relationship between the Tac antigen and the IL2 receptor, since it was suggested that the Tac antigen molecule defined by the binding of anti-Tac might not necessarily correspond to the IL2 receptor defined by IL2 binding, even though the Tac antigen carries the binding site for IL2 within the molecule.

ATL-2 cells (2 x 10^6) were incubated with 15 ng/ml of labelled IL2 or 250 ng/ml of labelled anti-Tac antibody, in the presence of cold IL2 or anti-Tac. When the amounts of added cold IL2 and anti-Tac were increased, labelled IL2 binding was inhibited by cold anti-Tac as well as by IL2; while labelled anti-Tac binding was not blocked by the addition to the concentration of enough cold IL2 to block the labelled IL2 biniing (Fig. 5). The same results were also observed when MT-1 and HUT-102 cells were used as target cells. These results indicate the accessibility of IL2 binding sites to anti-Tac and the lack of accessibility of the anti-Tac binding site ot the IL2 molecule. All of these results suggest that the Tac antigen defined by anti-Tac binding does not necessarily correspond to the IL2 receptor defined by IL2 binding, although the latter is far more relevant for IL2-driven immune responses triggered by an IL2 ligand-receptor interaction.

DISCUSSION

In this study, it was demonstrated that there exist discrepancies in the number of the IL2 and anti-Tac binding sites on HTL cells; and anti-Tac binding to ATL-2 cells was not blocked by IL2, whereas the same concentration of IL2 was enough to block IL2 binding. These observations immediately give rise to the question of the identity of the IL2 and the anti-Tac binding sites. There is considerable evidence suggesting the presence of the IL2 binding site in the Tac antigen.[6,7] Furthermore, Green's and Honjo's groups reported the expression of the cDNA clone coding the Tac antigen in Cos cells resulted in the expression of molecules on the cell surface capable of binding radiolabelled IL2 and anti-Tac.[8,9] Accordingly, there is no doubt as to the common nature of the Tac antigen and IL2 receptor genes.

The data obtained in the present study could be explained by supposing the presence of variations in the binding affinity of the IL2 receptor for IL2, since the Tac antigen has been found to consist of heterogeneous molecules, generated by post-translational modification including glycosylation. Consequently it may be possible that one of these post-translationally modified components contains the binding site for IL2 and the other the binding site for anti-Tac. The validity of this interpretation might be supported by the finding that the Tac antigen showed broad immunoprecipitation with anti-Tac antibody on polyacrylamide gel electrophoresis, whereas the band precipitated by IL2 was narrow.[6] Furthermore, the observation in the present study that anti-Tac binding to ATL-2 was inhibited by the addition of a large amount of IL2 suggests the presence of high- and low-affinity IL2-R on ATL-2. The low affinity

IL2 receptor might be unlikely to play any physiological role in IL2-mediated immune responses, since it was observed that 0.1 to 1.0 ng/ml of IL2 is sufficient to induce IL2-mediated responses, including the induction of normal activated T cell proliferation, the induction of cytotoxic T cells and the augmentation of natural killer cell activity.

On the other hand, it was found that the number of the IL2 binding sites on YT cells was around ten times higher than that of anti-Tac. This greater number of IL2 binding sites than of anti-Tac suggests the possibility that some IL2 receptor molecules on YT cells are not accessible by anti-Tac. Ortaldo et al. reported supportive evidence for this interpretation: anti-Tac did not reduce the IL2-mediated augmentation of natural killer cell activity.[10] However, further experiments may be necessary to define the biochemical and antigenic relationship between IL2 receptors and Tac antigens.

REFERENCES

1. Leonard, W.J., Depper, L. M., Uchiyama, T., Smith, K.A., Waldmann, T.A., and Green, W.C. (1982): A monoclonal antibody that appears to recognize the receptor for human T cell growth factor; partial characterization of the receptor. *Nature, 300*, 267.
2. Smith, K.A. (1980): T cell growth factor. *Immunol. Rev., 51*, 3377.
3. Robb, R.J., Munck, A. and Smith, K.A. (1981): T cell growth factor receptors. Quantitation, specificity and biological relevance. *J. Exp. Med., 154*, 1455
4. Tsudo, M., Uchiyama, T. Uchino, H. and Yodoi, J. (1983): Failure of regulation of Tac antigen/TCGF receptor on adult T cell leukemia cells by anti-Tac antibody. *Blood, 61*, 1014.
5. Wano, Y., Uchiyama, T. Fukui, K., Maeda, M. Haruo, H. and Yodoi, J. (1984): Characterization of human interleukin 2 receptor (Tac antigen) in normal and leukemic T cells: coexpression of normal and aberrant receptors on HUT-102 cells. *J. Immunol., 132*, 3005.
6. Robb, R.J. and Green, W.C. (1983): Direct demonstration of T cell growth factor binding protein and the Tac antigen. *J. Exp. Med., 158*, 1332.
7. Leonard, W.J., Depper, J.M., Robb, R.J., Waldmann, T.A. and Green, W.C. (1983): Characterization of the human receptor for T cell growth factor, *Proc. Natl. Acad. Sci., USA, 80*, 6957.
8. Leonard, W.J., Depper, J.M., Crabtree, G.R., Rudikoff, S., Pumphrey, J., Robb, R.J., Krönke, M., Svetlik, P.B., Peffer, N.J., Waldmann, T.A. and Green, W.C. (1984): Molecular cloning and expression of cDNAs for the human interleukin 2 receptor. *Nature, 311*, 626.
9. Nikaido, T., Shimizu, A., Ishida, N., Sabe, H., Teshigawara, K., Maeda, M., Uchiyama, T., Yodoi, J. and Honjo, T. (1984): Molecular cloning of cDNA encoding human interleukin 2 receptor. *Nature, 311*, 631.
10. Ortaldo, J. R., Mason, A. T., Gerard, J. P., Henderson, L. E., Farrer, W., Hopkins, R. F., III, Herberman, R. B. and Rabin, H. (1984): Effects of natural and recombinant IL2 on regulation of IFNγ production and natural killer activity: lack of involvement of the Tac antigen for these immunoregulatory effects. *J. Immunol., 133*, 779.

Relationships between chemotherapy and immunotherapy: A brief overview

Enrico Mihich

INTRODUCTION

During the past 30 years, cancer chemotherapy has achieved a measure of success. In fact, as a consequence of chemotherapeutic treatments, patients with certain types of neoplasia are now free of detectable disease five years or longer after diagnosis. Major limitations still hamper the successful utilization of chemotherapy in the management of cancer, particularly of the most common types of solid tumors. These limitations are mainly related to the lack of sufficient selectivity of the available agents and to the phenomenon of resistance.

Efforts are being made toward improving therapy through the development of new drugs and new combination treatments based on increased knowledge of the mode of action of drugs, the identification of new cellular sites for intervention, the prevention or elimination of resistance, the achievement of increased selectivity through improved and/or more specific drug delivery systems and the development of new treatment modalities such as those based on a favorable modification of biological responses to tumor.

In recent years, evidence has been obtained suggesting that effective antitumor host responses may occur in humans. The programmatic concept of Biological Response Modifiers (BRMs) reflects the expectation that these BRMs, which comprise a number of agents and approaches, can be exploited therapeutically.[1] A BRM treatment may augment effective antitumor host responses through their stimulation or modulation, it may provide natural or synthetic mediators adding to the host response, it may modify the tumor such that it becomes more sensitive to host defenses, it may promote the differentiation of tumor cells, or it may boost the defenses of the host against opportunistic infections resulting from the neoplastic disease and/or chemotherapy-induced immunosuppression. In this discussion only treatments with BRMs involving systems of host defense, namely, immunotherapy in a broad sense, are considered and some of their relationships to chemotherapy mentioned.

Comparison between immunotherapy and chemotherapy

To date, immunotherapy, particularly with immunoaugmenting agents, has proven to be of relatively little value in clinical practice as compared with the curative effects obtained with chemotherapy. One should recognize that overoptimistic and premature conclusions about the value of anticancer immunotherapy have elicited greater expectations than justified and have cast a measure of undeserved discredit on this approach. In fact, it is now apparent that certain types of immunotherapics do have clinical potential under certain conditions. Moreover, recent information on the mechanisms of immune responses and their regulation suggests that certain immunotherapeutic treatments may be optimally used in a given patient only under selective conditions during the evolution of the relationships between tumor and host defenses.

Therapeutic potential

The expected advantages of immunotherapy in comparison with chemotherapy reside in the potential specificity and selectivity of immunotherapy and in the fact that the mechanisms of its antitumor action appear to be rather unique in most cases and not directly related to the mechanisms of toxicity. Moreover, toxicity is usually rather limited and occurrence of resistance or cross-resistance unusual. In contrast, chemotherapy with cytotoxic agents is essentially limited in its antitumor selectivity because drug action on tumors is generally based on the same mechanisms which determine toxicity to normal tissues. Moreover, the development of resistance is a common phenomenon and cross-resistance among drugs occurs rather frequently. On the other hand, the limitations of immunotherapy are related to weak antitumor effectiveness in contrast to the powerful cytoreductive action of chemotherapy. In addition, in the past it has been difficult to obtain certain BRMs in pure form and in sufficient quantity; this limitation may be rapidly overcome through the utilization of recombinant DNA technology. The lack of sufficient knowledge of the basic phenomena underlying tumor immunity in humans is an important limitation on the optimal utilization of BRMs.

The limited antitumor potency of immunoaugmenting agents may be due to several factors, such as lack of effective preparations, weak immunogenicity of tumor, untoward effects of tumor-induced immune suppressor functions or other mechanisms of tumor escape.[2] Although it is generally assumed that immunotherapy may be effective only in the presence of a limited tumor mass, questions may be asked about the validity of this assumption in view of the rejection of even large allogenic tumor masses upon discontinuation of immunosuppressive treatments in patients with kidney transplants.[3] As knowledge of the mechanisms and regulation of antitumor host defenses increases, it should become possible to design more effective treatments based on immunoaugmentation and immunomodulation, thus fulfilling more effectively the potential for selectivity of antitumor action of this approach.

Toxicology

Fundamental differences must be recognized between the requirements for preclinical toxicological and Phase I studies of chemotherapeutic agents and those of BRMs. Because the effective antitumor and toxic dose-response curves for most chemotherapeutic agents are in parallel, maximum tolerated doses (MTD) must be determined in animals and during Phase I trials in order to identify doses and regimens to be used in Phase II and III clinical trials. In contrast, because for many BRMs the "BRM effective" dose-response curve is bell-shaped and BRM action may be optimal at doses much lower than the MTD, it is essential that the optimal BRM dose (OBRMD) be determined in animals and in Phase I trials based on measurements of the biological responses which are expected to be modified by the agent. The MTD should also be determined in animals, however, unless the BRM is species-specific or non-toxic up to reasonably high doses and antigen-specific. The need for identifying the OBRMD has been recognized since the inception of the BRM Program[1] and is now being increasingly accepted.

Clinical evaluation of antitumor activity

The clinical evaluation of the antitumor activity of cytotoxic anticancer drugs requires a rigorous quantitation of effects based on reduction of tumor size, remission induction, prolongation of disease-free interval and survival. The criteria for the evaluation of the antitumor action of BRM must be as rigorous but may have to be focussed on different and/or additional parameters. Duration of tumor-free interval and/or survival may be the parameters of choice when BRMs are given as adjuvants after "debulking" by chemotherapy or surgery, or following remission induction by chemotherapy or after radical surgery. Moreover, it is important that in each case the status of relevant tumor immunity, rather than that of irrelevant immunoreactivities, be measured before and during BRM treatments. Therapeutic effects should be correlated with BRM action. This correlation would provide a basis for further regimen optimization.

General approaches in cancer immunotherapy

The utilization of immunotherapeutic agents, and that of other types of BRMs, in the treatment of human cancer are at a primordial stage. In fact, this approach is somewhat similar in its stage of development to that of cancer chemotherapy in the early fifties, when new drugs started to be systematically studied in humans as single agents, and the concepts of both combination chemotherapy and treatment beyond complete remission induction had not yet been verified; indeed the very criteria for a definition of complete remission had not yet evolved. Thus thc doubts raised by some chemotherapists about the potentialities of BRMs in cancer therapeutics should be moderated by the awareness that similar doubts had been raised in relation to chemotherapy at a comparable level of sophistication. Whereas it is reasonable to predict that chemotherapy of cancer has not yet reached its limits, it is also reasonable to expect that improved uses of BRMs will provide additional opportunities for cancer eradication which should optimally be integrated with chemotherapy and other forms of treatment.

Based on what is known to date, it can be expected that the optimal use of immunotherapeutic agents can be fully achieved only when the status of antitumor immunity, its regulation and its evolution in the course of the disease, can be measured in individual patients with cancer; this is truly a tall order. At present, compromises and approximations based on generalizations about disease type-related phenomena are being adopted in the design of immunotherapies with the realization that semi-empirical approaches may nevertheless yield therapeutic advantages and provide further information on as yet unresolved basic issues.

In a broad sense, approaches in immunotherapy may be arbitrarily divided into antigen-dependent and antigen-independent, the latter involving effectors such as macrophages and natural killer cells (NK). This division is somewhat artificial; indeed questions are being asked, for instance, as to whether tumors truly devoid of immunogenicity can be inhibited by macrophages or whether antigenic tumors can be inhibited by macrophages in immune suppressed or incompetent hosts.[3] The possibility of exploiting therapeutically antigen-independent host defenses would seem to have promise in the face of tumor cell heterogeneity and related antigenic diversity, which may limit the usefulness of strictly antigen-dependent approaches.

Given the necessity for caution which transpires from the above considerations, one may divide possible approaches in cancer immunotherapy into three major groups, namely: a) immunomodulation which would modify existing host defense mechanisms by means of an intervention on tumor and/or host; b) exogenous supplementation of effectors such as antibodies, cells or lymphotoxins, which may augment the responses to tumor; and c) immunization with tumor associated antigens (TAA).

Immunomodulation

In a strict sense, the effectiveness of this approach is dependent on the presence on tumor cells of potentially immunogenic TAA against which modulated host responses may react in a therapeutically favorable manner. In a broader sense, however, so-called antigen-independent mechanisms may be included, given the reservations mentioned above.

Immunomodulation may be elicited by chemical agents, natural products, cytokines and antibodies. Several anticancer agents as well as chemically defined immunomodulators without direct anticancer activity have been shown to exert immunoaugmenting or modulating actions in a variety of animal model systems. Natural products have been used with different degrees of purification; many of these are currently under preclinical and clinical development, particularly in Japan. Cytokines include both lymphokines and the interferons (IFN); IFNα has been undergoing extensive clinical trials for several years while only recently has IFNγ been obtained through genetic engineering technology in Japan and elsewhere, and its systematic clinical trials are in progress or about to be initiated. Certain natural and recombinant DNA lymphokines are now becoming available and it can be expected that they will be studied systematically in humans in the near future. Monoclonal antibodies directed against T-cell specificities, especially T suppressor cell determinants, may be used to induce therapeutic immunomodulation.

Because of the limited scope of this discussion, only immunomodulation by certain anticancer agents and IFN is mentioned. Of the bacterial and related extraction products, only BCG is discussed, with emphasis on what was learned from its clinical use. The effects of muramyldipeptide derivatives, which are most promising agents, are mentioned elsewhere in this proceedings, as are those of certain lymphokines and antibodies.

Administration of effectors

This approach is not discussed to any extent herein. Suffice to say that effector supplementation is aimed at reducing deficiencies or insufficiencies in the antitumor immune effectiveness of the cancer patient without necessarily involving the participation of defenses of the recipient. This concept can be readily challenged, however, in view of such evidence as that suggesting that the adoptive transfer of immune T cells actually involves the transfer of T helper cells to which host T effector cells must be able to respond for the transfer to be effective,[4,5] or that antitumor monoclonal antibodies are not cytotoxic *per se* but mark the tumor cells for cytotoxicity by limiting host K cells through the mechanism of antibody-dependent cellular cytotoxicity.[3] The essential issues, however, are the presence on tumor cells of determinants with which the transferred effectors (or the effector-triggered mechanisms) may interact, and the capability of effectors to reach them. In this respect, it may be mentioned, for example, that anti-idiotypic antibodies against B-cell lymphoma antigen became effective only after most antigen circulating in blood had been bound.[6] Physiopathological characteristics of tumors such as those related to vascularization and intercellular spaces may also limit the accessibility of tumor cells to certain effectors.[7] It is conceivable that the passive administration of lymphotoxins or mediators of host cell cytotoxicity may represent one of the few procedures which may be truly independent of host defense mechanisms in the recipient patient; the possibility of carrying out systematic studies of lymphotoxins in animals and in humans is likely to become real in the foreseeable future with the expected availability of recombinant DNA products.[7]

Immunization with TAA

Active immunization with sufficiently pure TAA preparations has not yet been clinically accomplished. This approach represents a reasonable extension of the demonstration of TAA on human tumor cells. In experimental systems, active immunization with TAA[8] or modified TAA[8,9] has been successfully utilized. After sufficient amounts of purified human TAA preparations become available, it may be possible to answer several questions of practical relevance, such as those related to TAA immunogenicity, stimulation of antitumor effector cells, formation of immune complexes, sequestration by RES, and optimal mode of administration.

Immunomodulation: Anticancer drugs and IFN

Only a few examples related to the effects of adriamycin (ADM) and cyclophosphamide (Cy) and to those of IFNα are briefly discussed.

Immunomodulation induced by anticancer drugs

The possibility that certain anticancer agents may have antitumor immunoaugmenting effects through immunomodulation and may exert synergistic therapeutic effects in cooperation with host defense mechanisms has been repeatedly demonstrated in experimental model systems and amply discussed previously.[10–12] Such synergisms may have practical value in therapeutics, for instance, in developing optimal remission maintenance or adjuvant treatments.

The immunomodulating effects of ADM have been reviewed recently.[13–15] In short, the drug has been found to cause augmentation of splenic T cell responses to tumor alloantigens and to tumor isoantigens in mice. In allogeneic systems this augmentation is associated with augmentation of macrophage differentiation from precursor cells, this presumably providing the necessary accessory function for cytotoxic T cell development. Under conditions of limiting numbers of macrophages, the drug-induced reduction in the regulation of cytotoxic T cell development by T cells adherent to glass can be demonstrated. The anthracyclin also causes increased production (or release) of PGE_2 from spleen macrophages, this effect being consistent with the demonstrated inhibition of NK cells by the drug. The increased levels of interleukin 2 (IL2) found in conditioned medium from cultures of spleen cells from ADM-treated mice also appears to play a role in the drug-induced augmenting effect on cytotoxic T cell function.[15,16] These augmenting effects of ADM do not appear to be related to the formation of free radicals, a mechanism likely to be involved in other actions of the drug, because 5-iminodaunorubicin, an analog of ADM which does not form free radicals, also has immunoaugmenting effects similar to those of ADM.[17]

The immunomodulating effects of Cy have been studied extensively with emphasis on the selective inhibitory effects of this alkylating agent on suppressor functions.[18,19] Recently these effects of Cy have been examined in greater detail *in vitro* using 4-hydroperoxycyclophosphamide as a precursor of active Cy metabolites[18,20]: selective inhibition of precursors of T suppressor cells in both mouse and human systems was demonstrated. Tumors can stimulate T suppressor cells[2,3,19] and it is known that non-T cells may also exert this function as part of the tumor escape mechanisms which evolve during tumor progression.[2] The possibility of developing immunomodulation-mediated antitumor therapies through selective inhibition of suppressor functions is being explored in several laboratories,[19] as is the possibility of facilitating adoptive immunotherapy through elimination of tumor-induced suppressor cells.[21]

Immunomodulation and antitumor effects induced by IFN

It is well known that IFN causes a variety of effects on different components of host defense systems depending on the experimental conditions.[22–24] In addition, IFN has been found to induce the expression of certain antigens on tumor cells,[25,26] and this effect may also contribute to the immunomodulating effects of the agent.

Despite the diverse effects of IFN on the immune system demonstrated to date, it is not yet clear whether any of them is instrumental in determining the antitumor effects observed in animal models and in humans. The agent has direct "antitumor cell" effects and it is possible, although not proven, that these effects may be related to interference with cell regulatory phenomena.[7] Both effects on tumor cells and on host defenses against tumor may be involved in the antitumor effects seen *in vivo*, one perhaps predominating over the other depending on the conditions.

In general, it may be said that IFNα has shown objective antitumor activity in patients with such tumors as certain lymphomas, renal cell carcinoma, melanoma, myeloma, Kaposi's sarcoma, and hairy cell leukemia.[23] Although the effects have been modest, they have not been too different from those exhibited at analogous early stages of development by anticancer drugs now effectively used in combination treatments.

Immunoaugmentation by BCG

It is fair to state that therapeutic advantages of this treatment have been well documented only after injection of BCG into dermal metastases from malignant melanoma, in post-surgical adjuvant use in patients with stage I non-oat cell carcinoma of the lung and, by local instillation, in patients with superficial bladder cancer.[3]

Despite the apparent disproportion between the clinical efforts spent on studies of BCG and the clinical therapeutic advantages achieved, it is important to note that it has been possible to demonstrate that, under certain conditions, the presumably non-specific stimulation of host defenses, predominantly of macrophages, may induce measurable therapeutic effects in cancer patients. This conclusion is encouraging in the expectation that numerous other bacterial or extraction products that are currently at various stages of development will be studied in humans. Moreover, several lessons were learned from the BCG experience which should be invaluable in studies of other immunoaugmenting agents, indeed of BRM in general, as they clearly indicate what should be avoided in future clinical trials. The early clinical studies of BCG have been characterized by such undesirable characteristics as slow patient accrual, excessive diversification of goals, inconsistencies among the preparations used (which had not been purified to homogeneity), lack of patient stratification and randomization, and premature reporting of results. In addition, the fact that combinations of BCG with levamisole had reduced effects in patients with lung cancer[3] points at the need for caution in combining two or more immunoaugmenting agents. Indeed, as already mentioned, the design of clinical trials of BRMs should take into careful consideration what is known about the mode of action of the agent studied. Moreover, it seems extremely important that reproducible preparations, if possible purified to homogeneity, or better synthetic ones, be used in future studies aimed at the evaluation of BRM-related antitumor activity.

CONCLUSION

As mentioned above, the clinical use of BRMs in patients with cancer is still in its infancy. The experience gained in early immunotherapy studies using BCG or other bacterial products and current knowledge of basic immunopharmacology indicate that the clinical evaluation of this group of agents must include parameters different from those used in evaluating chemotherapeutic agents but must be carried out as rigorously in terms of study design and quantitation of results. In most cases, adequate knowledge of the basic phenomena related to tumor immunity in humans is lacking and approximations with compromises are made in the realization that semi-empirical studies may nevertheless contribute to therapeutic advantages and in fact to increased knowledge of basic phenomena. As mentioned above, the assumption that immunotherapy would be optimally effective only in the presence of small tumor masses may not be completely valid under all circumstances. A clarification of this issue is dependent on the acquisition of knowledge on the evolution of relationships between tumor and host defenses and on immunoregulation during disease progression; such a clarification would determine whether or not immunotherapy must necessarily be preceded or accompanied by cytoreductive treatment.

There are good reasons to expect that, with progress in basic knowledge and availability of better and more defined BRMs, immunotherapy taken as a whole will offer therapeutic advantages in the future. In fact, TAA have been demonstrated on human tumors and have been found to be immunogenic in some cases,[3] IFNs did cause objective clinical responses as single agents, the feasibility of attaining objective tumor responses in humans through the use of immunoaugmenting agents has been proven in some cases, and it is becoming increasingly possible to obtain by recombinant DNA technology amounts of biological factors and regulators in pure form. Moreover, the observation that certain anticancer agents can exert immunomodulating effects suggests the possibility that certain chemotherapeutic agents may be usefully combined with immunotherapy not only for their cytoreductive activity, but also by virtue of their potential immunomodulating effects.

In conclusion, cautious optimism is warranted in this new area of cancer therapeutics. The paucity of basic knowledge available to support the rational development of these agents should not be viewed as a reason for discouragement but rather as an opportunity and challenge to seek such knowledge so that related therapeutic gains may be achieved. Only then may it be possible to obtain definitive proof of major therapeutic activity for BRMs in human cancer.

REFERENCES

1. Mihich, E. and Fefer, A. (eds) (1983): Report on the Biological Response Modifiers by the Subcommittee of the DCT Board of Scientific Advisors. *J. Natl. Cancer Inst. Monogr.*, 63.
2. Ozer, H. (1982): Tumor immunity and escape mechanisms in humans. In: *Immunological Approaches to Cancer Therapeutics*, p. 39. Editor: E. Mihich. John Wiley and Sons, New York.
3. Mastrangelo, M.J., Berd, D. and Maguire, H.C. (1984): Current condition and prognosis of tumor immunotherapy: a second opinion. *Cancer Treat. Rep., 68*, 207.
4. Cheever, M.A., Greenberg, P.D., and Fefer, A. (1984): Lymphocyte transfer for cancer therapy: prerequisites for efficacy and the use of long-term cultured T lymphocytes. In: *Biological Responses in Cancer: Progress Toward Potential Applications, Vol 2*, p. 145. Editor: E. Mihich. Plenum Press, New York.
5. Fefer, A., Cheever, M.A. and Greenberg, P.D. (1982): Lymphocyte transfer as potential cancer immunotherapy. In: *Immunological Approaches to Cancer Therapeutics,* p. 333. Editor: E. Mihich. John Wiley and Sons, New York.
6. Miller, R.A., Maloney, D.G., Warnicki, E.R. et al. (1982): Treatment of B cell lymphoma with monoclonal anti-idiotype antibody. *N. Engl. J. Med., 306*, 517.
7. Mihich, E.: Biological Response Modifiers: potentialities and limitations in cancer therapeutics. *Clinical Investigation*, (In press).
8. Mihich, E. (1973): Tumor immunogenicity in therapeutics. In: *Drug Resistance and Selectivity*, p. 391. Editor: E. Mihich. Academic Press, New York.
9. Kobayashi, H. (1982): Modification of tumor antigenicity in therapeutics: increase in immunologic foreignness of tumor cells in experimental model systems. In: *Immunological Approaches to Cancer Therapeutics*, p. 405. Editor: E. Mihich. John Wiley and Sons, New York.
10. Mihich, E. (1978): Chemotherapy and immunotherapy as a combined modality of cancer treatment. In: *Advances in Tumour Prevention, Detection and Characterization, Vol. 4: Characterization and Treatment of Human Tumours;* Intl. Congress Series, No. 420, p. 113. Editors: W. Davis and K.R. Harrap. Excerpta Medica, Amsterdam.
11. Mihich, E. (1979): Drug specificity in the suppression of the immune response. In: *Drugs and Immune Responsiveness*, p. 25. Editor: J.L. Turk. Macmillan Press Ltd., London.
12. Ehrke, M.J. and Mihich, E. (1984): Immunological effects of anticancer drugs. In: *Clinical Chemotherapy, Vol. III: Antineoplastic Chemotherapy*, p. 475. Editors: B. Berkarda, K. Karrer and G. Mathe. George Thieme Publishers, Stuttgart.

13. Ehrke, M.J., Cohen, S.A. and Mihich, E. (1982): Selective effects of adriamycin on murine host defense systems. *Immunol. Rev.*, *65*, 55.
14. Ehrke, M.J. and Mihich, E. (1984): Immunoregulation by cancer chemotherapeutic agents. In: *The Reticuloendothelial System: A Comprehensive Treatise, Vol. 8: The Pharmacology of the Reticuloendothelial System*, p. 309. Editors : J.W. Hadden and J.R. Battisto. Plenum Press, New York.
15. Ehrke, M.J. and Mihich, E. (1984): Adriamycin and other anthracyclines. In: *Clinics in Immunology and Allergy, Vol. 4, No. 2: Immune Suppression and Augmentation*, p. 259. Editors: J. Fahey and M.S. Mitchell. W.B. Saunders, East Sussex, England.
16. Ehrke, M.J. and Mihich, E. (1984): The effect of adriamycin treatment of spleen donor mice on the production of "IL-2 like" activity. Abstracts, IUPHAR 9th International Congress of Pharmacology, London, Abstract 57.
17. Maccubbin, D., Ehrke, M.J., Taniguchi, N. and Mihich, E. (1984): 5-Iminodaunorubicin augments *in vitro* cell mediated cytotoxicity against alloantigen. *Proc. Am. Assoc. Cancer Res.*, *25*, 227.
18. Cowens, J.W., Ozer, H. and Ehrke, M.J. (1984): Inhibition of the development of suppressor cells in culture by 4-hydroperoxycyclophosphamide. *J. Immunol.*, *132*, 95.
19. North, R.J. (1984): Murine antitumor immune response and its therapeutic manipulation. In: *Advances in Immunology*, p. 89. Editors: H.G. Kunkel and F. J. Dixon. Academic Press. New York.
20. Ozer, H., Cowens, J.W., Colvin, M. et al. (1982): *In vitro* effects of 4-hydroperoxycyclophosphamide on human regulatory T subset function. I. Selective effects on lymphocyte function in T-B collaboration. *J. Exp. Med.*, *155*, 276.
21. North, R.J. (1982): Cyclophosphamide-facilitated adoptive immunotherapy of an established tumor depends on elimination of tumor-induced suppressor T cells. *J. Exp. Med.*, *55*, 1063.
22. Borden, E.C., Edwards, B.S., Hawkins, M.J. et al. (1982): Interferons: biological response modification and pharmacology. In: *Biological Responses in Cancer: Progress Toward Potential Applications, Vol. 1*, p. 169. Editor: E. Mihich. Plenum Press, New York.
23. Kirkwood, J.M. and Ernstoff, M.S. (1984): Interferons in the treatment of human cancer. *J. Clin. Oncol.*, *2*, 336.
24. Johnson, H.M. (1982): Modulation of the immune response by interferons and their inducers. In: *Immunological Approaches to Cancer Therapeutics*, p. 241. Editor: E. Mihich. John Wiley and Sons, New York.
25. Doyle, A., Gazdar, A., Martin, J. et al. (1984): The deficit in HLA expression in small cell lung cancer (SCLC) resides at the transcriptional level and is reversed by interferon. *Proc. Am. Soc. Clin. Oncol.*, *3.*, 52.
26. Houghton, A.N., Thomson, T.M., Gross, D. et al. (1984): Surface antigens of melanoma and melanocytes. *J. Exp. Med.*, *160*, 255-269.

Effect of lentinan against allogeneic, syngeneic and autologous primary tumors, and its prophylactic effect against chemical carcinogenesis

Tetsuya Suga, Noriko A. Uchida, Takashi Yoshihama, Tsuyoshi Shiio, Makoto Rokutanda, Jőszef Fachet, Yukiko Y. Maeda and Goro Chihara

SUMMARY

The antitumor effect of lentinan, a T-cell oriented immune adjuvant, in allogeneic, syngeneic and autologous tumor-host systems and its suppressive effect on carcinogenesis were confirmed using DBA/2, A/J and SWM/Ms mice. It is likely that these strains of mice are the most susceptible to delayed-type hypersensitivity and/or cytotoxic T cell responses in which T cells and lentinan play important roles. The tumor-host systems presented here provide good models in which lentinan retains inhibitory capacity in syngeneic and autochthonous hosts; such models offer possibilities for future studies on host defense mechanisms against cancer.

INTRODUCTION

Lentinan, a fully purified polysaccharide obtained from *Lentinus edodes*, has marked antitumor activity against various tumors. Immunologically, it can be characterized as a T cell oriented adjuvant in whose actions macrophages play some part.[1,2]

Previously, the authors reported that the activity of lentinan against sarcoma 180 varied significantly among different mouse strains: it was most effective in DBA/2, A/J and SWM/Ms and less effective in C3H/He and C57BL/6 hosts.[3]

This review discusses the strong effect of lentinan against syngeneic and even autochthonous tumors and its suppression of chemical carcinogenesis when using such high responder mouse strains. The differences in these effects seen in different strains are discussed.

EXPERIMENTAL FINDINGS

Effect of lentinan against sarcoma 180 in mice in different inbred strains and their F_1 hybrids

The results of assays of lentinan's activity against sarcoma 180 in different inbred strains and their F_1 hybrids of mice are shown in Table 1. Lentinan had a strong inhibitory effect on tumor growth in DBA/2, A/J and SWM/Ms mice. When lentinan was given to these strains in daily doses of 4 mg/kg i.p. for five days starting one day after subcutaneous tumor transplantation, almost all tumors underwent complete regression and the inhibition ratios of tumor growth were 100, 96.5 and 100% respectively. In contrast, C3H/He and C57BL/6 mice were weakly respon-

Table 1 Effect of lentinan against sarcoma 180 in different inbred strains and their F_1 hybrids

Parent strains		DBA/2	A/Jax	BALB/c	CBA	C3H/He	C57BL/6	SWM/Ms
DBA/2	I.R.(%)	100	98.7	96.6	90.7	64.3	87.5	
	C.R.	5/5	4/6	2/6	3/5	1/6	0/8	
	response	high	high	high	high	moderate	moderate	
A/Jax	I.R.		96.5	91.5	91.5	41.6	68.2	
	C.R.		6/7	1/5	0/6	0/7	0/6	
	response		high	high	high	low	moderate	
BALB/c	I.R.			80.6	75.7	36.6	43.4	
	C.R.			3/6	2/7	0/7	0/6	
	response			moderate	moderate	low	low	
CBA	I.R.				74.1	71.9	71.8	
	C.R.				0/6	0/5	0/6	
	response				moderate	moderate	moderate	
C3H/He	I.R.					36.2	58.8	
	C.R.					0/6	0/6	
	response					low	low	
C57BL/6	I.R.						51.8	
	C.R.						0/6	
	response						low	
SWM/Ms	I.R.							100
	C.R.							6/6
	response							high

I.R.: Inhibition ratio of tumor growth.
C.R.: Complete regression of tumors.
Antitumor assay: Dose of lentinan, 4 mg/kg i.p. daily for 5 days; tumor transplantation, s.c.

sive to lentinan treatment and no complete regressions were observed. BALB/c and CBA mice were moderately reactive.

The susceptibility of tumors in F_1 hybrids to lentinan treatment seems to be determined by the parent mice. For example, (DBA/2×A/J) F_1 hybrid mice were high responders and many complete regressions of tumors were observed, but (C3H/He×C57BL/6) F_1 mice were low responders and no complete regressions were observed. (DBA/2×C3H/He) mice were intermediate responders. In this context, DBA/2, A/J and SWM/Ms mice were the most suitable hosts for lentinan treatment.

Effect of lentinan against A/Ph. MC • S1 and DBA/2. MC. CS-1 fibrosarcomas in syngeneic hosts

Once it had been confirmed that DBA/2 and A/Ph or A/J mice were suitable hosts, an attempt was made to examine the effect of lentinan against syngeneic and autochthonous tumors using these strains of mice. Lentinan administered in a dose of 1 mg/kg/day i.p. for ten days caused complete regression of methylcholanthrene (MC)-induced A/Ph. MC. S1 fibrosarcoma in A/Ph (A/J) syngeneic hosts (Fig. 1).[4] A/Ph mice in which these tumors had regressed were also able to reject a secondary challenge with the same tumor.

Lentinan also had marked antitumor activity against the native and

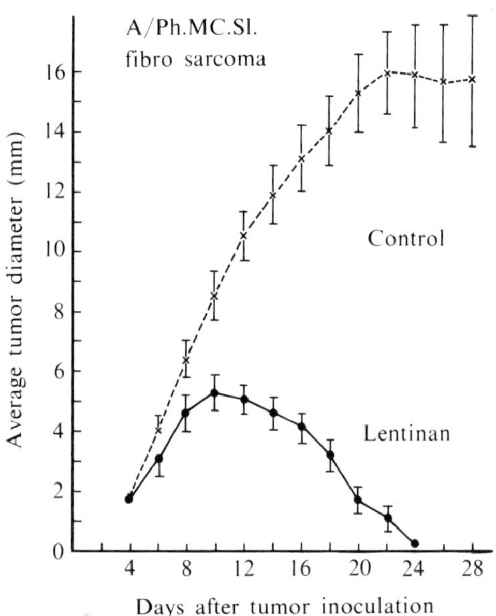

Fig. 1 Growth of 3-methylcholanthrene-induced A/Ph. MC. Sl fibrosarcoma in lentinan treated (1 mg/kg/day i.p.×10) and control A/Ph mice

Table 2 Effects of lentinan on growth of native and trypsinized DBA/2. MC.SC-1 fibrosarcoma in DBA/2 mice

DBA/2.MC.CS-1 fibrosarcoma	Treatment[d]	Dose	Dead/ Total mice	Average tumor weight (g)	Tumor inhibition ratio (%)	Number of complete regressions
Trypsinized	Lentinan	1 mg/kg × 10	0/7	0.47	76.5[e]	2/7
tumor [a]	control		0/7	2.00		0/7
Native tumor[b]	Lentinan	1 mg/kg × 10	0/6	2.19	54.0[e]	0/6
	control		0/6	4.76		0/6
Native tumor[b]	Lentinan	10 mg/kg × 1	0/6	2.99	47.3[e]	0/6
	control		0/6	5.67		0/6
Native tumor[c]	Lentinan	5 mg/kg × 4	0/5	0.84	57.4[e]	2/5
	control		0/6	1.97		0/6

[a] 2.4×10^6 tumor cells were transplanted s.c.

[b] 0.1 ml of tumor cell suspension (1 g of tumor tissue per 1 ml of saline), probably over 10^7 cells, was transplanted s.c.

[c] approximately 1×10^4 tumor cells were transplanted s.c.

[d] route: i.p.

[e] $p < 0.01$. Student's t-test as compared to the control group.

trypsinized DBA/2. MC. CS-1 fibrosarcoma established in our laboratory for these experiments (Table 2). As a trypsinized tumor cannot accurately be called syngeneic in the strict sense of the word, the native DBA/2. MC. CS-1 sarcoma was mainly used. When 0.1 ml of tumor cell suspension ($>10^7$ cells) of the native DBA/2. MC. CS-1 fibrosarcoma was transplanted subcutaneously into DBA/2 mice, the inhibition ratios of tumor growth induced by lentinan in doses of 1 mg/kg×10 and 10 mg/kg×1 were 54.0%and 47.3% respectively. Lentinan was more effective against this tumor when DBA/2 mice were implanted with a smaller dose (1×10^4 cells) of native DBA/2. MC. CS-1 fibrosarcoma: the tumor inhibition ratio was 57.4% and complete regression was observed in two out of five mice after four intraperitoneal injections of 5 mg/kg of lentinan.

In the case of trypsinized DBA/2. MC. CS-1 fibrosarcoma, the tumor inhibitory effect of lentinan was more striking. After ten 1 mg/kg doses of lentinan, the tumor inhibition ratio was 76.5%, and tumors underwent complete regression in two out of seven mice.

Effect of lentinan against 3-methylcholanthrene-induced autologous primary tumors

When DBA/2 mice were used, intraperitoneal injection of lentinan inhibited growth of MC-induced autochthonous primary tumors (Table 3). Tumors appearing and grown to 5 mm in diameter within 15 weeks of MC inoculation were markedly inhibited by the lentinan treatment. The

Table 3 Antitumor activity of lentinan against MC-induced primary tumors in DBA/2 mice

MC-induced primary tumor occurred:*	Treatment**	Dose†	Average tumor weight (g)	Tumor inhibition ratio (%)	Complete regressions of tumor
Within 15 weeks	Lentinan	1 mg/kg	0.58	80.5	2/5
of MC incoculation	Control		2.97		0/5
Between 16 and 36	Lentinan	1 mg/kg	2.75	40.5	0/4
weeks after MC inoculation	Control		4.79		0/4

* MC: 3-methylcholanthrene.

** Lentinan treatment was started when a primary tumor had reached 5 mm in diameter.

† i.p., daily for 10 days.

inhibition ratio of tumor growth was 80.5% and the primary tumors underwent complete regression in two out of five mice. On the other hand, the tumor inhibitory effect of lentinan against tumors appearing 16 to 36 weeks after MC-inoculation was 40.5% and no complete regressions were observed. This difference in effect may be due to the higher antigenicity of developing tumors early than of later occurring ones.[5]

Prophylactic effect of lentinan against 3-methylcholanthrene-induced carcinogenesis in DBA/2, BALB/c and SWM/Ms mice

The suppressive effect of lentinan on tumor occurrence in DBA/2 mice following MC inoculation is shown in Fig. 2. Eighty DBA/2 female mice about six weeks old were divided into two groups: 50 were treated with lentinan and 30 were used as a control group. After MC inoculation of both groups of mice, the lentinan-treated group was given 1 mg/kg of lentinan intraperitoneally daily for ten days from 2 weeks after MC inoculation. Lentinan effectively prevented MC-induced carcinogenesis (Fig. 2). The tumor occurrence rates in the lentinan-treated group were 0%, 21.6% and 36.1%, while those of the control group were 14.2%, 50.0% and 77.7%, at 8, 20 and 36 weeks after MC inoculation respectively.

The effect of lentinan on tumor occurrence in BALB/c mice after MC inoculation is shown in Fig. 3. Eighty BALB/c female mice about six weeks old were divided into two groups: 50 in the lentinan-treated group and 30 in the control group. The experiment on the preventive effect of lentinan against MC-induced carcinogenesis using BALB/c mice was performed in the same way as when studying DBA/2 mice. The tumor occurrence rate in the lentinan-treated group was 74.0% and that in the control group was 86.6% at the end of the 30th week. There was no statistical difference between the groups. Therefore this experiment

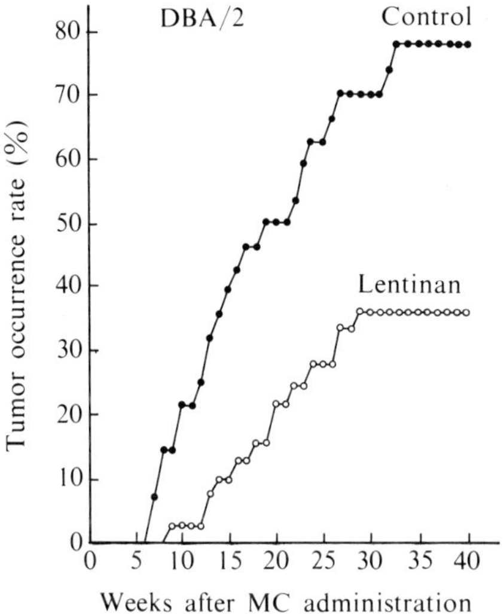

Fig. 2 Preventive effect of lentinan against MC-induced carcinogenesis in DBA/2 mice.

-●-●-●- : Controls (no lentinan injections).
-○-○-○- : Lentinan-treated mice. Injections (1 mg/kg/day i.p.×10) started 2 weeks after MC inoculation.

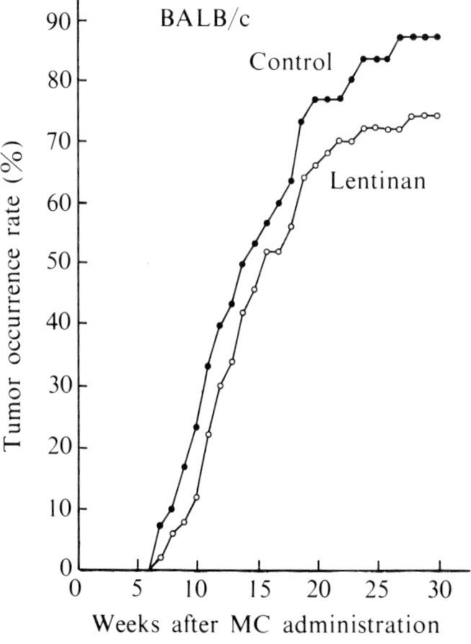

Fig. 3 Preventive effect of lentinan against MC-induced carcinogenesis in BALB/c mice.

-●-●-●- : Controls (no lentinan injections).
-○-○-○- : Lentinan-treated mice. Injections (1 mg/kg/day i.p.×10) started from 2 weeks after MC inoculation.

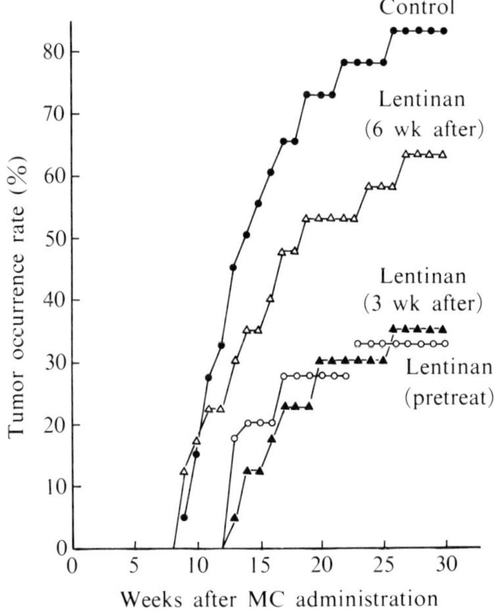

Fig. 4 Significance of timing of lentinan injections in prevention of MC-induced carcinogenesis in SWM/Ms mice.

-●-●-●- : Controls (no lentinan injections).
-○-○-○- : Lentinan injections begun 10 days before MC inoculation.
-▲-▲-▲- : Lentinan injections started three weeks after MC inoculation.
-△-△-△- : Lentinan injections started six weeks after MC inoculation.
Dose of lentinan, 1 mg/kg daily for ten days.

demonstrated no suppressive effect by lentinan in BALB/c mice.

In the preliminary experiments using C57BL/6 and C3H/He mice, lentinan treatment delayed the appearance of tumors, but the occurrence rate of tumors 35 weeks after MC inoculation was the same as in the control group. This strain difference in lentinan activity may provide a valuable insight into the mechanism of host defense against tumors.

In another experiment on the preventive effect of lentinan against chemical carcinogenesis, the timing of lentinan administration was examined using SWM/Ms mice, which were also high responders to lentinan treatment. About eighty six-week-old female SWM/Ms mice were inoculated with MC according to the same procedure as was used for DBA/2 and BALB/c mice. The MC-treated mice were divided into four groups of 20 mice each: three groups of lentinan-treated mice and one control group. The three lentinan-treated groups were injected with 1 mg/kg of lentinan intraperitoneally once a day for ten days from three weeks after, six weeks after, or ten days before MC inoculation respective-

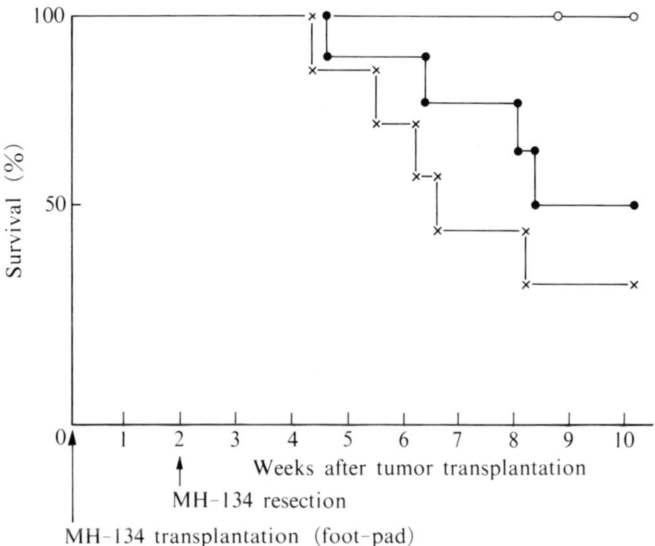

Fig. 5 Inhibition of post-operative MH-134 hepatoma metastasis by lentinan administration.
-×-×-×- : Controls (surgery only)
-●-●-●- : Surgery+Lentinan 1 mg/kg/day i.p.×10, from Days 1 to 14 after tumor resection
-○-○-○- : Surgery-Lentinan 1 mg/kg/day i.p.×10, from Days 15 to 28 tumor resection
MH-134 transplantation: foot-pad
MH-134 resection: 2 weeks after tumor transplantation

ly. The results are shown in Fig. 4. Tumor occurrence rates at the 30th week were 31% in the pretreated group and 33% in the group whose treatment began three weeks after MC inoculation; in those treated from six weeks after and in controls, the rates were 63% and 83% respectively. Thus lentinan was shown to be effective for prevention of chemical carcinogenesis when given within three weeks of MC inoculation.

This suggests that the smaller number of tumor cells occurring in the host within three weeks of MC inoculation are capable of being regressed by immunopotentiation induced by lentinan, but the larger number present by six weeks cannot be induced to regress by lentinan. Therefore, lentinan may be effective against micrometastases after surgical operations. In practice, the reappearance of MH-134 hepatoma by micrometastasis after surgery was completely prevented by the administration of lentinan (Fig. 5).[6]

Differences in antitumor activity by lentinan and host factors in different mouse strains

These results raise the question: Why are DBA/2, A/J and SWM/Ms mice such high responders and C57BL/6 and C3H/He mice such low responders to antitumor action by lentinan?

H-2 haplotypes

In contrast to a previous paper[7] which claimed that polysaccharide therapy increased the regression ratios of tumors in several strains of mice lacking the $H\text{-}2^d$ allele (homozygous and heterozygous), susceptibility to lentinan's action showed no relation to the mouse *H*-2 haplotypes in this study. The DBA/2 mice and their F_1 hybrids with A/J, BALB/c or CBA mice used in the present study have the $H\text{-}2^d$ allele, but were very high responders to lentinan treatment, as were A/J mice lacking $H\text{-}2^d$. On the other hand, C3H/He ($H\text{-}2^k$), C57BL/6 ($H\text{-}2^b$) and their F_1 hybrids lacking the $H\text{-}2^d$ allele were low responders and no lentinan-induced tumor regression was observed. The relationship between *H*-2 haplotypes and the antitumor effect of lentinan is shown in Table 4.

Fur-color gene

The fur-color genes of mouse strains also showed no relation to lentinan's action (Table 5). A/J (aabbcc) white mice and DBA/2 (aabbCC) chocolate mice were both high responders. With agouti mice, (DBA/2 × CBA) F_1 (AaBbCC) and (A/J × CBA) F_1 (AaBbCc) were high responders, but C3H/He (AABBCC) was a low responder. C57BL/6 (aaBBCC) black mice were also low responders to lentinan's action.

Host immune factors

Since it has no relationship with *H*-2 haplotypes, fur-color genes or allogeneicity between tumor and host, lentinan's differing action in different strains may be determined by certain host factors whose immune reactivity is regulated by lentinan.

This factor is almost certainly not natural killer (NK) cells, because NK-reactivity is deficient in the A/J and SWR/J (similar to SWM/Ms) strains,[8,9] and C3H/He mice, which have high NK reactivity, are the lowest responders to lentinan action. Furthermore, the doses of lentinan required to activate NK-reactivity in DBA/2 mice were relatively higher than the doses required for antitumor activity and for other immune

Table 4 Relationship between *H*-2 haplotypes and antitumor effect of lentinan

Parent strains		DBA/2	A/Jax	BALB/c	CBA	C3H/He	C57BL/6
DBA/2	*H*-2 haplotype	*dd*	*da*	*dd*	*dk*	*dk*	*db*
	Response	high	high	high	high	mod.	mod.
A/Jax	*H*-2 haplotype		*aa*	*ad*	*ak*	*ak*	*ab*
	Response		high	high	high	low	mod.
BALB/c	*H*-2 haplotype			*dd*	*dk*	*dk*	*db*
	Response			mod.	mod.	low	low
CBA	*H*-2 haplotype				*kk*	*kk*	*kb*
	Response				mod.	mod.	mod.
C3H/He	*H*-2 haplotype					*kk*	*kb*
	Response					low	low
C57BL/6	*H*-2 haplotype						*bb*
	Response						low

Table 5 Relationship between fur-color genes and antitumor effect of lentinan

Parent strains		DBA/2	A/Jax	BALB/c	CBA	C3H/He	C57BL/6
DBA/2	Gene	aabbCC	aabbCc	AabbCc	AaBbCC	AaBbCC	aaBbCC
	Color	chocolate	chocolate	chocolate	agouti	agouti	black
	Response	high	high	high	high	moderate	moderate
A/Jx	Gene		aabbcc	Aabbcc	AaBbCc	AaBbCc	aaBbCc
	Color		white	white	agouti	agouti	black
	Response		high	high	high	low	moderate
BALB/c	Gene			AAbbcc	AABbCc	AABbCc	AaBbCc
	Color			white	agouti	agouti	agouti
	Response			moderate	moderate	low	low
CBA	Gene				AABBCC	AABBCC	AaBBCC
	Color				agouti	agouti	agouti
	Response				moderate	moderate	moderate
C3H/He	Gene					AABBCC	AaBBCC
	Color					agouti	agouti
	Response					low	low
C57BL/6	Gene						aaBBCC
	Color						black
	Response						low

reactivities stimulated by lentinan.[2]

Phagocytic macrophage function also can have no relation to the strain differences, since lentinan was unable to activate the phagocytic action of macrophages in CD-1/ICR and SWM/Ms mice.[10] Phagocytic functions in DBA/2 and A/J are weak, as demonstrated by their inability to control bacterial proliferation following infection with a sublethal dose of *Lysteria monocytogenes*, in contrast to C57BL/6 mice which showed characteristic resistance after infection with a comparable dose of this bacterium.[11,12]

The most likely possibility is that the strain difference in lentinan reactivity depends on the T cell capability of the mouse strain. SWM/Ms, in contrast to C3H/He mice, showed a strong delayed-type hypersensitivity (DTH) reaction,[13] which is able to inhibit the growth of syngeneic and autochthonous tumors in animal models.[14,15] A/Ph (similar to A/J) mice also showed a strong DTH reaction.[16,17]

DBA/2 mice showed a strong cytotoxic T-lymphocyte (CTL) reaction. Lentinan augmented CTL responses *in vitro* and *in vivo* when DBA/2 mice were used,[18,19] and activation of CTL induced by Ia^+ macrophage-dependent IL-2 has been proposed as a possible mechanism for lentinan's antitumor action.[2]

The relationship between susceptibility to lentinan's antitumor action and the capability of various host factors, DTH, CTL, NK and phagocytic macrophages, in inbred mouse strains is summarized in Table 6.

In general, multiple changes were detected in lentinan-treated animals, depending on the experimental system employed. The DTH and/or CTL responses seem to be the most important mechanisms for the antitumor action of lentinan in syngeneic and autochthonous hosts, of which DBA/2, A/J and SWM/Ms mice are the most suitable strains.

CONCLUSION

It is indisputable that lentinan has marked antitumor activity in syngeneic and even autochthonous hosts as well as allogeneic hosts, and suppresses carcinogenesis when used with suitable strains of mice. This is the first time that systemic effectiveness of an immunomodulator against autologous primary tumors has been found.

The use of the DBA/2, A/J and SWM/Ms strains known to be very responsive to T-cell adjuvant lentinan affords the best opportunity of

Table 6 Relationship between susceptibility to lentinan's antitumor action and capability of DTH, CTL, NK and phagocytic macrophages in inbred mouse strains

	ATS	DTH	CTL	NK	Mϕ
DBA/2	high		high		low
A/Jax	high	high		low	low
SWM/Ms	high	high		low	low
BALB/c	moderate			low	
C3H/He	low	low		high	high
C57BL/6	low			moderate	high

ATS: Susceptibility to lentinan's antitumor effect.
DTH: Delayed-type hypersensitivity.
CTL Cytotoxic T-lymphocyte reactivity.
NK: Natural killer cell activity.
Mϕ: Macrophage phagocytic activity.

determining host defense mechanisms in syngeneic and autochthonous tumor-host systems including those involved in the prevention of carcinogenesis.

REFERENCES

1. Chihara, G., Hamuro, J., Maeda, Y.Y., Arai, Y. and Fukuoka, F. (1970): Fractionation and purification of the polysaccharides with marked antitumor activity, especially lentinan, from *Lentinus edodes* (Berk.) Sing. (an edible mushroom). *Cancer Res.*, *30*, 2776.
2. Hamuro, J. and Chihara, G. (1984): Lentinan, a T-cell oriented immunopotentiator: its experimental and clinical applications and possible mechanism of immune modulation. In: *Immune Modulation Agents and Their Mechanisms,* p. 409. Editors: R.L. Fenichel and M.A. Chirigos. Marcel Dekker, New York.
3. Suga, T., Shiio, T., Maeda, Y.Y. and Chihara, G. (1984): Antitumour activity of lentinan in murine syngeneic and autochthonous hosts, and its suppressive effect on 3-methylcholanthrene-induced carcinogenesis. *Cancer Res., 44,* 5135.
4. Zakany, J., Chihara, G. and Fachet, J. (1980): Effect of lentinan on tumour growth in murine allogeneic and syngeneic hosts. *Int. J. Cancer, 25,* 371.
5. Klein, G., Sjögren, O., Klein, E. and Hellström, K.E (1960): Demonstration of resistance against methylcholanthrene-induced sarcoma in the primary autochthonous host. *Cancer Res., 20,* 1956.
6. Shiio, T. and Yugari, Y. (1981): The antitumour effect of lentinan and tumor recognition in mice. In: *Manipulation of Host Defense Mechanisms,* p. 29. Editors: T. Aoki, I. Urushizaki and E. Tsubura. Excerpta Medica, Amsterdam.
7. Tarnowski, G.S., Mountain, I.M. and Stock, C.C. (1973): Influence of genotype of host on regression of solid and ascitic forms of sarcoma 180 and effect of chemotherapy on the solid form. *Cancer Res., 33,* 1885.
8. Kiessling, R., Karre, K. and Klein, G. (1980): Genetic control of *in vitro* NK reactivity and its relationship to *in vivo* tumor resistance. In: *Genetic Control of Natural Resistance to Infection and Malignancy,* p. 389. Editors: E. Skamene, P.A.L. Kongshavn and M. Landy. Academic Press, New York.
9. Klein, G.O., Klein G. and Kiessling, R. (1980): Hybrid resistance to parental tumours: influence of host and tumour genotype and derivation. In: *Genetic Control of Natural Resistance to Infection and Malignancy,* p. 467. Editors: E. Skamene, P.A.L. Kongshavn and M. Landy. Academic Press, New York.
10. Maeda, Y.Y. and Chihara, G. (1973): The effect of neonatal thymectomy on the antitumour activity of lentinan, carboxymethypachymaran and zymosan, and their effects on various immune responses. *Int. J. Cancer, 11,* 153.
11. Mackaness, G.B. (1962): Cellular resistance to infection. *J. Exp. Med., 116*, 381.
12. Stevenson, M.M., Kongshavn, P.A.L. and Skamene, E. (1980): Macrophage inflammatory response in *Listeria*-resistant and *Listeria*-sensitive mice. In: *Genetic Control of Natural Resistance to Infection and Malignancy,* p. 565. Editors: E. Skamene, P.A.K. Kongshavn and M. Landy. Academic Press, New York.
13. Nakamura, R.M. and Tokunaga, T. (1980): Genetic control of delayed-type hypersensitivity to *Mycobacterium bovis* BCG infection in mice. In: *Genetic Control of Natural Resistance to Infection and Malignancy,* p. 185. Editors: E.

Skamene, P.A.L. Kongshavn and M. Landy. Academic Press, New York.
14. Hoy, W.E. and Nelson, D.S. (1969): Delayed-type hypersensitivity in mice after skin and tumor allografts and isografts. *Nature (Lond.), 222,* 1001.
15. Waksman, B.H. (1979): Cellular hypersensitivity and immunity: conceptual changes in last decade. *Cell. Immunol., 42,* 155.
16. Zákány, J., Chihara. G. and Fachet, J. (1980): Effect of lentinan on the production of migration inhibitory factor induced by syngeneic tumor in mice. *Int. J. Cancer, 26,* 783.
17. Zákány, J., Jánossy, T., Németh, P., Chihara, G., Fachet, J. and Petri, G. (1983): Mechanism of the A/Ph. MC. Sl tumor graft rejection in syngeneic mice. *Gann, 74,* 712.
18. Hamuro, J., Wagner, H. and Röllinghoff, M. (1978): β (1→3) Glucan as a probe for T-cell specific immune adjuvant: enhanced *in vitro* generation of cytotoxic T-lymphocytes. *Cell. Immunol., 38,* 328.
19. Hamuro, J., Röllinghoff, M. and Wagner, H. (1978): β (1→3) Glucan-mediated augmentation of alloreactive murine cytotoxic T-lymphocytes *in vivo. Cancer Res., 38,* 3080.

Combination therapy with antitumor polysaccharides in mice

Shigeru Abe, Masatoshi Yamazaki and Den'ichi Mizuno

SUMMARY

The effective tumor-spectrum of combination therapy with lentinan and lipopolysaccharide (LPS), named LL therapy, was expanded by two additional immunological manipulations. When the growth of MM46 carcinoma, which is highly immunogenic and susceptible to LL therapy, was inhibited by LL therapy, the delayed hypersensitivity reaction (DHR) of the hosts to MM46 antigens was augmented. Experiments on the transfer of ^{51}Cr-labeled spleen cells revealed that the antitumor DHR caused assembly of normal spleen cells at sites injected with the MM46-antigen fraction. Winn-type assay showed that tumor growth was inhibited non-specifically at the sites eliciting the antitumor DHR. Thus, it is concluded that the antitumor DHR, which was observed as local inflammation, has an important role in the mechanism of tumor rejection of LL therapy. On the other hand, with weakly immunogenic tumors such as MH134 hepatoma and Lewis lung carcinoma, LL therapy did not cause tumor rejection and did not enhance the antitumor DHR. To make LL therapy effective against these tumors, two additional types of immunological manipulation were tested:

1. Augmentation of the antitumor DHR by inhibition of suppressor mechanisms with cyclophosphamide.
2. Induction of local inflammation by a *Streptococcus* preparation, OK432.

It was found that combination of LL therapy and these manipulations strongly inhibited growth of weakly immunogenic tumors such as MH134 hepatoma, colon 38 adenocarcinoma and Lewis lung carcinoma.

INTRODUCTION

The authors are studying combination therapy with immunomodulators to obtain higher antitumor activity against murine transplantable tumors. They have reported previously that immunomodulators can be classified according to the extent to which they increase LB, a serum protein in mice, and that many combinations of different types of immunomodulators are effective therapeutically.[1] One especially effective combination is of lentinan, a type II agent which increases the level of LB slowly, with bacterial lipopolysaccharide (LPS), a type I agent which increases the LB level rapidly.[2] The combination of lentinan plus LPS (LL) has strong antitumor activity against some strongly immunogenic tumors, such as MM46 mammary carcinoma and allogeneic Ehrlich carcinoma. However, this therapy is not effective against some weakly immunogenic tumors, such as MH134 hepatoma.[3]

Thus, for more effective combination therapy, the tumor spectrum must be expanded. Therefore, the authors tried to make LL therapy effective against weakly immunogenic tumors by applying additional manipulations. This paper summarizes their studies on experimental combination therapy against some tumors. The importance of the induction of inflammation in tumor lesions is discussed.

MATERIALS AND METHODS

Tumors and animals

MM46 mammary carcinoma and MH134 hepatoma in male C3H/He mice, and Lewis lung carcinoma and colon 38 adenocarcinoma in male C57BL/6 mice were used. All mice were purchased from Shizuoka Agricultural Cooperative Association for Laboratory Animals, Hamamatsu, Japan.

Agents

Lentinan was kindly provided by Dr. G. Chihara of the National Cancer Center Research Institute, Tokyo and Ajinomoto Co., Kawasaki, Japan. OK432 was from Chugai Pharmaceutical Co., Tokyo. Lipopolysaccharide (LPS) from *E. coli* 0127, B8 was purchased from Difco Lab., Detroit, Mich, and cyclophosphamide (CY) from Shionogi and Co., Ltd., Osaka, Japan.

Antitumor test

Tumor cells were implanted subcutaneously into the right flank or intradermally (i.d.) into the abdomen of mice. Lentinan, LPS or CY in 0.2 ml of saline was administered intraperitoneally. OK432 in 0.1 ml of saline was injected into five sites in tumor lesions.

Assay of the delayed hypersensitivity reaction (DHR) against tumor antigens

The DHR was assayed by the footpad test described previously.[3,4] Antigen fractions of tumor cells were prepared by sonication of tumor cells.[3] The tumor specificity of footpad swelling has been confirmed previously.[3]

RESULTS

Role of the DHR to tumor antigens in the antitumor mechanism of LL therapy

The authors reported previously that administration of a combination of lentinan and LPS on Day 12 after subcutaneous tumor inoculation caused complete regression of MM46 and allogeneic Ehrlich carcinomas in 60% to 90% of the mice tested.[2] In this combination therapy (LL therapy), the optimal doses of lentinan and LPS were 6.25 mg/kg and 0.3 to 0.5 mg/kg respectively, and repeated injections were more effective than a single one.

Mice in which MM46 had regressed after LL therapy were resistant to a second challenge with MM46 tumor. This suggested that some immunological mechanism was involved in this therapy.[2] It was found previously that in a MM46-C3H/He mouse system, antibody-dependent macrophage-mediated cytotoxicity is an effector mechanism and that no killer cells could be detected,[5] but that DHR lymphocytes to MM46 antigens have some part in the antitumor actions of some polysaccharides.[6]

On the basis of these findings, the immunological state of tumor-bearing mice after LL therapy was tested. Table 1 shows that LL therapy caused a rapid and long-lasting increase in the antitumor DHR. No correlation was found between the level of antitumor antibodies and the antitumor activity of LL therapy (data not shown).

The role of the antitumor DHR was then analyzed. Table 2 shows that the anti-MM46 DHR was transferred locally to normal C3H/He mice by peritoneal exudate cells (PEC) from MM46-immune mice and that the transferred DHR caused not only swelling but also accumulation of non-specific host cells at the site of antigen injection.[7] Furthermore, MH134 hepatoma, which did not cross-react antigenically with MM46, showed inhibited growth at sites eliciting an anti-MM46 DHR (Fig. 1).

Table 1 Augmentation of the anti-MM46 footpad response by lentinan plus LPS (LL)

	DHR to MM46 antigens		Tumor diameter (mm) on Day 30
	Day 20	Day 29	
Control	–	–	15
Lentinan	+	+	11
LPS	+	–	10
Lentinan+LPS	++	++	5

Lentinan (6.25 mg/kg) and LPS (0.5 mg/kg) were administered i.p. on Day 12 after s.c. inoculation of 4×10^6 MM46 cells. Increase in foot thickness (IFT) was measured 24 hours after injection of 600 μg of protein from MM46 antigen fraction.
The strength of the DHR is indicated as follows: –: IFT<0.05 (mm); +: 0.05≦IFT<0.10; ++: IFT≧0.10.

Table 2 Local inflammation induced by passive transfer of anti-MM46 DHR or injection of OK432

Injection		Increase in foot thickness	Accumulation of ^{51}Cr-spleen cells
Right foot [R]	Left foot [L]	[R]–[L]±SD (mm)	[R]– [L]±SD (%)
Exp. 1			
MM46-immune PEC +MM46 antigen fraction	MM46-immune PEC	0.86±0.12	0.29±0.04
Normal PEC+MM46 antigen fraction	Normal PEC	0.02±0.04	–0.01±0.03
Exp. 2 OK432 (1 KE)	–	0.62±0.13	0.25±0.10
Dextran (1 mg)	–	0.11±0.01	0.03±0.01

^{51}Cr-labeled spleen cells were prepared from normal C3H/He mice and injected i.v. into all test mice 3 to 5 hours after injections of the indicated samples into the footpads.[7,8] Footpad swelling was measured 13 to 15 hours later; the feet were then amputated to determine the percentage accumulation of ^{51}Cr-spleen cells (counts in foot/total counts injected×100).
In Exp. 1, peritoneal exudate cells from normal or MM46-immunized mice with or without MM46 antigen fractions were injected into the footpads of normal C3H/He mice. In Exp. 2, OK432 or dextran, as a negative control, was injected.

Therefore, it was concluded that the inflammation of tumor lesions induced by antitumor DHR is important in the antitumor mechanism of LL therapy.

LL therapy alone did not induce regression of weakly immunogenic tumors such as MH134 hepatoma and Lewis lung carcinoma, or augment the antitumor DHR of the host with these tumors. Two ways to make LL therapy effective against these tumors seemed theoretically possible:
1. Augmentation of the antitumor DHR by addition of a third component to the LL therapy.
2. Combination of LL therapy with induction of local inflammation in

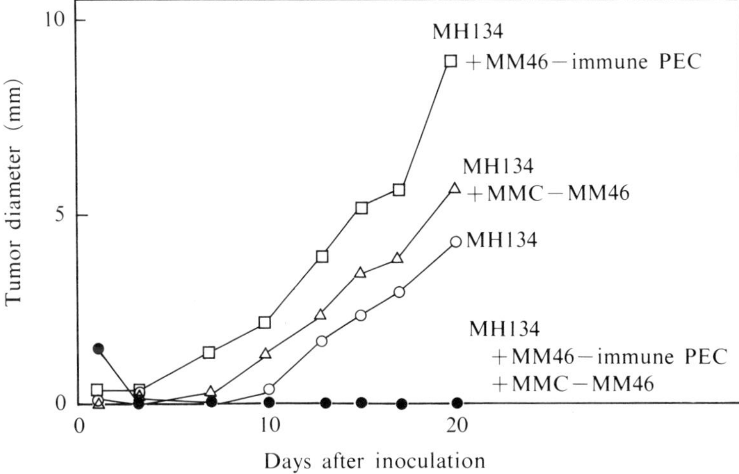

Fig. 1 Growth inhibition of MH134 hepatoma at sites eliciting locally transferred DHR against MM46 carcinoma. MH134 hepatoma cells (3×10^5 cells) were mixed with peritoneal exudate cells (1×10^7 cells) of MM46-immunized mice and/or mitomycin C (MMC)-treated MM46 tumor cells (1×10^6 cells), and injected into the footpads of normal C3H/He mice.[7]

tumor lesions, which may replace the role of antitumor DHR.

Combination of LL therapy and cyclophosphamide (CY) treatment

Immune suppressor systems have been reported to enhance growth of various types of tumors and to make the tumors resistant to immunological manipulations.[9] The authors reported previously that the DHR to MM46 antigens is weakened by specific suppressor T cells in tumor-bearing mice and that suppressor cells are inhibited by administration of 100 to 150 mg/kg of cyclophosphamide (CY).[10]

Therefore, the authors tried to augment the antitumor DHR by CY treatment in combination with LL therapy. Table 3 shows that in MH134-bearing mice, the antitumor DHR was greater with a combination of LL and CY treatments than with either alone.

This combination of the three components caused complete tumor regression in about 60% of the animals inoculated with MH134 cells; all three components were needed for maximal antitumor activity. Growth of colon 38 adenocarcinoma was also inhibited by this combination therapy.[3]

Combination of LL therapy and intralesional administration of OK432

The effect of additional induction of local inflammation was also tested as a method for expanding the effective tumor spectrum of LL therapy.

Table 3 Antitumor activity of combination therapy with cyclophosphamide (CY) and augmentation of the anti-MH134 footpad response

Treatment	Tumor diameter ±SD (mm) (Day 30)	Increase in foot thickness±SE (mm) (Day 23)	Cured/tested (Day 70)
Control	17.8±2.4	0.06±0.02	0/10
Lentinan+LPS	16.3±1.2	0.07±0.01	0/8
CY	12.2±1.8	0.09±0.03	0/10
Lentinan+LPS+CY	6.1±2.5	0.18±0.03	5/9

Lentinan (6.25 mg/kg), LPS (0.5 mg/kg) and CY (100 mg/kg) were administered i.p. on Days 12, 18 and 24 after s.c. inoculation of 5×10^5 MH134 cells. Increase in foot thickness represents the DHR to MH134 antigens.

Injections of some immunomodulators are known to induce local inflammation resembling the DHR.[8]

The authors previously examined the extent of inflammation induced by intraperitoneal injections of more than ten immunomodulators, finding that a *Streptococcus* preparation, OK432 (2 KE), induced very strong inflammation with accumulation of polymorphonuclear leukocytes (PMN $>2.0\times10^7$ cells) and macrophages ($>1.0\times10^7$ cells) in the peritoneal cavity of C3H/He mice.[11]
Table 2 shows that injection of OK432 into the footpads induced not only footpad swelling but also accumulation of transferred ^{51}Cr-labeled spleen cells, as observed in the antitumor DHR in the MM46 system.

Table 4 shows that combination therapy comprising injection of OK432 into the lesions and then intraperitoneal administration of LL caused almost complete regression of MH134 hepatomas and that all three components were needed for maximal antitumor activity. The cured mice were resistant to rechallenge with MH134;[4] their acquired resistance might be explained by their augmented DHR[4] and by antitumor antibodies which showed cytotoxicity dependent on macrophages (unpublished data).

Combination therapy against Lewis lung carcinoma

Lewis lung carcinoma in C57BL/6 mice is highly metastatic. Its regression could not be induced by any of the combination therapies described above. The effect of combining all four components (OK432, CY, lentinan and LPS) was therefore tested.

Table 5 shows that this combination caused complete regression in more than 50% of animals. It should be noted that with this therapy the timing of the administration of LL was important for antitumor activity: LL was effective when administered after CY, as will be reported elsewhere.

Table 4 Antitumor activity of combination therapy with OK432 against MH134

Treatment	Tumor diameter ±SD (mm)	Cured/tested
Control	19.1±3.1	0/8
Lentinan+LPS	14.6±3.9	0/8
OK432	13.5±4.4	1/8
OK432+lentinan	8.3±7.9	4/6
OK432+LPS	6.9±5.9	3/8
OK432+lentinan+LPS	4.3±5.4	7/8

OK432 (1 KE/mouse) was injected into the tumor on Day 5 after i.d. inoculation of 2.0×10^5 MH134 cells.[4]
Lentinan (6.25 mg/kg) and LPS (0.5 mg/kg) were administered i.p. on Day 12. Tumor diameter and tumor regression were examined on Day 27.

Table 5 Antitumor activity of combination therapy against Lewis lung carcinoma

Treatment			Survivors on Day 60/ tested mice	Survival ratio (%)
Lentinan plus LPS	OK432	CY		
−	−	−	0/14	0
−	+	−	0/12	0
−	−	+	0/12	0
+	−	+	2/12	17
+	+	−	0/8	0
−	+	+	4/12	33
+	+	+	7/12	58

C57BL/6 mice were inoculated i.d. with 3×10^5 Lewis lung cells on Day 0; OK432 (3 KE/head) was injected into the tumor on Days 4, 7 and 10. The mice then received i.p. injections of CY (100 mg/kg) on Days 12, 16 and 20, and lentinan (6.25 mg/kg) and LPS (0.5 mg/kg) on Days 20, 24 and 28.

DISCUSSION

The results presented in this paper show that the effective tumor spectrum of LL therapy can be expanded by combined treatments with CY and OK432. It is known that the susceptibility of tumors to antitumor polysaccharides depends on the immunogenicity of the tumors[12] and that Lewis lung carcinoma, which is weakly immunogenic, is not cured effectively by immunological manipulations. Consequently, the results presented here provide a model for use in development of immunological manipulations against weakly immunogenic tumors.

The present combination therapy is based on two types of approach known to augment intratumoral inflammation. One is augmentation of the antitumor DHR by inhibition of suppressor mechanisms with CY (Table 3). The other is induction of local inflammation directly by injection of OK432 into the tumor (Table 2). The authors think that these two agents have a therapeutic effect through augmentation of intratumoral inflammation, because antigen-nonspecific inhibition of tumor growth was observed in sites with inflammation (Fig. 1). However, other actions by these agents should also be taken into account, as has been discussed previously.[3,4]

To make this combination therapy even more useful, the authors are now attempting to exclude toxic LPS from the combination.

REFERENCES

1. Yoshioka, O., Abe, S., Masuko, Y. and Mizuno, D. (1981): Typing of immunomodulators in terms of their effects on the electrophoretic pattern of serum proteins and antitumor combination therapy based on this typing. *Gann*, *72*, 471.
2. Abe, S., Yoshioka, O., Masuko, Y., Tsubouchi, J., Kohno, M., Nakajima, H., Yamazaki, M. and Mizuno, D. (1982): Combination antitumor therapy with lentinan and bacterial lipopolysaccharide against murine tumors. *Gann*, *73*, 91.
3. Abe, S., Tsubouchi, J., Takahashi, K., Yamazaki, M. and Mizuno, D. (1982): Combination therapy of murine tumors with lentinan plus lipopolysaccharide plus cyclophosphamide. *Gann*, *73*, 961.
4. Abe, S., Takahashi, K., Tsubouchi, J., Yamazaki, M. and Mizuno, D. (1983): Combination therapy of murine tumors with lentinan, bacterial lipopolysaccharide and a *Streptococcus* preparation, OK432. *Gann*, *74*, 273.
5. Yamazaki, M., Shinoda, H. and Mizuno, D. (1976): Antibody-dependent macrophage-mediated cytolysis in a murine syngeneic tumor system. *Gann*, *67*, 651.
6. Masuko, Y., Nakajima, H., Tsubouchi, J., Yamazaki, M., Mizuno, D. and Abe, S. (1982): Changes of antitumor immunity of hosts with murine mammary tumors regressed by lentinan: potentiation of antitumor delayed hypersensitivity reaction. *Gann*, *73*, 790.
7. Abe, S., Takahashi, K., Yamazaki, M. and Mizuno, D. (1984): Assembly of transferred normal spleen cells *in situ* at sites eliciting the delayed hypersensitivity reaction to tumor antigen in mice. *Gann*, *75*, 442.
8. Abe, S., Takahashi, K., Tsubouchi, J., Aida, K., Yamazaki, M. and Mizuno, D. (1984): Differential local therapeutic effects of various polysaccharides on MH134 hepatoma in mice and its relation to inflammation induced by the polysaccharides. *Gann*, *75*, 459.
9. Fujimoto, S., Green, M.I. and Sehon, A.H. (1976): Regulation of immune response to tumor antigens. I. Immunosuppressor cells in tumor-bearing hosts. *J. Immunol.*, *116*, 791.
10. Nakajima, H., Abe, S., Masuko, Y., Tsubouchi, J., Yamazaki, M. and Mizuno, D. (1981): Elimination of tumor-enhancing cells by cyclophosphamide and its relevance to cyclophosphamide therapy of a murine mammary tumor. *Gann*, *72*, 723.
11. Morikawa, K., Kikuchi, Y., Abe, S., Yamazaki, M. and Mizuno, D. (1984): Early cellular responses in the peritoneal cavity of mice to antitumor immunomodulators. *Gann*, *75*, 370.
12. Abe, S., Yamazaki, M. and Mizuno, D. (1978): Correlation of differences in

antigenicity of four 3-methylcholanthrene-induced tumors in syngeneic mice with susceptibility of tumors to an immunopotentiator, PS-K. *Gann*, *69*, 223.

Synergistic effect of lentinan and surgical endocrine therapy on the growth of DMBA-induced mammary tumors of rats and of recurrent human breast cancer

Akio Kosaka, Yuuichi Hattori, Atsuko Imaizumi and Akira Yamashita

SUMMARY

The synergistic effects of lentinan, an immunomodulator polysaccharide extract from *Lentinus edodes*, and surgical endocrine therapy were studied in rats with 7,12-dimethyl benzanthracene (DMBA)- induced mammary turors and in patients with recurrent breast cancer.

Surgical endocrine therapy alone (adrenalectomy+ovariectomy, ovariectomy, or adrenalectomy) resulted in a partial inhibition of tumor growth in rats bearing palpable mammary tumors. Multiple injections of lentinan following surgical endocrine therapy induced a much greater regression of tumor growth than that produced by surgery alone. No significant changes in body weight, survival rate or histamine sensitivity response were observed in rats treated with lentinan compared with those of saline-treated controls. These quantitative findings were confirmed by a histological study showing that the degree of growth or degeneration of adenocarcinoma fitted well with the quantitative data in each experimental group, and also that lentinan treatment accelerates degeneration of tumor cells and induces an infiltration into the stroma surrounding adenocarcinomatous foci of cells consisting mainly of lymphocytes, macrophages and inflammatory cells.

The efficacy of lentinan treatment of patients with recurrent breast cancer who had previously undergone bilateral adrenalectomy and ovariectomy was evaluated in a randomized controlled study. Patients treated with lentinan showed longer disease-free intervals and survival times, and a much higher survival rate than controls. No severe side effects were caused by lentinan treatment.

These data indicate that lentinan might be a useful and safe agent for treatment of mammary tumors in combination with surgical endocrine therapy.

INTRODUCTION

There is a good deal of evidence that lentinan, a polysaccharide isolated from *Lentinus edodes*, has marked antitumor activity *in vivo* and plays an effective role in host resistance against cancer as an immunomodulator.[1,2] Two distinct mechanisms of action of lentinan have been suggested, one hormonal and one immunological.[1,2] It is therefore important to investigate whether lentinan exerts an antitumor action on hormone-dependent tumors *in vivo*.

It is well documented that DMBA-induced mammary tumors are biologically and histologically malignant and have characteristics that resemble those of some human breast cancers, because they involve adjacent tissues, end the life of the host, and are extremely hormone dependent.[3,4] In an animal experiment using a DMBA-induced autochthonous tumor system, the authors determined whether lentinan therapy is synergistic with surgical endocrine therapy. In addition, the clinical efficacy and safety of lentinan for the treatment of human patients with recurrent breast cancer who have previously undergone adrenalectomy and ovariectomy were evaluated in a 6-year randomized controlled study.

The biological and histological studies provided evidence that lentinan treatment results in a marked regression of mammary tumor growth both in rats and human patients when combined with surgical endocrine therapy.

EXPERIMENTAL STUDY

Materials and Methods

Animals

Female nulliparous Sprague-Dawley (SD) rats, 40 to 50 days old, were used for these experiments. All rats were maintained in an air-conditioned room at a temperature of 24 ± 1°C and a relative humidity of 60 to 70%, offered a standard diet, and given tap water *ad libitum*. After adrenalectomy/ovariectomy, tap water was replaced by normal saline.

Adrenalectomy and ovariectomy

Bilateral adrenalectomy was performed under ether anesthesia by the dorsal approach. Bilateral ovariectomy and adrenalectomy were performed simultaneously by the abdominal approach. Sham operations were performed on the control group.

Experimental protocol

As Fig. 1 shows, 40- to 50-day-old SD rats received a single intravenous injection of a fat emulsion containing 0.5% DMBA (30 mg/kg body weight); they were examined for palpable mammary tumors every five days thereafter. Fifty to sixty days after DMBA administration, when palpable tumors reached about 1 cm in diameter, these rats were divided into four groups. One group, the control group, underwent sham operations. The other three groups, each consisting of 16 to 20 animals, served as surgical endocrine therapy groups as follows: a bilateral adrenalectomized (AX) group, an ovariectomized (OVX) group and an adrenalectomized and ovariectomized (AX+OVX) group. Starting two weeks after operation, each group was given an intravenous injection of lentinan (1 mg/kg body weight) or 0.85% saline solution (0.2 ml) daily for 10 days. General condition, body weight and tumor size were observed for four

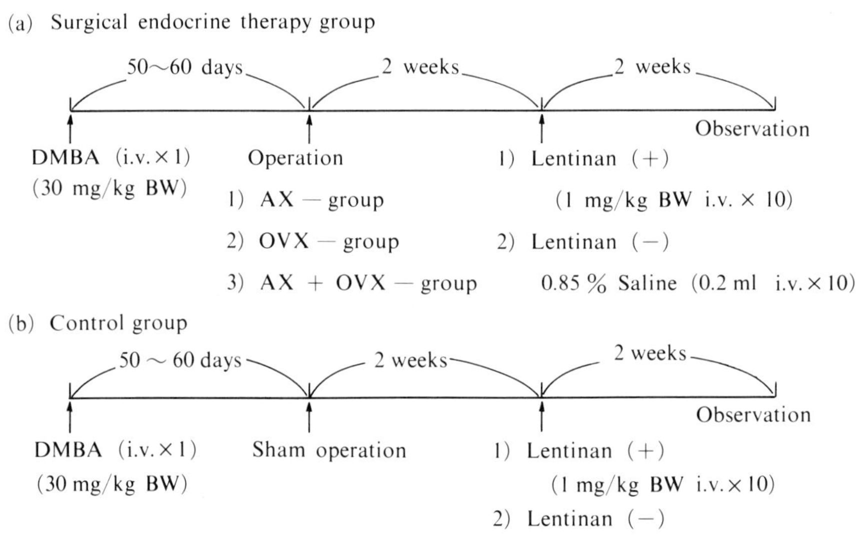

Fig. 1 Experimental protocol for combination treatment of DMBA-induced rat mammary tumor with lentinan and surgical endocrine therapy.

weeks after the operation. Tumor size was measured by calipers and expressed as the mean logarithmic value per rat, calculated by Geran's formula (greatest diameter × shortest diameter^2 × ½).[5] Six days after the last injection, all rats were tested for histamine sensitivity and then decapitated. Mammary tumors were removed immediately, fixed in Carnoy's fixative and stained with hematoxylin-eosin. Sections were observed under a light microscope.

Determination of histamine sensitivity

The vascular permeability response of skin to histamine was determined by the method described by Leme et al.[6] In the present study, Evans blue was used instead of methylene blue.

Reagents

DMBA was dissolved in a fat emulsion. Lentinan, a β (1→3) glucan isolated from *Lentinus edodes* (Berk.) Sing., an edible mushroom growing in Japan, was supplied by Ajinomoto Co., Ltd., Kawasaki, Japan.

Results

Vascular permeability response to histamine

In rats given an injection of saline solution, the degree of histamine sensitivity was markedly greater in all of the surgical endocrine therapy groups than in the control group. Sensitivity in the AX+OVX group and the AX group was greater than in the OVX group (Fig. 2). Lentinan injection resulted in a further augmentation of the elevated sensitivity, not only in all of the surgical endocrine therapy groups but also in the control group (Fig. 2). The AX group given the lentinan injection showed an extremely high degree of sensitivity.

Changes in body weight and survival rate

No significant differences in body weight were found between any groups (Fig. 3). Furthermore, the high survival rate (over 90% in all groups, data not shown) indicates that lentinan treatment caused no deaths. No episodes of shock or convulsion followed lentinan injections.

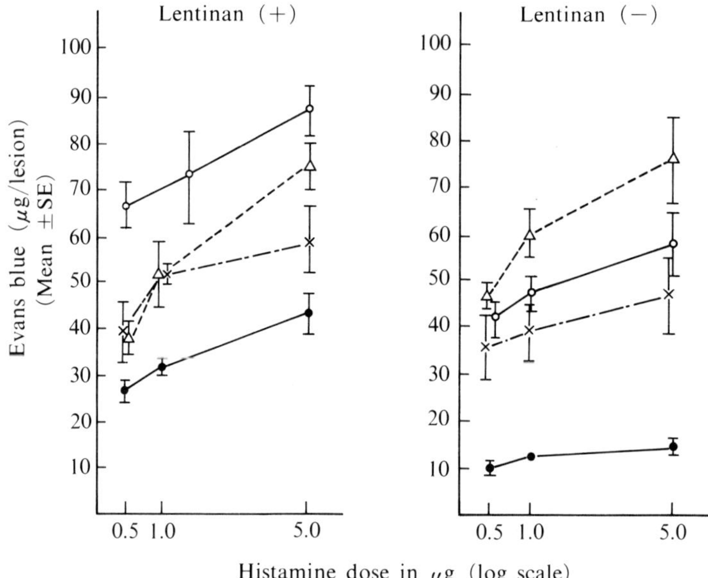

Fig. 2 Effect of lentinan injection on the vascular permeability response to histamine. The strength of the permeability response is expressed by the mean volume (μg) of Evans blue per lesion. ●——●: Control group; ○——○: Adrenalectomized (AX) group; ×—·—·—×: Ovariectomized (OVX) group; △----△: AX+OVX group.

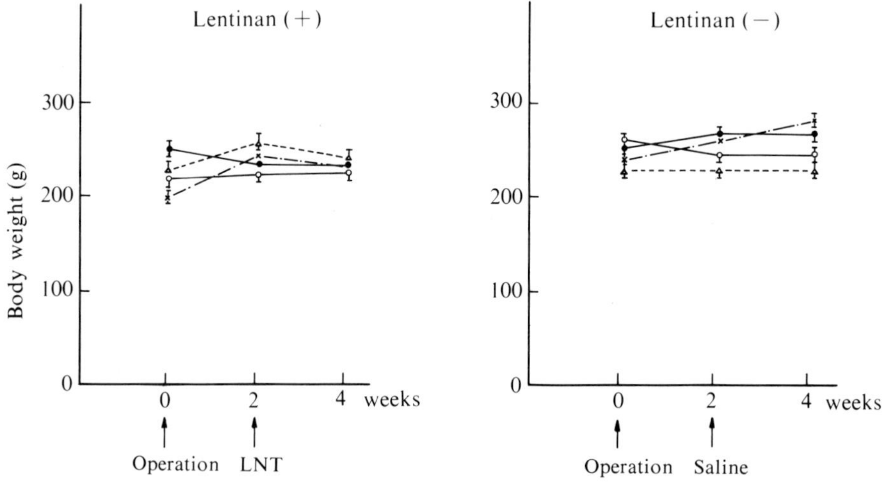

Fig. 3 Effect of lentinan (LNT) injection on body weight. Body weight in each group is expressed as the mean value of 6 to 8 measurements. ●——●: Control group; ○——○:AX group: ×—-—×:OVX group; △----△: AX+OVX group.

Tumor response to combined therapy

The mean volume of tumor per rat was measured in all groups at specified intervals after operation. Mammary tumors in the control group given the saline injection grew linearly after DMBA administration. Tumor growth in all of the surgical endocrine therapy groups was partially suppressed after operation compared with controls; there was no difference in the degree of suppression among these groups. On the other hand, tumor growth was slightly retarded after lentinan injection, compared with growth in the saline-injected group, suggesting that lentinan alone can exert some suppressive effect on tumor growth (Fig. 4). In the OVX and AX+OVX groups which received lentinan injections, much greater reduction of tumor volume was seen than in the saline-injected group (Fig. 4).

These quantitative data were supported by the histological study. Table 1 shows the summarized histological findings on mammary tumors in all groups four weeks after operation. The degree of growth, degeneration or atrophy of adenocarcinoma fitted well with the quantitative data

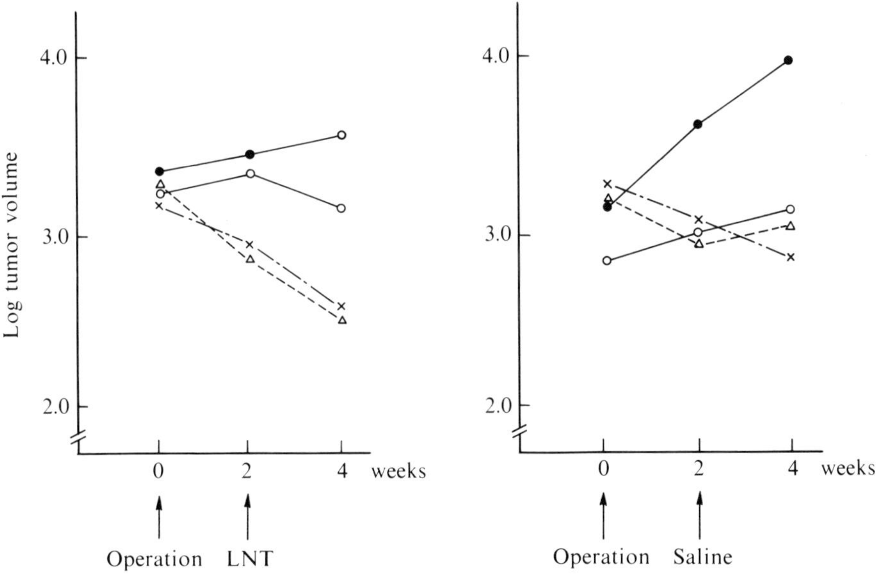

Fig. 4 Synergistic effect of lentinan (LNT) injections and surgical endocrine therapy on the growth of DMBA-induced mammary tumors in rats. Total tumor volume per rat is expressed as the mean logarithmic value of 5 to 6 examinations. ●——●: Control group; ○——○: AX group; ×—-—×: OVX group; △----△: AX+OVX group.

Table 1 Histological changes in DMBA-induced mammary tumors in rats treated with immuno-endocrine therapy*

Experimental group	Mammary tumor cells		Degree of cell infiltration**			
	Growth**	Degeneration**	Lymph.	Mϕ	PMN	Mast
DMBA → (−)	+++	−	+	+	±	++
DMBA → AX	+++	−	+	+	±	++
DMBA → OVX	++	+	+	+	+	±
DMBA → Lentinan (LNT)	++	+	++	++	+	+
DMBA → AX+LNT	++	+	++	++	+	++
DMBA → OVX+LNT	+	++	+++	+	+	±
DMBA → AX+OVX+LNT	+	+++	++	+	++	±

* Histological changes in mammary tumors (same size in each group: 10 to 15 mm in diameter) from each group were observed light microscopically four weeks after operation.

** −: absent; ±: very weak; +: weak; ++: moderate; +++: massive. Lymph., lymphocytes; Mϕ, macrophages; PMN, polymorphonuclear leukocytes; Mast, Mast cells.

given above. In the OVX and AX+OVX groups given the lentinan injection, suppression of tumor growth was much greater than that in other groups (Table 1). It is of interest that in the lentinan-injected groups adenocarcinomatous foci which showed marked atrophy were surrounded by stroma which was infiltrated intensely with a number of lymphocytes, macrophages and other inflammatory cells. Figure 5a shows a representative mammary tumor from the AX+OVX group given the lentinan injection. In contrast, well-differentiated adenocarcinoma was observed in the AX group given the saline injection (Fig. 5b).

CLINICAL STUDY

Patients and Methods

Over a period of 6 years, beginning in March 1978, the authors performed a randomized controlled study of lentinan treatment on 32 consecutive female patients with recurrent breast cancer who had previously been treated by bilateral adrenalectomy and ovariectomy in Shimizu City Hospital. Figure 6 shows the protocol of the clinical study, which used the so-called envelope method. The 32 patients showed complete response (CR), partial response (PR) or no change (NC); they were divided into a control group (N=17) and a lentinan group (N=15). Patients showing progressive disease (PD) were excluded from this study. The lentinan group was given an intravenous injection of 1 mg of lentinan twice weekly during their period of hospitalization and 5 mg of lentinan twice

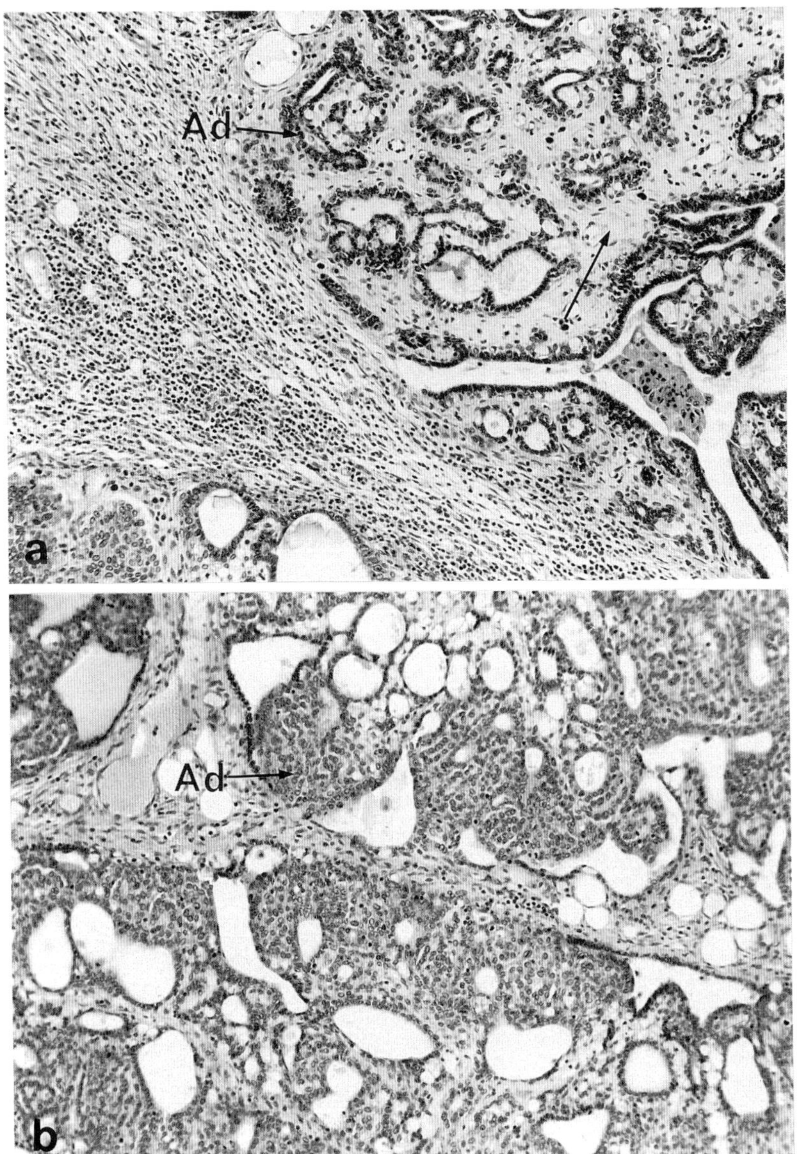

Fig. 5 Histological findings on DMBA-induced mammary tumors in rats treated with lentinan-endocrine therapy. (a) Mammary tumor of a rat treated with lentinan injections and AX+OVX. Marked atrophy of adenocarcinomatous foci (Ad) with a varying degree of replacement by connective tissue (arrow) is present. Massive diffuse cell infiltration consisting mainly of lymphocytes, macrophages and other inflammatory cells can be seen in the stroma around small adenocarcinomatous foci. (b) Mammary tumor of a rat treated with adrenalectomy alone. A number of large foci of well-differentiated adenocarcinoma (Ad) can be seen. There is a slight degree of cell infiltration in the stroma. (a) and (b), HE ×180

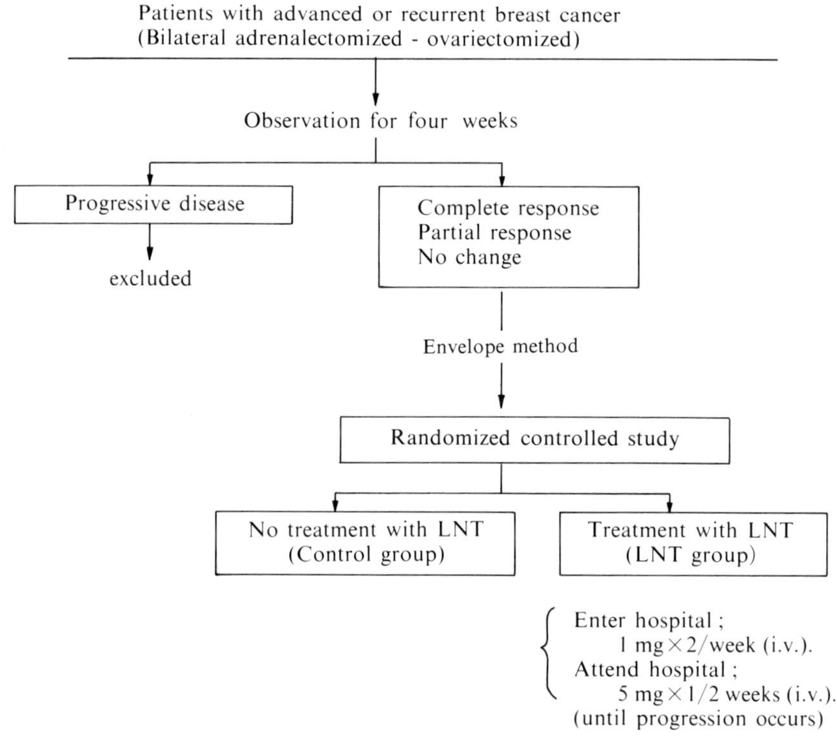

Fig. 6 Protocol for the randomized controlled study of lentinan treatment of patients with breast cancer.

Table 2 Background factors of patients with breast cancer in the randomized controlled study

Group	Age			Condition		Menopause		Site of metastasis				Stage			
	<39	40–59	>60	Advanced	Recurrent	Before	After	Lung	Liver	Bone	Local	I	II	III	IV
Control	4	6	7	1	16	7	10	3	0	10	4	0	5	10	2
Lentinan	4	9	2	1	14	11	4	1	0	12	1	0	2	13	0
Total	8	15	9	2	30	18	14	4	0	22	5	0	7	23	2

monthly as out-patients until they exhibited signs of disease progression. No other drugs or irradiation were administered during the study. The background factors of the patients are shown in Table 2. The mean age of the patients was 49.5 years, with a range of 35 to 69 years. Most metastases were found in bone and lung. Most patients had stage 3 disease. There were no differences between the background factors of the lentinan group and the control group. Survival rate was measured by the Kaplan-Meier method.[7] For the statistical analysis of prolongation of life-span, the generalized Wilcoxon test[8] was used.

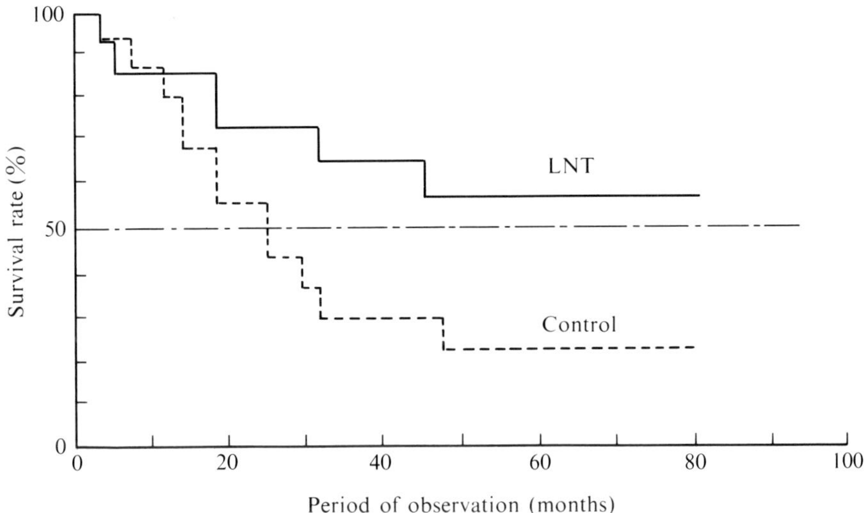

Fig. 7 Effect of lentinan (LNT) treatment on the survival rate of patients with breast cancer.
———: Lentinan-treated group; ------: Control group.

Results

Figure 7 shows the effect of lentinan treatment in combination with the surgical endocrine therapy on the survival rate of patients with breast cancer. The fifty per cent survival periods of the control and lentinan groups were 25 months and over 80 months respectively. Moreover, life span was greater in the lentinan group than the control group (Fig. 7); the difference was probably significant ($z = -1.6607$, $0.05 < p < 0.01$). The histogram of the survival times of individual patients also shows that lentinan treatment tended to prolong the disease-free interval and survival period, and also to increase the survival rate (Fig. 8). The survival rates of the control and lentinan groups were 24% and 53% respectively.

Only 3 of 15 patients who received multiple injections of lentinan showed side effects; these were a feeling of pressure in the breast, facial flushing and lumbar pain. These were mild and transient. No shock, allergic reactions or edema were observed in any of the patients studied during this trial.

DISCUSSION

This study demonstrated the efficacy and safety of lentinan treatment in

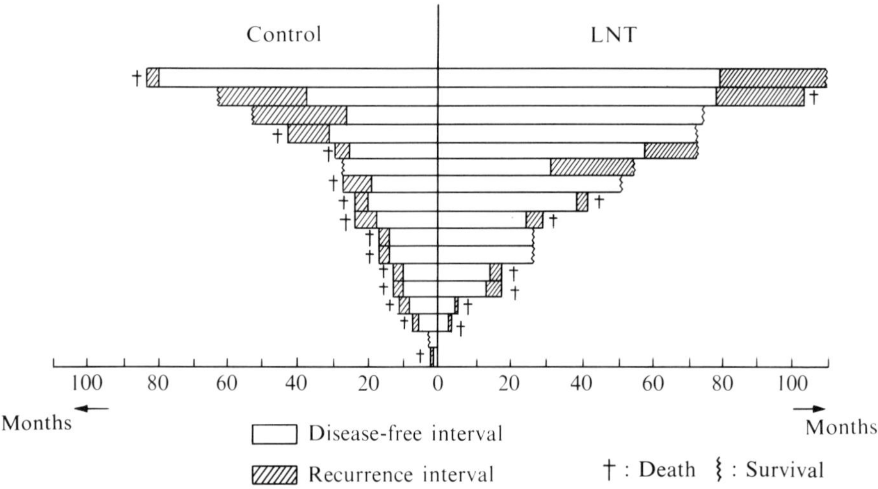

Fig. 8 Histogram of survival times of individual patients in the control and lentinan groups.

combination with surgical endocrine therapy for mammary tumor-bearing animals and patients with recurrent breast cancer.

A serious concern was risk of death due to shock, allergic reaction or an increase in histamine sensitivity response. Maeda et al.[1] reported that most adrenalectomized female ICR mice die of shock accompanied by convulsions very similar to the shock caused by histamine, after intraperitoneal injection of lentinan (1 mg/kg BW). Moreover, Honma et al.[9] found that lentinan increases the histamine sensitivity of ddY mice. However, in the present study, no animal deaths from shock with convulsions or decrease of survival rate were observed, although the study was performed using mammary tumor-bearing rats under almost the same experimental conditions as pertained to the above studies. Moreover, lentinan treatment caused no severe side effects in patients with breast cancer.

These findings indicate that lentinan may be a safe agent for adrenalectomized animals and patients who have previously received surgical endocrine therapy. However, the elevated degree of histamine sensitivity following surgical endocrine operation was further augmented by lentinan treatment (Fig. 2). Moreover, tumor-bearing rats tend to be more sensitive to histamine or some histamine sensitizing agents than normal rats.[10] Thus, in the clinical use of lentinan for hormone dependent tumors which have previously been treated by the surgical endocrine therapy, one should always consider the possibility of the occurrence of shock resulting from a marked increase in histamine sensitivity.

The mechanism of lentinan treatment in combination with surgical endocrine therapy was not elucidated in the present study. Recently, the authors observed that prior treatment of the host with lentinan results in a reduction in the incidence of DMBA-induced mammary tumors, and decreases significantly the serum level of prolactin (paper in preparation). Nagasawa et al.[11,12] have reported that the administration of *Nocardia rubra* cell wall skeleton exerts a similar effect on mammary tumors in mice and rats. Thus, it is possible that lentinan's action on tumors is mediated by hormonal activity, in particular by the hypothalamo-hypophyseal system. On the other hand, the present histological study (Table 1, Figs. 5 and 6) showed that, in the AX+OVX and OVX groups receiving lentinan treatment, adenocarcinomatous foci were greatly atrophied and surrounded by stroma that was intensely infiltrated by lymphocytes, macrophages and inflammatory cells. Lentinan injection alone resulted in massive infiltration of lymphocytes and macrophages, but not in so much degeneration of tumor cells, indicating that lentinan may induce a mobilization of immunocompetent cells into foci of tumor cells. Thus, these data indicate that lentinan exerts an antitumor effect through both immunological and hormonal mechanisms synergistic with surgical endocrine therapy, although the precise mechanisms remain obscure.

In the clinical study, the efficacy and safety of lentinan treatment of patients with recurrent breast cancer in combination with surgical endocrine therapy (AX+OVX) were demonstrated by the 6-year randomized controlled study (Figs. 7 and 8). However, in order to evaluate the statistical significance of this benefit, many more cases need to be observed over a longer period than was possible in the present study.

REFERENCES

1. Maeda, Y.Y., Hamuro, J., Yamada, Y., Ishimura, K. and Chihara, G. (1974): The nature of immunopotentiation by the anti-tumor polysaccharide lentinan and the significance of biogenic amines in its action. In: *Immunopotentiation, Ciba Found. Symp.*, p. 259. New Series, 18. Associated Scientific Publications, Amsterdam.
2. Akiyama, Y. and Hamuro, J. (1981): Effect of antitumor polysaccharides on specific and nonspecific immune responses and their immunological characteristics. *Protein, Nucleic acid and Enzyme, 26*, 208 (in Japanese).
3. Huggins, C. and Yang, W.C. (1962): Induction and extension of mammary cancer. *Science, 137*, 257.
4. Sterental, A., Dominguez, J.M., Weissman, C. and Pearson, O.H. (1963): Pituitary role in the estrogen dependency of experimental mammary cancer. *Cancer* Res., 23, 481.
5. Geran, R.I., Greenberg, N.H., MacDonald, M.M., Schumacher, A.M. and Abbott, B.J. (1972): Protocols for screening chemical agents and natural products

against animal tumors and other biological systems. *Cancer Chemother. Rep., 3*, 51.

6. Leme, J.G. and Wilhelm, D.L. (1975): The effects of adrenalectomy and corticosterone on vascular permeability responses in the skin of the rat. *Br. J. Exp. Path., 56*, 402.
7. Kaplan, E.L. and Meier, P. (1958): Nonparametric estimation from incomplete observations. *J. Am. Stat. Assoc., 53*, 457.
8. Gehan, E. (1965): A generalized Wilcoxon test for comparing arbitrarily singly-censored samples. *Biometrika, 52*, 203.
9. Honma, R. and Kuratsuka, K. (1973): Histamine sensitizing activity of lentinan and antitumor polysaccharide. *Experientia, 29*, 290.
10. Kosaka, A., Wani, T., Hattori, Y. and Yamashita, A. (1982): Effect of lentinan on the adrenalectomized rats and human patients with breast cancer. *Jpn. J. Cancer Chemother., 9*, 1474 (In Japanese).
11. Nagasawa, H., Yanai, R. and Azuma, I. (1979): Inhibitory effect of *nocardia rubra* cell wall skeleton on carcinogen-induced mammary tumorigenesis in the rats. *Eur. J. Cancer, 16*, 387.
12. Nagasawa, H., Yanai, R. and Azuma, I. (1978): Suppression by *nocardia rubra* cell wall skeleton of mammary DNA synthesis, plasma prolactin level, and spontaneous mammary tumorigenesis in mice. *Cancer Res., 38*, 2160.

End-point result of a randomized controlled study on the treatment of gastrointestinal cancer with a combination of lentinan and chemotherapeutic agents

Tetsuo Taguchi, Hisashi Furue, Tadashi Kimura, Tatsuhei Kondo, Takao Hattori, Ichiji Ito and Nobuya Ogawa

SUMMARY

To investigate the efficacy of lentinan in prolonging survival, a long-term follow-up study was carried out on the subjects of a clinical trial performed between August 1979 and September 30, 1980, in which patients with advanced or recurrent gastric or colorectal cancer were given lentinan in combination with mitomycin C (MMC) plus 5-fluorouracil (combination: MF), or with tegafur (FT). The following conclusions were reached:
(1) A statistically significant prolongation of life span was observed in the lentinan-treated groups, the results showing the same tendency as was seen at the conclusion of the clinical study.
(2) Higher rates of survival, according to analysis using life-expectancy tables, were observed in the lentinan-treated groups, especially in cases of gastric cancer in which lentinan was used in combination with tegafur. The following survival rates were observed: in patients with gastric cancer, 12.97% ($p<0.05$) at two years after the beginning of lentinan treatment, 9.51% at three years ($p<0.05$), and 3.81% at four years; in patients with colorectal cancer, 9.10% and 4.55% at two and three years respectively.

INTRODUCTION

A report has already been published on the results of a randomized controlled Phase III study on the efficacy of lentinan administered in combination with mitomycin C (MMC) plus 5-fluorouracil (combination: MF) or with tegafur (FT) in advanced or recurrent carcinoma of the stomach or large intestine.[1]

The results from the period of the above study, which ran from August 1979 to September 30, 1980, demonstrated statistically significant prolongation of life in the lentinan-treated groups compared with those that did not receive lentinan, and direct antitumor effect in cases of stomach cancer was reinforced by combined administration of lentinan and FT, the difference from the group given only FT again being significant. Moreover, although there were no significant differences among the other groups, strong reinforcement of antitumor action was observed in all groups treated with lentinan in combination with other drugs.

No reports have hitherto been published in which a controlled study of patients with advanced or recurrent cancer of the digestive tract has been succeeded by a follow-up study in which the final results were analyzed statistically. Since the authors considered that it is unsatisfactory from the viewpoint of treatment evaluation to try to discuss the effectiveness of a cancer therapy without examining the final outcome, we carried out a follow-up survey to the above-mentioned Phase III study, and re-examined the results published in the previous report in order to assess the usefulness of lentinan in combination with chemotherapeutic agents.

PARTICIPATING INSTITUTIONS AND PERIOD OF SURVEY

This follow-up survey of the outcome of cases as of May 1, 1984, and of the treatment in the interim was performed at the 32 institutes listed in the footnote at the end of the article. The subjects were those cases surviving when the controlled clinical study ended, on September 30, 1980.

METHODS OF TREATMENT

The treatment methods used in the study are shown in Table 1. The control groups were treated with MF or FT alone, and the treatment groups were given lentinan in combination with one of these agents. After the conclusion of the Phase III study, i. e., after October 1, 1980, treatment methods were not restricted in any way and were dependent on the judgement of the physician concerned.

Table 1 Protocols used during the clinical study

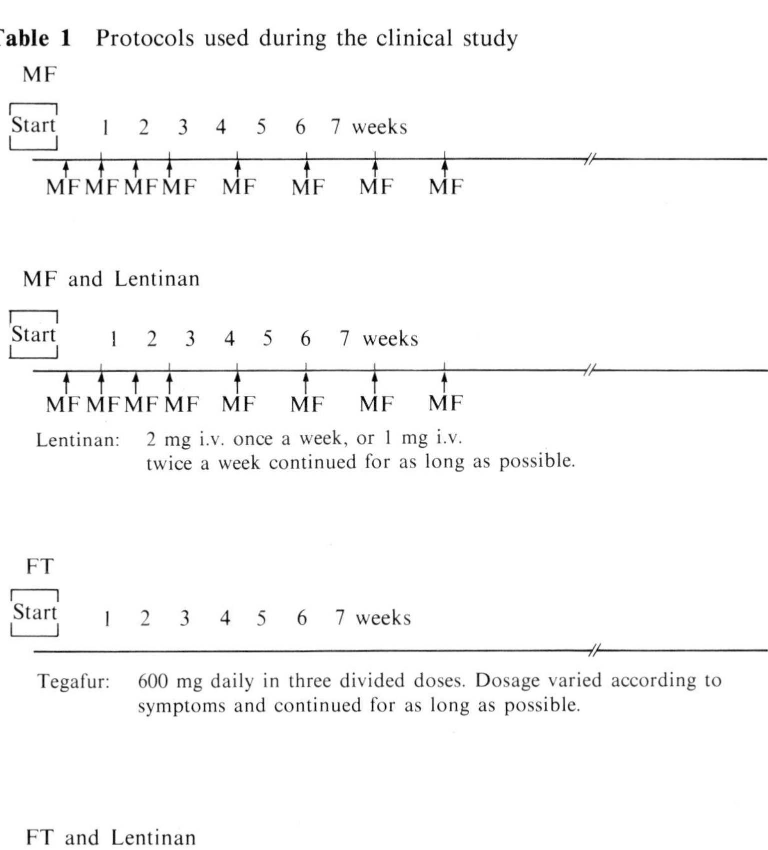

ASSESSMENT OF LIFE PROLONGATION

The life-prolonging action of lentinan was assessed by applying the generalized Wilcoxon test to the survival curves obtained by the Kaplan-Meier method. In addition, a controlled study was carried out by calculating the survival rates for each year by means of analysis using life expectancy tables.

Table 2 Revisions to the previous classification of cases[1] and to the number of subjects

<table>
<tr><th colspan="2" rowspan="2"></th><th colspan="4">Original report</th></tr>
<tr><th>Subjects</th><th colspan="4">Excluded cases</th></tr>
<tr><td rowspan="3">Present survey</td><td>Subjects</td><td></td><td colspan="4">Two cases not included in original subject group on grounds of insufficient washout period. These patients were included in the present study as it was discovered that their washout periods had in fact been satisfactory</td></tr>
<tr><td>Excluded cases</td><td>1. Patients who had undergone surgery as treatment for the cancer since the clinical trial: 4 cases
2. Washout period found to have been insufficient: 1 case</td><td colspan="4"></td></tr>
<tr><td>Withdrawn cases</td><td>1. Patients found to have been switched to another drug during clinical trial: 4 cases
2. Curative surgery performed during clinical trial: 1 case</td><td colspan="4"></td></tr>
<tr><td colspan="2">Site of cancer</td><td></td><td colspan="2">Stomach</td><td colspan="2">Colon</td></tr>
<tr><td colspan="2">Basic treatment</td><td></td><td>MF</td><td>FT</td><td>MF</td><td>FT</td></tr>
<tr><td colspan="2">Number of cases:</td><td>Control group</td><td>59 (60)</td><td>68 (72)</td><td>19 (19)</td><td>17 (17)</td></tr>
<tr><td colspan="2"></td><td>Treatment group</td><td>74 (76)</td><td>77 (77)</td><td>31 (31)</td><td>22 (23)</td></tr>
</table>

( ): in original report.

RESULTS

Cases

For the present study, there were some small alterations in the cases included compared with the previous report[1]: there were a total of ten cases among the subjects of the previous study who were either ineligible or withdrawn (Table 2). It was found afterwards that, at the time of inclusion in the study, four patients had had adjuvant therapy in the form of curative or non-curative excision of tumor; there was one patient who had undergone curative excision during the trial; and five patients had taken an inadmissible drug during the period of the trial.

Table 3 Age and sex of subjects (367 cases)

	Background factor	Stomach MF treatment C* 59	Stomach MF treatment L* 74	Stomach FT treatment C 68	Stomach FT treatment L 77	Colon MF treatment C 19	Colon MF treatment L 31	Colon FT treatment C 17	Colon FT treatment L 22
Age range (years)	Up to 20	1	0	0	0	0	0	0	0
	21 to 30	1	3	1	1	1	1	1	0
	31 to 40	5	5	6	4	1	2	0	2
	41 to 50	7	8	5	12	5	3	1	2
	51 to 60	20	20	10	19	4	8	3	8
	61 to 70	18	25	23	20	4	12	9	6
	71 to 80	7	13	23	21	4	5	3	4
	Significance	$t=0.9561$		$t=1.2592$		$t=0.7202$		$t=1.0216$	
	(U-test)	$p=0.3390$		$p=0.2079$		$p=0.4714$		$p=0.3070$	
Sex	Male	44	47	50	49	10	19	10	9
	Female	15	27	18	28	9	12	7	13
	Significance	$x^2=1.3826$		$x^2=1.2069$		$x^2=0.0942$		$x^2=0.6192$	
	(x^2-test)	$p=0.2397$		$p=0.2719$		$p=0.7589$		$p=0.4314$	

*C=Control group; L=Treatment group.

Table 4 Zubrod performance status (PS) of subjects

		Stomach MF treatment C* 59	Stomach MF treatment L* 74	Stomach FT treatment C 68	Stomach FT treatment L 77	Colon MF treatment C 19	Colon MF treatment L 31	Colon FT treatment C 17	Colon FT treatment L 22
	0	2	1	4	3	2	0	1	2
	1	8	9	11	14	2	7	5	5
PS	2	24	39	20	29	7	10	7	7
	3	22	23	30	31	8	14	3	8
	4	3	2	3	0	0	0	1	0
	Significance	$t=0.5860$		$t=0.8586$		$t=0.2357$		$t=0.3998$	
	(U-test)	$p=0.5579$		$p=0.3905$		$p=0.8137$		$p=0.6893$	

*C=Control group; L=Treatment group.

Background factors

As in the previous report,[1] there was no bias in age or sex (Table 3). In addition, in relation to the Zubrod performance status of cases at the time of entry to the study, a factor which greatly affects recuperation, no bias that would affect evaluation was found (Table 4).

Treatment following conclusion of the clinical trial

Table 5 presents a summary of the drugs administered to the patients after the Phase III study had ended. The majority of patients to whom treatment was given received combinations of lentinan, mitomycin C (MMC),

Table 5 Treatment after conclusion of clinical trial

	Nature of treatment	Stomach MF		Stomach FT		Colon RF		Colon FT	
		C*	L*	C	L	C	L	C	L
	No treatment	12	4	3	15	3	8	0	1
Chemotherapy	FT			8	7	1		2	3
	5FU	2	2		1	1	1		1
	MMC+5FU	3	2			1			
	MMC+FT			1					
	MMC						1		
	Combination of above drugs,or other drugs		2	1	2	1	2	1	
	Subtotals	5	6	10	10	4	4	3	4
LNT+Chemotherapy	LNT*		4		1		1		1
	FT+LNT		2	1	13		1		2
	MF or 5FU+LNT		5		1		2		
	Combination of above drugs, or other drug+LNT		2		3		1		5
	Subtotals	0	13	1	18	0	5	0	8
Not determined		0	0	0	0	1	0	1	2
Totals		17	23	14	43	8	17	4	15

*C=Control group; L=Treatment group; LNT=Lentinan.

FT, and 5-fluorouracil (5FU); in other words, in general, they remained on the same treatment as they had been having during the trial. In addition, there was a comparatively large number of patients (five out of 12) among the colorectal cancer patients treated with FT in combination with lentinan during the trial who took drugs other than the above. There five were given OK-432 (a streptococcal preparation), PSK (a protein-bound polysaccharide from *Coriolus versicolor*) or cyclophosphamides as well as lentinan, MMC and FT.

The number of patients on whom surgery was carried out was small. Six in all, they were distributed as follows: in the stomach cancer patients treated with MF, none among the controls, but one among those given lentinan, who died on the 568th day; in the stomach cancer patients treated with FT, one among the controls, who died on the 178th day, and three among those given lentinan, who died on the 345th, 469th and 991st days; in the colorectal cancer patients treated with the MF, none among the controls, but one among those given lentinan, who died on the 179th day; and in the colorectal cancer patients treated with FT, none either in the control group or in the lentinan group. In all cases included in the present study, the operations were palliative procedures.

Testing of survival curves

Survival curves at end of the clinical trial

The survival curves to September 30, 1980, for the cases included in the present survey are shown in Figs. 1 and 2; these are compared with the previously published data in Table 6. No significant differences were found between the present curves and those from the previous study. In both analyses, significant life prolongation was observed in the groups that were treated with lentinan for stomach cancer, whether combined with MF or with FT; for colorectal cancer, lentinan prolonged survival in combination with FT.

Survival curves for the follow-up survey

The survival curves as of May 1, 1984, are shown in Figs. 3 and 4. A comparison of generalized Wilcoxon test values and of 50% survival periods at the end of the trial and the time of the survey was performed (Table 7). Significant prolongation of survival was still evident in three

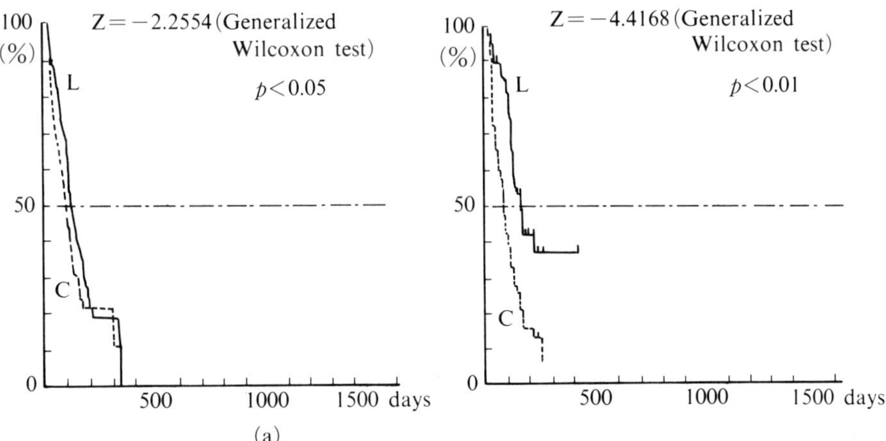

Fig. 1 Stratified survival curves of stomach cancer patients as of September 30, 1980.
(a) MF treatment; 133 cases.
C: control group (MF alone); 59 cases; 50% survival, 98 days.
L: lentinan + MF; 74 cases; 50% survival, 125 days.
(b) FT treatment; 145 cases.
C: control group (FT alone); 68 cases; 50% survival, 96 days.
L: lentinan + FT; 77 cases; 50% survival, 163 days.

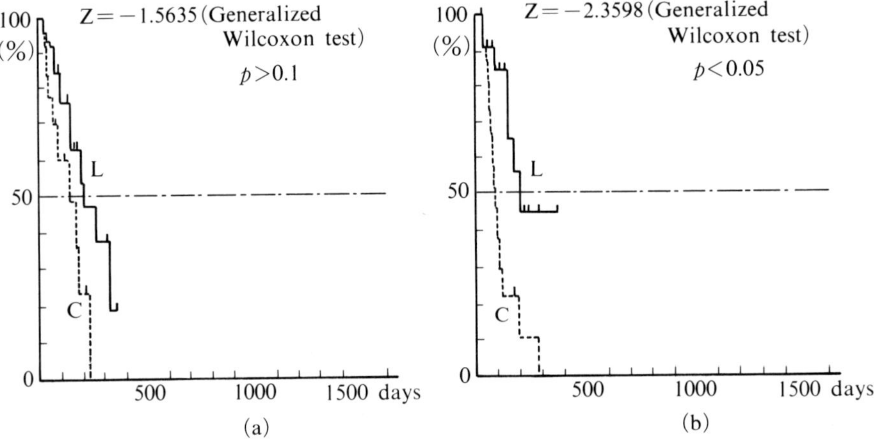

Fig. 2 Stratified survival curves of colorectal cancer patients as of September 30, 1980.
(a) MF treatment; 50 cases.
C: control group (MF alone); 19 cases; 50% survival, 147 days.
L: lentinan+MF; 31 cases; 50% survival, 209 days.
(b) FT treatment; 39 cases.
C: control group (FT alone); 17 cases; 50% survival, 94 days.
L: lentinan+FT; 22 cases; 50% survival, 200 days.

Table 6 Revision of survival curve at end of treatment period as result of alteration of study population

Site of cancer	Treatment Group	Results of present revisions			Original published values		
		Number of cases	50% survival period (days)	Statistical evaluation	Number of cases	50% survival period (days)	Statistical evaluation
Stomach	MF	59	98	$Z = -2.2554$ $p < 0.05$ (Fig 1)	60	101	$Z = -2.1985$
	MF+LNT	74	125		76	129	$p < 0.05$
	FT	68	96	$Z = -4.4168$ $p < 0.001$ (Fig 1)	72	105	$Z = -3.7771$
	FT+LNT	77	163		77	163	$p < 0.01$
Colon	MF	19	147	$Z = -1.5635$ $p > 0.1$ (Fig 2)	19	147	$Z = -1.5635$
	MF+LNT	31	209		31	209	$p > 0.1$
	FT	17	94	$Z = -2.3598$ $p < 0.05$ (Fig 2)	17	94	$Z = -2.4814$
	FT+LNT	22	200		23	200	$p < 0.05$

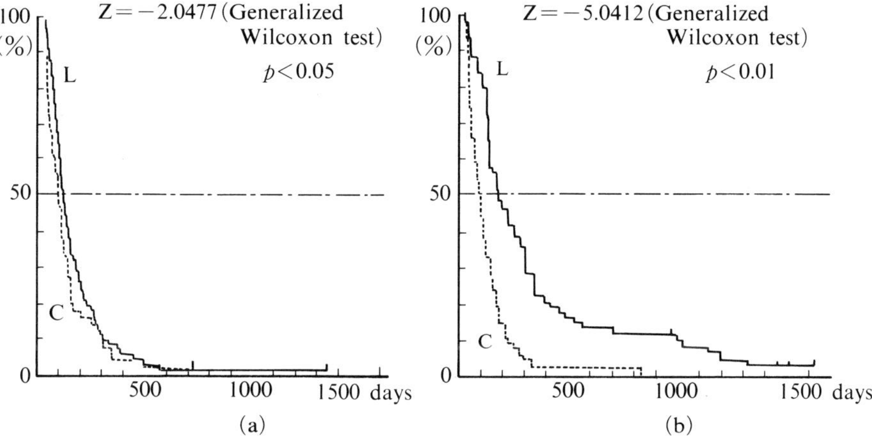

Fig. 3 Stratified survival curves of stomach cancer patients as of May 1, 1984.
(a) MF treatment; 133 cases.
C: control group (MF alone); 59 cases, 50% survival, 105 days.
L: lentinan+MF; 74 cases; 50% survival, 125 days.
(b) FT treatment; 145 cases.
C: control group; 68 cases; 50% survival, 92 days.
L: lentinan+FT; 77 cases; 50% survival, 173 days.

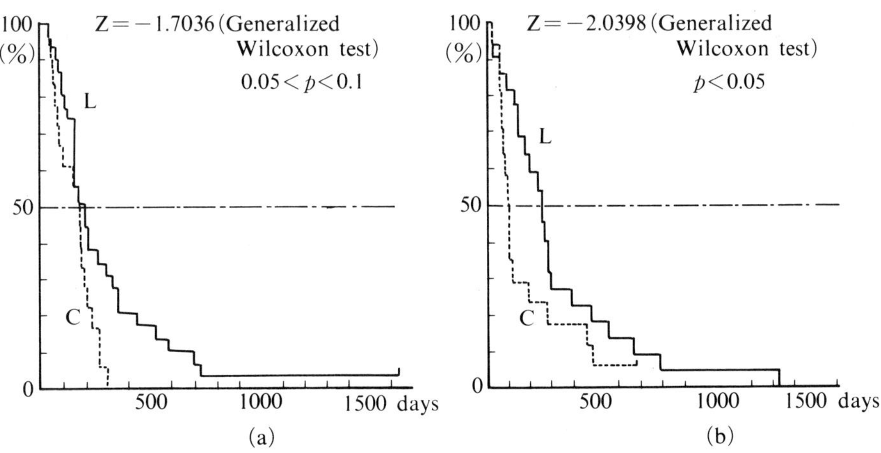

Fig. 4 Stratified survival curves of colorectal cancer patients as of May 1, 1984.
(a) MF treatment; 50 cases.
C: control group (MF alone); 19 cases; 50% survival, 175 days.
L: lentinan+MF; 31 cases; 50% survival, 199 days.
(b) FT treatment; 39 cases.
C: control group (FT alone); 17 cases; 50% survival, 98 days.
L: lentinan+FT; 22 cases; 50% survival, 250 days.

Table 7 Comparison of survival curves at May 1, 1984

Site of cancer	Treatment group	Results of follow-up, May 1, 1984.			Results at end of treatment period		
		Number of cases	50% survival period (days)	Statistical evaluation	Number of cases	50% survival period (days)	Statistical evaluation
Stomach	MF	59	105	$Z=-2.0477$ $p<0.05$ (Fig 3)	59	98	$Z=-2.2554$ $p<0.05$ (Fig 1)
	MF+LNT	74	125		74	125	
	FT	68	92	$Z=-5.0412$ $p<0.01$ (Fig 3)	68	96	$Z=-4.4168$ $p<0.01$ (Fig 1)
	FT+LNT	77	173		77	163	
Colon	MF	19	175	$Z=-1.7036$ $0.015<p<0.10$ (Fig 4)	19	147	$Z=-1.5635$ $p>0.1$ (Fig 2)
	MF+LNT	31	199		31	209	
	FT	17	98	$Z=-2.0398$ $p<0.05$ (Fig 4)	17	94	$Z=-2.3598$ $p<0.05$ (Fig 2)
	FT+LNT	22	250		22	200	

of the four groups receiving combined treatment: in the stomach cancer, lentinan plus MF-treated group ($p<0.05$), in the stomach cancer, lentinan plus FT-treated group ($p<0.01$), and in the colorectal cancer, lentinan plus FT-treated group($p<0.05$). In the other group (colorectal cancer, MF treatment), a probably significant trend in the same direction was found ($0.05<p<0.10$). The results of the follow-up survey are similar to those obtained at the end of the clinical trial (Table 7); thus, the efficacy of lentinan in prolonging life when given in combination was confirmed by this survey.

Analysis of survival rates using life-expectancy tables

Using life-expectancy tables, an analysis of cases from the initiation of the trial in August 1979 to May 1, 1984, the period covered by the present survey, was performed. The overall results of these calculations are shown in Table 8.

Table 8 shows that the survival rate for each year after the start of the trial was higher in the lentinan-treated groups than in the control groups in almost every case. This was particularly true in the stomach cancer groups treated with FT, in which administration of lentinan brought about a significantly raised survival rate. More specifically, the survival rates for each of years 1 to 4 were: 24.32% ($p<0.01$), 12.97% ($p<0.05$), 9.51% and 3.81% respectively.

An analysis of the survival rates was made by Fisher's direct method

Table 8 Comparison of survival rates based on analysis using life-expectancy tables

Site of cancer	Treat-ment	Patients surviving at Day 365 Survival rate (%)	Statistical evaluation	Patients surviving at Day 730 Survival rate (%)	Statistical evaluation	Patients surviving at Day 1095 Survival rate (%)	Statistical evaluation	Patients surviving at Day 1460 Survival rate (%)	Statistical evaluation
Stomach	MF	6.09	$p>0.1$	2.03	$p>0.1$	0	—	0	—
	MF+LNT	9.59		1.60		1.60		1.60	
	FT	3.07	$p<0.01$	3.70	$p<0.05$	0	$p<0.05$	0	—
	FT+LNT	24.32		12.97		9.51		3.81	
Colon	MF	2.70	$p<0.05$	0	—	0	—	0	—
	MF+LNT	21.31		3.55		3.55		3.55	
	FT	17.65	$p<0.1$	3.53	$p<0.1$	0	—	0	—
	FT+LNT	27.27		9.10		4.55		0	

Table 9 Comparison and statistical testing of survival rates of different treatment groups (Fisher's direct method)

Site of cancer	Treatment group	More than 1 year Survival rate	Statistical evaluation	More than 2 years Survival rate	Statistical evaluation	More than 3 years Survival rate	Statistical evaluation
Stomach	MF	2/59 (3.4%)	$p=0.30$	0/59 (0%)	$p=1.00$	0/59 (0%)	$p=1.00$
	MF+LNT	6/74 (8.1%)		1/74 (1.4%)		1/74 (1.4%)	
	FT	2/68 (2.9%)	$p<0.01$	2/68 (2.9%)	$p=0.10$	0/68 (0%)	$p=0.06$
	FT+LNT	15/77 (19.5%)		8/77 (10.4%)		5/77 (6.5%)	
Colon	MF	0/19 (0%)	$p=0.07$	0/19 (0%)	$p=1.00$	0/19 (0%)	$p=1.00$
	MF+LNT	6/31 (19.4%)		1/31 (3.2%)		1/31 (0%)	
	FT	3/17 (17.6%)	$p=0.70$	0/17 (0%)	$p=0.49$	0/17 (0%)	$p=1.00$
	FT+LNT	6/22 (27.3%)		2/22 (9.1%)		1/22 (4.5%)	

and a comparison of the results is presented in Table 9. The same trends as were found by analysis using life-expectancy tables can be seen here. Thus, the two-year survival rate from the time the trial began showed high values in the groups treated with lentinan plus FT: 10.4% for stomach and 9.1% for colorectal cancer.

Survivors at May 1, 1984

At the time of the follow-up survey, there were no survivors in the control groups, but three in the lentinan-treated groups: two in the stomach cancer, FT-treated group and one in the colorectal cancer, MT-treated group.

One of the cases in the former group was a 68-year-old woman with advanced cancer of the stomach (initial occurrence) which at the start of the trial had already metastasized to the left lobe of the liver and to the hepatic lymph nodes. Histologically, the cancer was identified as well-differentiated tubular adenocarcinoma. Since curative surgery was impossible, the patient was treated with oral FT, 600 mg daily in three divided doses, and intravenous lentinan, 1 mg twice a week. Three months of this treatment reduced the size of the solid tumor from 7.8 x 7.9 cm to 6.5 × 6.5 cm; therefore, the same treatment was maintained. When the patient's stomach was X-rayed after the conclusion of the trial on October 10, 1980, the tumor was found to have disappeared. Then, on June 15, 1981, an abdominal CT scan failed to reveal metastases either in the liver or in the hepatic lymph nodes. Subsequently, in July of the same year and again one year later, no tumor was found on endoscopic examination, and biopsies were negative for cancerous tissue. At the time of writing (July 22, 1984), she is alive and well. The amount of lentinan administered since the end of the study was 44 mg over a period of 26 months; 516.6 g of FT was given over 33 months. On May 1, 1984, the patient had survived for 1542 days since admission to the trial.

The other case in the stomach cancer, FT-treated group was a recurrent case. The patient was a 47-year-old man who had undergone curative excision of a tumor in July 1977. However, in March 1980, recurrence of the cancer was found in the abdominal wall and he was included in the trial. Histology identified a well-differentiated tubular adenocarcinoma. Treatment of this case was initiated with oral FT, 600 mg daily in three divided doses, and intravenous lentinan, 2 mg once a week.

Five months of this treatment reduced the size of the solid tumor from 2 × 2 cm to 1 × 1 cm. Combined treatment with lentinan and FT was continued until September 1980, and the total amount of lentinan given was 46 mg. After the end of the clinical trial, the patient received only FT. The tumor was found to continue its reduction in size, and by the end of December 1980 had disappeared. Thereafter no recurrence was observed and the patient's condition remained good. In April 1984, the patient was healthy and medication was withdrawn. His survival time at May 1, 1984, was 1572 days.

The third survivor was a recurrent case in the MF-plus-lentinan-treated colorectal cancer group. This patient was a 71-year-old woman who had had the right half of her colon removed together with the ileocecum on January 10, 1979, for treatment of ileocecal cancer. At laparotomy in November of that year, the patient was found to have not only a recurrent tumor at the point of surgical anastomosis, but also mesenteric metastases. Histologically the cancer was identified as tubular adenocarcinoma. When lentinan, 2 mg twice a week, and MF treatment was initiated on November 13 of the same year, the diameter of the tumor was 11 cm. By the following January, it had increased in size to 17.5 x 12.5 cm, but two months later (March 1980) the diameter had decreased to 12 cm. By May 1980 it had disappeared, and since then no tumor has reappeared. The direct efficacy on the solid tumor during the trial was rated as "partial response". The total amount of lentinan administered during the trial was 80 mg, that of MMC 80 mg and that of 5FU 10 g. Since the end of the trial, this patient has received 96 mg of lentinan (overall total, 176 mg), 128 mg of MMC (overall total, 208 mg), and 16 g of 5FU (overall total, 26 g). May 1, 1984, was the patient's 1684th day of survival and she is in good health.

DISCUSSION

In a follow-up survey of the subjects of a controlled clinical trial of lentinan, the same trend was observed in the results as in the original trial: administration of lentinan yielded significant life-prolonging effects. The groups treated with lentinan also showed high survival rates two or more years after their treatment began. Table 10 presents data from Kurihara et

Table 10 Survival times of gastric cancer patients given chemotherapy in studies of 25 or more cases conducted in Japan

Author	Year of publication	Number of cases	Type of chemotherapy	One-year survival rate (total cases)	Two-year survival rate (total cases)
Konda	1968	35	FAMT	12.3%	—
Saito	1973	4,020 (total for all of Japan)	Various	—	0.8%
Saito	1984	13,137	Various		0.8%
Murakami	1976	136	Various, combined with radiotherapy	6.6%	1.5%
Yokoyama	1978	306	Various	2%	0.6%
Kurihara	1980	105*	Various	14.3%	—
	1980	97**	Various	14.4%	—

(From: Kurihara, M., Chemotherapy of Gastric Carcinoma, p. 155)
* Subjects of the Tokyo Cancer Chemotherapy Research Association
** Koyama-Saito criteria

al.'s survey of studies of treatment of gastric cancer with chemotherapy. From their figures, it can be seen that the survival rates in the present study are high. For example, in the studies they reviewed, two-year survival rates ranged from 0.6 to 1.5%; Saito et al.[2] reported a survival rate of 0.8% in such patients in his nationwide survey of 4020 patients performed in 1971. Their report of a survey of a population of 13,137 subjects also gave the figure of 0.8%.[2] However, in the present survey, the long-term survival in stomach cancer patients treated with combined lentinan and FT were 12.97% at two years ($p<0.05$), 9.01% at three years ($p<0.05$), and 3.81% at four years. Moreover, a similar result was seen in the crude survival rate. When these figures are compared with those reported so far for chemotherapeutic agents used alone, the combined use of lentinan with such agents is shown to be useful in the treatment of cancer.

Up to the present, in ordinary clinical trials of chemotherapeutic agents against advanced and recurrent cancer of the digestive tract, the direct antitumor effect has been employed as an index of usefulness. There have been few controlled clinical studies of antitumor effect, and no reports have been published on final survival periods. In the controlled clinical study referred to in this report,[1] the antitumor effect was investigated and found to be powerful in cases where lentinan was used in combination with other chemotherapeutic agents, and a life-prolonging effect was observed with this combined treatment.

It has been recommended[3] that assessment of activators of host defense mechanisms be performed as follows: The subjects should only be patients who have undergone curative excision and the efficacy of the adjuvant treatment should be evaluated in terms of prolongation of the disease-free interval or survival. However, the results of the present investigation show that these agents can also be meaningfully studied in cases where surgery has not been performed. Given that the efficacy of combining chemotherapy with curative excision is still being studied,[4] it is in any case not yet possible to reach definitive conclusions on each of these treatments. The usefulness of activators of host defense mechanisms should be investigated in any area where chemotherapy in known to be effective. The present study is an example of the latter approach. Even in studies of advanced or recurrent cancer such as this where survival periods are short, evaluation of treatment is possible not only in terms of direct antitumor effects but also of prolongation of survival, and by conducting a long-term follow-up study. In relation to lentinan's effect of activating the defense mechanisms of the host, several detailed investigations have been performed. Reports have been published on the mechanism of action of lentinan in man by Aoki et al.,[5] and recently, Miyakoshi et al.[6,7] have contributed a dynamic analysis of conditions after the administration of lentinan. Lentinan has been shown to induce interferon production and natural killer cell activity.[6,7] In addition, Herlyn et al.[8] have confirmed that the combined administration of monoclonal antibody 17-1A (IgG 2a) and lentinan against colonic cancer in man causes marked enhancement of antibody-dependent macrophage cytotoxicity to human colonic cancer cells *in vitro*. Therefore, this combination should be investigated clinically, as a new approach to cancer treatment.

Since lentinan is a host defense mechanism activator, it deserves further clinical investigation, particularly in the treatment of other solid tumors, leukemias and infectious diseases, both viral and bacterial.

REFERENCES

1. Furue, H., Ito, I., Kimura, T., Kondoh, T., Hattori, T., Ogawa, N. and Taguchi, T. (1981): Phase III Study on Lentinan. *Jpn. J. Cancer Chemother., 8,* 944.
2. Saito, T., Yokoyama, M. and Nakao, I. (1984): Results on life prolongation by cancer chemotherapy : comparison of the results of two surveys carried out seven years apart. Sci. Rep. Res. Inst. Tohoku Univ. Series C (Medicine), *The Report of the Research Institute for Tuberculosis and Cancer, 31*, 42.
3. Sakurai, Y. (1980): Method and evaluation of studies of immunological cancer drugs. *Jpn. J. Cancer Chemother., 7*, 1725.
4. Moertel, C.G. and Gastrointestinal Tumor Study Group (1984): Adjuvant therapy of colon cancer - Results of a prospectively randomized trial. *N. Engl. J. Med., 310,* 737.
5. Aoki, T., Urushizaki, I., Miyakoshi, H. and Ishitani, K. (1981): Enhancement of host immune response and removal of immunosuppressive substance by using augmenting agents. In: *Prospects of Manipulation of Host-Tumor Relationship.* Editors: J.C. Salmon and L. Israël. INSERM, Paris.
6. Miyakoshi, H. and Aoki, T. (1984): Acting mechanisms of lentinan in human-I. Augmentation of DNA synthesis and immunoglobulin production of peripheral mononuclear cells. *Int. J. Immunopharm., 6*, 365.
7. Miyakoshi, H., Aoki, T. and Mizukoshi, M. (1984): Acting mechanisms of lentinan in human-II. Enhancement of non-specific cell-mediated cytotoxicity as an interferon inducer. *Int. J. Immunopharm.,* 6, 373.
8. Herlyn, D., Kaneko, Y., Powe, J., Aoki, T. and Koprowski, H. (1985): Monoclonal antibody dependent murine macrophage mediated cytotoxicity against human tumors is stimulated by lentinan. *Gann, 76*, 37.

Footnote Institutions participating in the follow-up study

Name of Institution and Group	Leader
First Internal Medicine Group, Sapporo Medical College	Akira Yachi, Katsumi Sato
Fourth Internal Medicine Group, Sapporo Medical College	Ichiro Urushizaki, Jun Ibayashi
First Department of Surgery, Sapporo Medical College	Hiroshi Hayasaka
First Surgery Group, Hokkaido University	Yoichi Kasai
Second Surgery Group, Hokkaido University	Toshio Isomatsu
Internal Medicine Group, National Sapporo Hospital	Fumio Nagahama
First Surgery Group, Hirosaki University	Hisaaki Koie
Second Surgery Group, Tohoku University	Morio Kasai
The Research Institute for Tuberculosis and Cancer, Tohoku University	Akira Wakui
Surgery Group, National Sendai Hospital	Kaneo Kikuchi
Second Surgery Group, Gunma University	Masaru Izumio
Department of Internal Medicine, Saitama Prefectural Hospital	Seiichi Yoshida, Koichi Futatsuki
Surgery Group, Keio University,	Osahiko Abe, Kyuya Ishibiki
Second Department of Surgery, Teikyo University	Hisashi Furue
Departmant of Internal Medicine, National Medical Center	Noritsugu Umeda
Departmant of Surgery, Hiratsuka Municipal Hospital	Akahito Aoki
Department of Internal Medicine, Chigasaki Municipal Hospital	Kijuto Nomura
Second Surgery Group, Nagoya University	Tatsuhei Kondo, Hideo Kamei
First Department of Surgery, Mie University	Ryuji Mizumoto
Department of Surgery, Wakayama Medical College	Masaharu Katsumi
First Department of Surgery, Shinshu University	Shiro Hayashi
First Internal Medicine Group, Kanazawa University	Nobu Hattori
Second Surgery Group, Kanazawa University	Itsuo Miyazaki, Koichi Miwa
Department of Surgery, National Kyoto Hospital	Toru Yasutomi
First Surgery Group, Osaka University	Kazuyasu Nakao
Second Surgery Group, Osaka City University	Katsuji Sakai
Osaka Cancer Chemotherapy Research Association Group	Tetsuo Taguchi
Department of Internal Medicine, The Center for Adult Diseases, Osaka	Shigeru Okuda
Fourth Departmant of Internal Medicine, Hyogo Medical College	Takashi Shimoyama
First Surgery Group, Okayama University	Kunzo Orita
Surgery Group, National Kyushu Cancer Center	Motonosuke Furusawa
Second Departmant of Surgery, Kumamoto University	Masanobu Akagi

Lentinan treatment of Japanese cases infected with human T-lymphotropic retroviruses (HTLV-I and -III)

Tadao Aoki, Hideo Miyakoshi, Yoshimaru Usuda, Robert C. Y. Ting and Robert C. Gallo

SUMMARY

Although the presence in Japan of patients with acquired immunodeficiency syndrome (AIDS) or patients with signs or symptoms which precede AIDS (pre-AIDS) was not recognized by many Japanese medical doctors, antibody to human T-lymphotropic retrovirus type 3 (HTLV-III) or lymphadenopathy virus (LAV) was detected in the serum of a 57-year-old female with operated mammary carcinoma. This Case 1 did not show the typical clinical course of AIDS or pre-AIDS, but antibodies to HTLV-I and -III in serum, and HTLV-I p24 antigen in short-term cultured peripheral blood lymphocytes (PBL) were found and dysfunction of or a decrease in the number of helper T-lymphocytes ($OKT4^{+}$) appeared. The Case 2, a 42 year-old-male, suffered from high fever for over one month, diarrhea, and lymphadenopathy associated with marked leukopenia, especially a decrease in $OKT4^{+}$ lymphocytes, and thrombopenia. Antibodies to HTLV-I and HTLV-I p24 antigen were detected in serum and short-term cultured PBL of this patient, respectively. These findings provide evidence for the existence in Japan of HTLV-III and pre-AIDS. These HTLV antibodies and antigens disappeared by the injection of a biological response modifier, lentinan.

INTRODUCTION

There is at present disagreement over the presence in Japan of patients with acquired immunodeficiency syndrome (AIDS) or who show signs or symptoms which typically precede AIDS (pre-AIDS), even though one Japanese patient suspected to have AIDS was reported.[1,2] Some are suspicious of such presence, while others deny it. Such denials have come despite the existence of patients with adult T-cell leukemia (ATL), which has been proven to be caused by human T-lymphotropic retrovirus type 1 (HTLV-I).[3–6] Afterwards, an additional subgroup of HTLV was isolated from human hairy-cell leukemia, called HTLV type 2 (HTLV-II).[7] These two subgroups of HTLV mainly relate to the etiology of T-cell leukemia or lymphoma. In addition, the isolation of a novel retrovirus subgroup HTLV type 3 (HTLV-III),[8–11] or what is identically the same, lymphadenopathy virus (LAV),[12] from lymphocytes of AIDS patients, and the establishment of HTLV-III-producing cell lines, make it easy to diagnose AIDS or pre-AIDS and carriers of this retrovirus. Accordingly, this HTLV-III has been well characterized and frequently isolated from patients with AIDS or pre-AIDS and from people at risk of AIDS. However, these three subgroups of HTLV belong to one retrovirus family (HTLV), and HTLV-I also has been considered to be a causative virus of AIDS and pre-AIDS in addition to ATL.[13]

Recently, we have found two Japanese cases which showed absolute lymphopenia and reduced subpopulation of helper T-lymphocytes ($OKT4^+$) and which were etiologically related to HTLV. The treatment of these cases with a biological response modifier, lentinan, seemed to affect their immunosuppressed status.

PATIENTS AND METHODS

Two patients were admitted to Shinrakuen Hospital, Niigata, Japan, in January, 1984. Both have no history of promiscuity, homosexuality, or intravenous drug abuse. Besides regular clinical and laboratory examinations, the investigations of blood features and lymphocyte functions such as the DNA synthesis, natural killer (NK) activity, $OKT4^+$ lymphocyte population, $OKT4^+/OKT8^+$ ratio, antibodies to HTLV-I and -III, interferon (IFN) titers, etc., were periodically conducted.

The DNA synthesis in peripheral blood lymphocytes (PBL), which were collected from heparinized venous blood by the Ficoll-Conray method, was measured as follows: these PBL were cultured with phytohemagglutinin P (PHA, Difco Laboratories, Detroit, Mich) for 72 hours and with Staphage Lysate (SPL stimulates both B cells and T cells; Delmont Laboratories, Swarthmore, Pa)[14] or concanavalin A (Con A, Pharmacia Fine Chemicals AB, Uppsala, Sweden) for 120 hours. Then, the incorporation of tritiated methyl thymidine (^3H-TdR) was measured with a liquid scintillation spectrometer.

For the NK activity assay of PBL, an established human myeloid cell line K562 was used as target cells to measure the ^{51}Cr release from these cells after incubation at 37°C for 6 hours at the mixture ratio of target cells to attacker cells of 1:20.

The titers of antibodies to HTLV-I and -III were measured by indirect immunofluorescence microscopy (IFM) and/or enzyme-linked immunosorbent assay (ELISA) using acetone-fixed HTLV-producing cells and purified HTLV.[17] For these tests, sera from French and American AIDS patients and from Japanese ATL patients were used as positive controls, and sera from healthy donors were used as negative controls.

One milligram of lentinan (Ajinomoto Co., Inc., Tokyo), which is a glucan extracted from the mushroom, *Lentinus edodes*,[15,16] was drip-infused intravenously in solution with, e.g., saline, glucose solution, and multiple vitamin solution.

International units of IFN were measured by the original method using cytopathic effects of vesicular stomatitis virus on FL cells.

RESULTS

Case 1

This is a 57-year-old female who had been surgically treated for right mammary carcinoma III on November 7, 1983, in another hospital. During this surgical operation, she was transfused with whole blood and injected with mitomycin C and 5FU. After the operation, radiation-therapy was achieved with cobalt for one month. Since these conventional cancer therapies progressively weakened the patient, she was admitted to our hospital on January 4, 1984, for the nonspecific immunotherapy with biological response modifiers. At that time, although no clinical symptoms suggesting AIDS or pre-AIDS (Table 1) were observed, the white blood cell count was 3,100/mm^3 including 35% lymphocytes with no changes in the red blood cell (RBC) count, total serum protein and its fractions (Table 2). Antibodies to HTLV-I and -III in serum were detected by IFM and/or ELISA (Fig. 1). HTLV-I p24 antigen in short-term cultured PHA-stimulated PBL was detected on acetone-fixed cells by IFM using goat hyperimmune serum to HTLV-I p24. The OKT4$^+$/OKT8$^+$ ratio of PBL was 0.92 and gradually decreased to 0.37 by May 22, 1984, and the mitogen-induced DNA syntheses of PBL also dropped in spite of lentinan administration (Fig. 1).
However, lentinan administration did improve general conditions, and NK activity was increased to normal (Fig. 1). It is difficult to judge whether this case is only a carrier of HTLV-I and -III or possessed signs

Table 1 Clinical signs

	Case 1 (57-year-old female)		Case 2 (42-year-old male)	
	Lentinan administration		Lentinan administration	
	Before (Jan. 5, 1984)	After (May 22, 1984)	Before (Jan. 27, 1984)	After (Apr. 3, 1984)
Fever	(−)	(−)	38C°−40C°	36.8C°−37.3C°
Lymphadenopathy	(−)	(−)	(++)	(−)
Diarrhea	(−)	(−)	(+)	(−)
Skin lesions	(−)	(−)	(−)	(−)
Complications	Mammary carcinoma		Pulmonary tuberculosis	

Table 2 Laboratory findings except for WBC system

Items tested	Case. 1 (57-year-old female)		Case 2 (42-year-old male)	
	Lentinan administration		Lentinan administration	
	Before (Jan. 5, 1984)	After (May 22, 1984)	Before (Jan. 27, 1984)	After (Apr. 3, 1984)
RBC ($\times 10^4$/mm^3)	364	418	394	388
Hematocrit (%)	33.5	37.0	35.0	34.5
Platelets ($\times 10^4$/mm^3)	11.1	26.9	6.0	18.0
CRP test	−	−	+	−
Total serum protein (g/dl)	6.7	7.4	6.3	7.1
Protein fractions (%)				
Albumin	57.5	57.8	60.6	60.5
Globulin $\alpha 1$	3.4	3.6	3.3	3.6
$\alpha 2$	8.4	8.4	8.2	7.0
β	10.1	11.5	9.0	10.5
γ	20.2	18.4	18.7	18.2
Albumin/Globulin	1.35	1.37	1.53	1.53

of pre-AIDS. These antibodies and the HTLV-I p24 antigen disappeared from serum and PBL by lentinan administration, even though IFN has not become detectable in serum. Since this patient received blood transfusion during the surgical operation mentioned above, HTLV-I and -III may have been transmitted from the blood donors.

Case 2

This patient is a 42-year-old male, married, and has two children. He was born in Sado Island, Niigata Prefecture, which is an HTLV-I endemic area.[17] His father and wife also possess antibody to HTLV-I at the titers 1:5 and 1:10 respectively by IFM. Since the end of December 1983, the patient had suffered from high fever, 38°C to 40°C, of unknown origin, several swollen lymph-nodes (1 cm in diameter) in the right neck and the left inguinal region, and from unexplained diarrhea, which had persisted for more than one month (Table 1). He was admitted to our hospital on

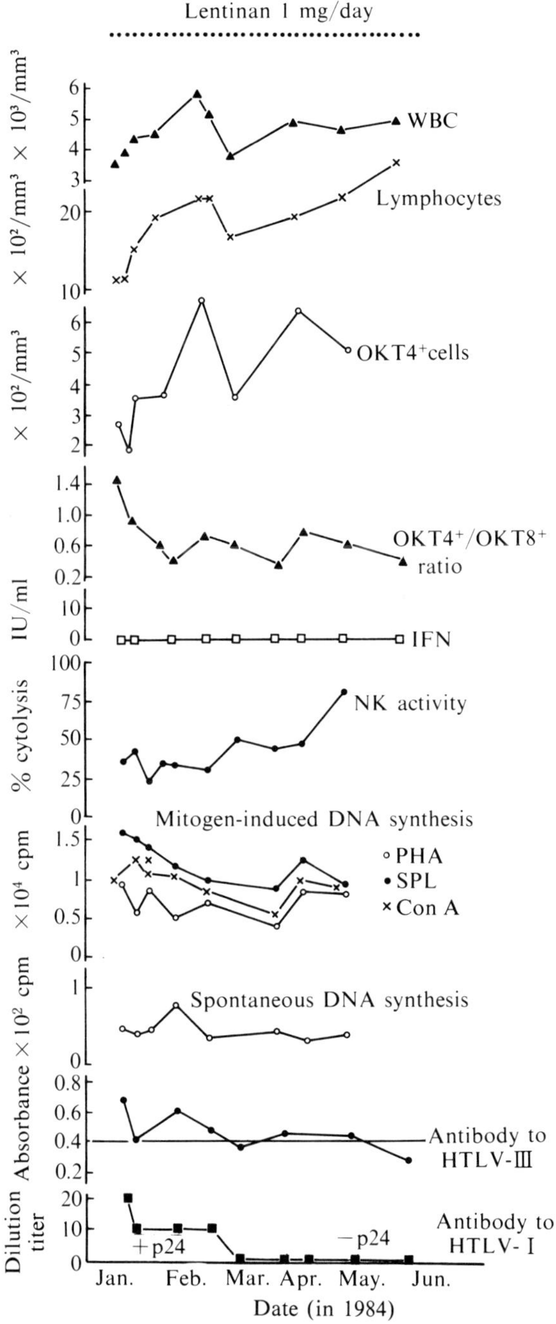

Fig. 1 Changes in immune status of Case 1. +24, 21% positive MT-2 cells by IFM with goat anti-HTLV-I p24 serum; and −p24, 0% positive cells.

January 26, 1984, without a conclusive diagnosis. In addition to the above clinical signs, the characteristic clinical findings (Table 2 and Fig. 2) were leukopenia involving helper T-lymphocytes ($OKT4^+$), $OKT4^+/OKT8^+$ ratio 0.73, thrombopenia, CRP test (+), and NK activity. At this time, his serum contained antibodies to HTLV-I-related antigens at the titer 1:20 according to by IFM. However, this was not supported by ELISA. HTLV-I p24 antigen was also detected in short-term cultured PBL. No other abnormal clinical findings such as anemia, hypoglobulinemia (Table 2), or abnormal shadows on the X-ray photograph of the chest, were found except for slight acceleration of erythrocyte sedimentation rate (ESR) to 17 mm/hr. For one week after the admission, high fever continued despite a temporary suppression by administration of an antipyretic. One milligram per day of lentinan was drip-infused intravenously twice a week as an IFN inducer. Simultaneously, 2,500 mg/day of serum immunoglobulin preparation (Glovenin, Takeda Chemical Industries, Ltd., and Nihon Seiyaku Co., Ltd., Osaka, Japan) were daily drip-infused intravenously for one week. During these treatments, high fever had gradually decreased to 37.5°C, but not completely to normal. For the next week, only lentinan injections were performed, and the fever fluctuated between 37.1°C and 37.5°C. However, leukopenia, lymphopenia, $OKT4^+/OKT8^+$ ratio, thrombopenia, CRP test, ESR, and NK activity had improved to some extent. After daily drip-infusion of Glovenin during the following week, these clinical indicators further improved, as described in Table 2 and Fig. 2. Again, antibody to HTLV-I as well as HTLV-I p24 antigen disappeared from serum and PBL. Just before and after the initiation of lentinan injections, IFN appeared very quickly in the peripheral blood circulation and gradually dropped beyond detectability. Finally, since the body temperature dropped to between 36.8°C and 37.3°C, the patient was discharged under the continuous treatment with lentinan as an outpatient.

During this whole clinical course, absolutely no trace of HTLV-III antibody was detected by ELISA. However, pre-AIDS was diagnosed according to the above clinical and laboratory findings.

Early in the beginning of May 1984, high fever of between 38°C and 39°C reappeared, and so the patient was again admitted. After the second admission, slight leukocytosis (WBC, 8,600/mm^3), acceleration of ESR to 36 mm/h and CRP test (++) were detected. An inflammatory shadow appeared suddenly on the upper area of the left lung on X-ray photograph, and spread rapidly. Since *Mycobacterium tuberculosis* was found in sputum, pulmonary tuberculosis was diagnosed with certainty. The clinical course has readily improved by anti-tuberculosis drug administration.

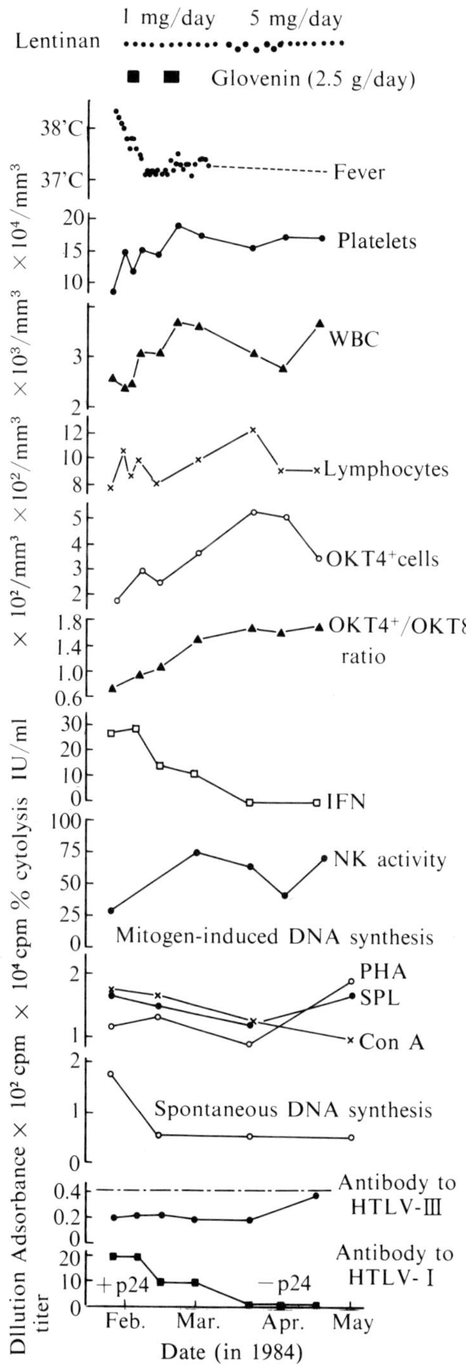

Fig. 2 Changes in immune status of Case 2. +p24, 34% of positive MT-2 cells by IFM with goat anti-HTLV-I p24 serum; and −p24: 0% positive cells.

DISCUSSION

The existence of patients with AIDS or pre-AIDS in Japan has not been officially recognized by Japanese physicians since the initial report of AIDS as a separate disease entity in 1981. Now, the presence of HTLV-III, or LAV, in Japan became evident by the detection of antibodies to HTLV-III and LAV in serum of Case 1. In Case 2, although antibody to HTLV-I and HTLV-I p24 antigen were detected instead of antibody to HTLV-III, it does not seem deniable that HTLV-I may be a causal factor of pre-AIDS or AIDS.[13] At least it is certain that HTLV-III exists in Japan as observed Case 1. So far, the Japanese patients with AIDS or pre-AIDS may have been missed because of lack of definite diagnostic criteria. Presently the conclusive diagnosis of these patients has become achievable by the detection of antibody to HTLV-III, its antigens or retrovirus itself. In addition, the carriers of HTLV also are easily detected by screening antibodies to HTLV.

Based on the clinical signs and the clinical course, particularly dysfunction of helper T-lymphocytes $OKT4^+$, Case 2 indicated a characteristic features of pre-AIDS. In terms of pulmonary tuberculosis in this patient, *M. tuberculosis* might have infected him in a latent form during this pre-AIDS stage, and its clinical manifestation took place afterwards. The clinical development of pulmonary tuberculosis was abrupt and rapidly advanced due to the immunodeficiency. However, its improvement also has been quite dramatic due to the relative recovery from the immunosuppressed status.

The retrovirus infection in Case 2 native in HTLV-I endemic area, Sado Island, would be vertically and/or horizontally derived from his father who was also born in Sado Island and positive for HTLV-I antibody in the serum. In contrast, the retrovirus in Case 1 has an uncertain origin; perhaps the source is the patient's husband, who might have been infected during a stay in Kyushu, well known to be the most HTLV-I endemic area in Japan.[18–20] Due to the long interval since the divorce of the patient and her husband, however, serum of the ex-husband was unable to be studied. Nevertheless, the coventional chemotherapy and radiation therapy may have suppressed the host immunity to the extent that HTLV-I and -III was activated to decrease further the $OKT4^+/OKT8^+$ ratio of her lymphocytes. Alternatively, the lowered immunity perhaps was induced by a prolonged HTLV infection. During this period, the mammary carcinoma might have been caused by some other oncogenic factor(s). In any case, it is of great interest that both patients related in some way to HTLV-I endemic areas in Japan.

The administration of lentinan eliminated antibodies to HTLV-I and/or -III and HTLV-I p24 antigen from sera and PBL of both patients. This seems to be an effective treatment for patients with AIDS or pre-AIDS or for HTLV-carriers. The acting mechanisms of lentinan[21-23] appear to affect the general conditions of these patients as well as their immunosuppressed status. However, the efficacy of lentinan should be decided by long-term observation of many patients or HTLV carriers.

In addition to lentinan, immunoglobulin was injected intravenously into Case 2, resulting in an increase in white blood cell count, particularly lymphocytes, and blood platelets. Therefore, it may be also important to study a role of immunoglobulin treatment in therapeutic effects on HTLV-infected patients.

ACKNOWLEDGEMENT

The authors thank Miss H. Abe for her excellent preparation of the manuscript.

ADDENDUM

The essence of this paper has been described in the *Lancet*: Aoki, T., Miyakoshi, H., Usuda, Y., Chermann, Jean-Claude, Barré-Sinoussi, F., Ting, R.C. and Gallo, R.C. (1984): Antibodies to HTLV-I and -III in sera from two Japanese patients, one with possible pre-AIDS. *Lancet ii*, 936-937.

REFERENCES

1. Miyoshi, I., Kobayashi, M., Yoshimoto, S., Fujishita, M., Taguchi, H., Kubonishi, I. and Ohtsuki, Y. (1983): ATLV in Japanese patient with AIDS. *Lancet*, *ii*, 275.
2. Kobayashi, M., Yoshimoto, S., Fujishita, M., Yano, S., Niiya, K., Kubonishi, I., Taguchi, H. and Miyoshi, I. (1984): HTLV-positive T-cell lymphoma/leukemia in an AIDS patient. *Lancet*, *i*, 1361.
3. Poiesz, B. J., Ruscetti, F. W., Gazdar, A. F., Bunn, P.A., Minna, J.D. and Gallo, R.C. (1980): Detection and isolation of type C retrovirus particles from fresh and cultured lymphocytes of a patient with cutaneous T-cell lymphoma. *Proc. Natl. Acad. Sci. U.S.A.*, *77*, 7415.
4. Poiesz, B.J., Ruscetti, F.W., Reitz, M. S., Kalyanaraman, V.S. and Gallo, R.C. (1981): Isolation of a new type C retrovirus (HTLV) in primary uncultured cells of a patient with Sézary T-cell leukemia. *Nature*, *294*, 268.
5. Hinuma, Y., Nagata, K., Hanaoka, M., Nakai, M., Matsumoto, T., Kinoshita, K., Shirakawa, S. and Miyoshi, I. (1981): Adult T-cell leukemia: Antigen in an ATL cell line and detection of antibodies to the antigen in human sera. *Proc. Natl. Acad. Sci. U.S.A.*, *78*, 6476.
6. Yoshida, M., Miyoshi, I. and Hinuma, Y. (1982): Isolation and characterization of retrovirus from cell lines of human adult T-cell leukemia and its implication in the disease. *Proc. Natl. Acad. Sci. U.S.A.*, *79*, 2031.

7. Kalyanaraman, V.S., Sarngadharan, M.G., Robert-Guroff, M., Miyoshi, I., Blayney, D., Golde, D. and Gallo, R.C. (1982): A new subtype of human T-cell leukemia virus (HTLV-II) associated with a T-cell variant of hairy cell leukemia. *Science, 218*, 571.
8. Popovic, M., Sarngadharan, M.G., Read, E. and Gallo, R.C. (1984): Detection, isolation, and continuous production of cytopathic retrovirus (HTLV-III) from patients with AIDS and pre-AIDS. *Science, 224*, 497.
9. Gallo, R.C., Salahuddin, S.Z., Popovic, M., Shearer, G.M., Kaplan, M., Haynes, B.F., Palker, T.J., Redfield, R., Oleske, J., Safai, B., White, G., Foster, P. and Markham, P.D. (1984): Frequent detection and isolation of cytopathic retroviruses (HTLV-III) from patients with AIDS and at risk for AIDS. *Science, 224*, 500.
10. Schüpbach, J., Popovic, M., Gilden, R. V., Gonda, M.A., Sarngadharan, M.G. and Gallo, R.C. (1984): Serological analysis of a subgroup of human T-lymphotropic retrovirus (HTLV-III) associated with AIDS. *Science, 224*, 503.
11. Sarngadharan, M.G., Popovic, M., Bruch, L., Schüpbach, J. and Gallo, R.C. (1984): Antibodies reactive with human T-lymphotropic retroviruses (HTLV-III) in the serum of patients with AIDS. *Science, 224*, 506.
12. Barrē-Sinoussi, F., Chermann, J.C., Rey, F., Nugeyre, M.T., Chamaret, S., Gruest, J., Dauguest, C., Axler-Blin, C., Vēnzinet-Brun, F., Rouzioux, C., Rozenbaum, W. and Montagnier, L. (1983): Isolation of a T-lymphotropic retrovirus from a patient at risk for acquired immune deficiency syndrome (AIDS). *Science, 220*, 868.
13. Gallo, R.C., Sarin, P.S., Gelmann, E.P., Robert-Guroff, M., Richardson, E., Kalyanaraman, V.S., Mann, D., Sidhu, G.D., Stahl, R.E., Zolla-Pazner, S., Leibowitch, J. and Popovic, M. (1983): Isolation of human T-cell leukemia virus in acquired immune deficiency syndrome (AIDS). *Science, 220*, 865.
14. Miyakoshi, H., Aoki, T. and Mizukoshi, M. (1981): Mitogenic substances in staphage lysate. *Biomed. Res., 2*, 629.
15. Chihara, G., Maeda, Y., Hamuro, J., Sasaki, T. and Fukuoka, F. (1969): Inhibition of mouse sarcoma 180 by polysaccharides from *Lentinus edodes* (Berk.) Sing. *Nature, 222*, 687.
16. Chihara, G., Hamuro, J., Maeda, Y. Y., Arai, Y. and Fukuoka, F. (1970): Fractionation and purification of the polysaccharides with marked anti-tumor activity, especially Lentinan, from *Lentinus edodes* (Berk.) Sing. (an edible mushroom). *Cancer Res., 30*, 2776.
17. Aoki, T., Miyakoshi, H., Koide, H., Yoshida, T., Ishikawa, H., Sugisaki, Y., Mizukoshi, M., Tamura, K., Misawa, H., Hamada, C., Ting, R.C., Robert-Guroff, M. and Gallo, R.C. (1985): Seroepidemiology of human T-lymphotropic retrovirus type 1 (HTLV-I) in residents of Niigata Prefecture, Japan–Comparative studies by indirect immunofluorescence microscopy and enzyme-linked immunosorbent assay-. *Int. J. Cancer*, *35*, 301.
18. Hinuma, Y., Komoda, H., Chosa, T., Kondo, T., Kohakura, M., Takenaka, T., Kikuchi, M., Yunoki, K., Sato, I., Matsuo, R., Takiuchi, Y., Uchino, H. and Hanaoka, M. (1982): Antibodies to adult T-cell leukemia associated antigen (ATLA) in sera from patients with ATL and controls in Japan: a nation-wide seroepidemiologic study. *Int. J. Cancer, 29*, 631.
19. Tajima, K., Tominaga, S., Suchi, T., Kawagoe, T., Komoda, H., Hinuma, Y., Oda, T. and Fujita, K. (1982): Epidemiological analysis of the distribution of antibody to adult T-cell leukemia-virus-associated antigen: possible horizontal transmission of adult T-cell leukemia virus. *Gann, 73*, 893.

20. Maeda, Y., Furukawa, M., Takehara, Y., Yoshimura, K., Miyamoto, K., Matsuura, T., Morishima, Y., Tajima, K., Okochi, K. and Hinuma, Y. (1984): Prevalence of possible adult T-cell leukemia virus-carriers among volunteer blood donors in Japan: a nation-wide study. *Int. J. Cancer, 33*, 717.
21. Aoki, T., Miyakoshi, H., Horikawa, Y., Shibata, A., Aoyagi, Y. and Mizukoshi, M. (1982): Interaction between interferon and natural killer cells in human after administration of immunomodulating agents. In: *NK Cells and Other Effector Cells*, p 1297. Editor: R.B. Herberman. Academic Press, New York.
22. Miyakoshi, H., Aoki, T. and Mizukoshi, M. (1984): Acting mechanisms of Lentinan in human-II. Enhancement of non-specific cell-mediated cytotoxicity as an interferon inducer. *Int. J. Immunopharum., 6*, 373.
23. Aoki, T. (1984): Lentinan. In: *Immune Modulation Agents and Their Mechanisms*, p 63. Editors: R.L. Fenichel and M.A. Chirigos. Marcel Dekker, Inc., New York.

The UV-irradiated mouse as a model for testing biological response modifiers

Margaret L. Kripke

SUMMARY

In addition to inducing primary cancers of the skin, ultraviolet (UV) radiation produces specific impairments in the immune system that contribute to the growth and pathogenesis of these skin cancers. The cellular basis for the immunological alterations induced in mice by UV radiation has been studied and characterized over the past ten years. It is now possible to make use of this system to study the activity and mode of action of biological response modifiers. The advantages of this system are that it employs primary hosts, which may respond quite differently from normal animals bearing a transplanted tumor, it closely parallels several specific situations relevant to human cancer, and it may be useful in establishing the mechanism of action of certain agents. Studies in which biological response modifiers have been used in conjunction with the UV carcinogenesis model are reviewed.

INTRODUCTION

It has been known for many years that ultraviolet (UV) radiation induces skin cancers in humans and in laboratory animals.[1] In addition to its carcinogenic activity, UV irradiation of mice also interferes with host defense mechanisms in a manner that contributes to skin cancer development.[2] Over the past ten years, the effects of UV radiation on host immunity, and in particular on the host response to skin cancers, has been extensively studied and characterized. Because much is known about the mechanisms by which UV radiation modifies host immunity, the UV carcinogenesis system in mice provides an excellent model for studying the mode of action of biological response modifiers (BRMs). In addition, because this system employs the primary host, it has many more parallels to the situations encountered with human cancer than do systems involving tumors transplanted into normal animals.

Interest in the immunological aspects of UV carcinogenesis stemmed from studies on the antigenicity of UV-induced skin cancers of mice. Many of these tumors are so antigenic that they are immunologically rejected upon transplantation to normal, syngeneic recipients.[3] This observation raised the intriguing question of how these tumors could escape immunological destruction during their development in the primary host. Studies addressing this question revealed that a brief series of exposures to UV radiation produced a systemic alteration in mice that left them unable to reject highly antigenic, UV-induced skin cancers.[4] This impairment not only prevented the rejection of tumors transplanted subcutaneously,[4] but also interfered with host resistance to pulmonary metastases[5] and to primary skin cancers.[6] The specificity of the systemic alteration is restricted in that immune responses to many other antigens are unaffected.[2] Analysis of the alteration indicated that it is mediated, at least partially, by suppressor T lymphocytes.[7–9] UV-irradiated mice have suppressor cells in their spleen and lymph nodes that prevent the induction of an immune response against developing UV-induced tumors.[6]

Having established that there is an important immunological component to the induction of skin cancers by UV radiation, we can ask whether BRMs can be used in the prevention or treatment of skin cancers. Specific questions of interest are the following: 1) Can treatment of UV-irradiated mice with BRMs increase their resistance to the growth and metastasis of transplanted skin cancers? 2) Will the treatment of mice with BRMs during UV carcinogenesis reduce the incidence of primary skin cancers? 3) Can treatment of UV-irradiated mice with BRMs activate macrophages to kill UV-induced tumors? 4) Can the induction of suppressor T cells by UV irradiation be prevented by administration of BRMs? In this paper, studies relevant to these questions are reviewed.

MATERIALS AND METHODS

Mice

Specific-pathogen-free mice of the inbred strain C3H/HeN (MTV^-) were supplied by the Animal Production Area of the NCI-Frederick Cancer Research Facility.

UV-irradiation

The UV radiation source was a bank of six Westinghouse FS40 sunlamps, which delivered an average dose rate of approximately 2.8 $J/m^2/sec$, over the wavelength range 280-340 nm. This range includes approximately 80% of the total energy output of the lamps. The mice were housed five per cage on a shelf 20 cm below the bulbs, and the cage order was systematically rotated to compensate for the uneven lamp output along the shelf. The dorsal fur of the animals was removed with electric clippers once per week. For chronic irradiation, 8- to 12-week old mice were exposed to UV radiation for one hour, three times per week. For acute irradiation, the animals were placed in individual compartments and given a single exposure to UV radiation for three hours.

UV tumors

Fibrosarcomas induced by the chronic UV irradiation protocol described above were used in these studies.[10] They were maintained in cell culture as described previously.[11]

Collection of mouse macrophages

Peritoneal exudate cells (PEC) were induced by an intraperitoneal injection of 3 ml thioglycolate. After five days, PEC were collected aseptically by washing the peritoneal cavity with Hanks' balanced salt solution (HBSS) containing 5 U heparin/ml. The PEC were washed; resuspended in Eagle's minimal essential medium containing 10% fetal bovine serum, 100 U penicillin/ml, 100 μg streptomycin/ml, 2 mM glutamine, sodium bicarbonate, and 5 mM HEPES buffer (complete minimal essential medium, CMEM); and plated in 60-mm culture dishes at a concentration of 1×10^5 or 1×10^6 cells per dish. Alveolar macrophages were collected by tracheobronchial lavage and plated in CMEM at a concentration of 1×10^5 cells per well of a microtest II plate.[12] After 30 to 40 minutes, the macrophage monolayers were washed to remove non-adherent cells.

In vitro activation of PEC

PEC monolayers were incubated with rat macrophage activating factor (MAF) for 48 hours or with 20 μg/ml of lipopolysaccharide (LPS) for 24 hours prior to the addition of target cells. MAF was prepared as described by Norbury et al.[13]

Cytotoxicity assay

Target tumor cells were labeled for 24 hours with either ^{125}I-iododeoxyuridine or ^{3}H-thymidine. After extensive washing, the cells were added to macrophage monolayers. Twenty-four hours later, the cultures were washed to remove non-adherent cells. The cultures were washed and the remaining cells were lysed with NaOH after five days of incubation for PEC or three days of incubation for alveolar macrophages. The residual radioactivity was measured, and the per cent cytotoxicity was calculated from the formula: per cent cytotoxicity = [(cpm of target cells with normal macrophages minus cpm of target cells with activated macrophages) ÷ cpm of target cells with normal macrophages] × 100.

BRM treatments

Pyran copolymer (NSC 46015) was obtained from the Cancer Chemotherapy National Service Center, Bethesda, Md. It was diluted in sterile, pyrogen-free saline to a concentration of 1 mg/ml immediately before use. Mice were injected with 0.5 ml of the solution every other week for the duration of the experiment. Muramyl dipeptide (MDP)-liposomes were injected intravenously in a volume of 0.2 ml. The liposomes were multilamellar vesicles composed of phosphatidylcholine and phosphatidylserine at a 7:3 molar ratio, and were administered at a dose of 2.5 μmol/mouse. MDP (Ciba-Geigy) was entrapped within the liposomes and administered at a dose of 2.5 μg/mouse.[12] Azimexon (BM 12.531; Boehringer Mannheim) was dissolved in phosphate buffered saline (PBS) and injected intraperitoneally at a dose of 100 mg/kg body weight.

Contact hypersensitivity (CHS)

To induce CHS, mice were shaved on the ventral side with a razor blade and painted with 100 μl of 3% TNCB in acetone. Six days later, their ears were painted with 1% TNCB in acetone (5 μl per ear surface). Ear thickness was measured with a spring-loaded micrometer before and 24 hours after ear challenge to determine the amount of ear swelling.

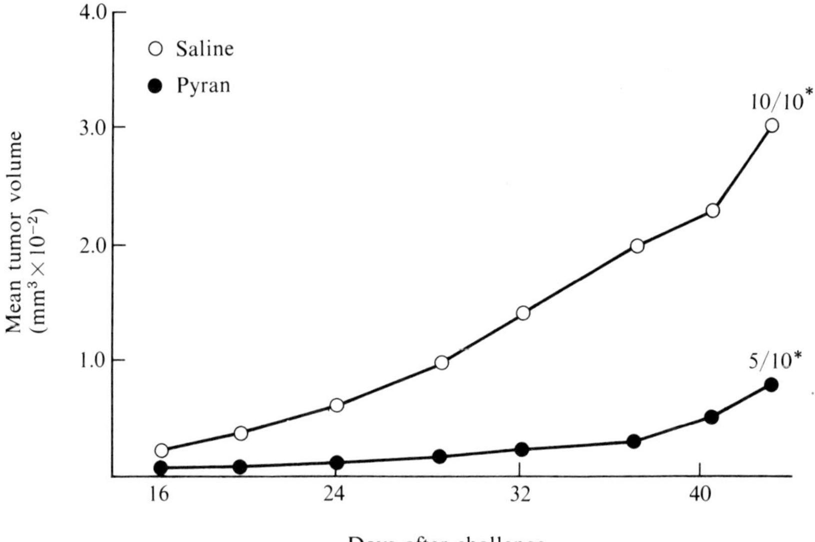

Fig. 1 Growth of UV-induced fibrosarcoma (UV-2446) in UV-irradiated mice treated with pyran copolymer or saline. Mice were exposed to UV radiation for 1 hr, 3 times per week for 12 weeks. Tumor cells from cell culture were injected s.c. on the ventral side at a concentration of 5×10^5 cells in 0.1 ml.[14] *Number of tumor-bearing mice/number implanted with tumor.

Table 1 Induction of primary skin cancers with UV radiation in mice treated with pyran copolymer[14]

Treatment*	Incidence of primary skin cancers(%)**	Average latency
Saline	22/25 (88)	32 weeks
Pyran copolymer, 1 mg/ml	13/25 (52)†	40 weeks

* 0.5 ml i.p. every other week for 70 weeks, beginning 2 days after the first UV exposure.

** At 70 weeks. Mice were exposed to UV radiation for one hour, 3 times per week for 16 weeks. More than 90% of tumors were fibrosarcomas.

† $p < 0.01$ versus saline-treated group.

RESULTS

Increased resistance of UV-irradiated mice to UV-induced tumors

UV-induced tumors grow progressively in UV-irradiated mice, leading eventually to the death of the animals. It appears that certain BRMs may

Table 2 *In vitro* activation of PEC from UV-irradiated mice by rat MAF or LPS[13]

Target tumor	Ratio PEC:tumor	PEC donor	Residual cpm* Control	MAF	% Cytotoxicity
UV-2343	20 : 1	Normal	4512	482	89
		UV**	4874	602	88
			Control	LPS	
UV-2343	50 : 1	Normal	2720	570	79
		UV**	2230	640	71

* ^{3}H-thymidine after a 5-day incubation.
** One hour, 3 times per week for 12 weeks.

have the potential to modify this course of events.[14] One example is given here: Repeated intraperitoneal treatment of mice with pyran copolymer during a 12-week course of UV irradiation reduced both the incidence and growth rate of a UV-induced tumor that was injected subcutaneously (Fig. 1). Furthermore, this treatment reduced the incidence of primary skin cancers induced by chronic UV irradiation (Table 1).

The mechanism by which BRMs can modify host resistance to transplanted and primary skin cancers is not known. One possibility is that activated macrophages are involved in the destruction of tumors *in vivo*. Another possibility is that treatment with BRMs prevents the induction of suppressor T cells by UV radiation. Experiments addressing these two possibilities are summarized below.

Activation of macrophages from UV-irradiated mice

To determine whether macrophages from UV-irradiated mice were capable of being activated to kill syngeneic UV-induced tumor cells *in vitro,* PEC were incubated *in vitro* with LPS or rat concanavalin A (Con A)-induced MAF.[13] The cytotoxicity of such PEC from normal and UV-irradiated mice is illustrated in Table 2. No difference was observed between the activity of PEC from normal mice and that of PEC from UV-irradiated animals. This demonstrates that macrophages from UV-irradiated mice can be activated *in vitro* with BRMs to kill cells from UV-induced tumors.

In vivo activation of the macrophages in UV-irradiated mice can also be achieved.[11] Intravenous injection of mice with MDP-liposome preparations activates alveolar macrophages, rendering them cytotoxic to syngeneic and allogeneic tumor cells (Table 3). A similar level of activation was observed with alveolar macrophages from UV-irradiated and non-irradiated animals.

Table 3 In vivo activation of alveolar macrophages (AM) in UV-irradiated mice by Liposome-MDP[12]

Target tumor	Ratio AM : tumor	AM donor	Residual cmp* Liposome-HBSS	Residual cmp* Liposome-MDP**	% Cytotoxicity
UV-2237	10 : 1	Normal	2378	1444	39
		UV†	2153	1450	33
B 16	10 : 1	Normal	1445	909	37
Melanoma		UV†	1448	791	45

* ^{125}I-iododeoxy-uridine after a 3-day incubation.
** Injected i.v. 24 hours before AM harvest. MDP dose: 2.5 μg/mouse.
† One hour, 3 times per week for 8 weeks.

Table 4 Effect of BRMs on UV-induced suppression of CHS to TNCB

Treatment group*	△Ear swelling**	% Suppression
Normal	24.6	
UV	6.2	75
UV-MDP (1)	10.9	56
UV-MDP (4)	7.7	67
Normal	15.0	
Normal-AZI (3)	18.9	
UV	4.2	72
UV-AZI (3)	4.7	69

* UV=a single 3-hour exposure to FS40 sunlamps on Day 0; MDP=muramyl dipeptide, 10 μg, encapsulated in liposomes, injected i.v. on the day indicated in parentheses; AZI=azimexon, injected i.p. in PBS at 100 mg/kg body weight on Day 3.
** Ear swelling of sensitized minus ear swelling of unsensitized mice. For sensitization, mice were painted on shaved abdominal skin with 100 μl of 3% TNCB in acetone, 8 days after UV treatment. Six days after sensitization, these mice and unsensitized controls were challenged by painting 5 μl of 1% TNCB on each ear surface. Ear swelling was measured at 24 hours after challenge. (Kripke and Morison, unpublished data.)

Effect of BRMs on suppression of CHS by UV radiation

In addition to suppressing tumor rejection, UV radiation also interferes with the induction of CHS reactions. Application of a contact-sensitizing hapten to the ventral skin of mice previously given a single dorsal exposure to UV radiation leads to the induction of hapten-specific suppressor T lymphocytes instead of CHS.[15] The mechanism by which UV radiation induces these suppressor cells is thought to be similar to that underlying the induction of the suppressor cells that prevent tumor rejection. To determine whether BRMs could prevent the induction of suppressor cells and reverse the depression of CHS, mice were treated with azimexon or MDP-liposomes. Treating mice with these agents after UV irradiation and before contact sensitization with TNCB did not reverse the UV-induced immunosuppression completely, although MDP-liposome treatment increased the CHS reaction (Table 4). This result suggests that azimexon probably does not prevent suppressor cell induction. On the other hand, MDP-liposomes may reduce the induction of suppressor cells, in addition to causing macrophage activation.

DISCUSSION

Although these studies leave many questions unanswered, they serve to illustrate the potential usefulness of the UV carcinogenesis system for studying BRMs. In this context, there are at least three different questions that can be addressed. The first question is whether a BRM can offer protection against developing or established cancers and their metastases in a primary host. This is important because the primary host may be quite different in its response, both to the tumor and to the BRM, from normal animals bearing a transplanted tumor. Second, because there is detailed information available concerning the cellular basis for UV-induced immunosuppression, the system can be used to explore the mechanism of action of a particular BRM. For example, specific tests can be performed in order to determine whether or not a BRM inhibits the formation of suppressor T lymphocytes.

Finally, the system may provide the means to develop preventive or therapeutic approaches for specific types of human cancer. For example, there are genetic diseases associated with a high risk of developing sunlight-induced skin cancers and melanomas that may be sunlight-associated. Preventive measures using BRMs might be useful in these instances, and this possibility can be explored with the UV carcinogenesis model. Also, sunlight-induced skin cancers in humans often occur as multiple primary tumors, and local recurrence and metastasis can be a significant problem in a certain percentage of cases. The UV carcinogenesis system could be used to design approaches for treating these specific situations, using BRMs or a combination of BRMs and specific immunization.

REFERENCES

1. Blum, H.F. (1959): *Carcinogenesis by Ultraviolet Light.* Princeton Univ. Press, N.J.
2. Kripke, M.L. (1981): Immunologic mechanisms in UV radiation carcinogenesis.

Adv. Cancer Res., 34, 69.

3. Kripke, M.L. (1974): Antigenicity of murine skin tumors induced by ultraviolet light. *J. Natl. Cancer Inst., 53*, 1333.
4. Kripke, M.L. and Fisher, M.S. (1976): Immunologic parameters of ultraviolet carcinogenesis. *J. Natl. Cancer Inst., 57*, 211.
5. Kripke, M.L. and Fidler, I.J. (1980): Enhanced experimental metastasis of ultraviolet light-induced fibrosarcomas in ultraviolet light-irradiated syngeneic mice. *Cancer Res., 40*, 625.
6. Fisher, M.S. and Kripke, M.L. (1982): Suppressor T lymphocytes control the development of primary skin cancers in ultraviolet-irradiated mice. *Science, 216*, 1133.
7. Fisher, M.S. and Kripke, M.L. (1977): Systemic alteration induced in mice by ultraviolet light irradiation and its relationship to ultraviolet carcinogenesis. *Proc. Natl. Acad. Sci. U.S.A., 74*, 1688.
8. Daynes, R.A. and Spellman, C.W. (1977): Evidence for the generation of suppressor cells by ultraviolet radiation. *Cell. Immunol., 31*, 182.
9. Fisher, M.S. and Kripke, M.L. (1978): Further studies on the tumor-specific suppressor cells induced by ultraviolet radiation. *J. Immunol., 121*, 1139.
10. Kripke, M.L. (1977): Latency, histology, and antigenicity of tumors induced by ultraviolet light in three inbred mouse strains. *Cancer Res., 37*, 1395.
11. Kripke, M.L., Gruys, E. and Fidler, I.J. (1978): Metastatic heterogeneity of cells from an ultraviolet light-induced murine fibrosarcoma of recent origin. *Cancer Res., 38*, 2962.
12. Fidler, I.J. (1981): The *in situ* induction of tumoricidal activity in alveolar macrophages by liposomes containing muramyl dipeptide is a thymus-independent process. *J. Immunol., 127*, 1719.
13. Norbury, K.C., Kripke, M.L. and Budmen, M.B. (1977): *In vitro* reactivity of macrophages and lymphocytes from UV-irradiated mice. *J. Natl. Cancer Inst., 59*, 1231.
14. Norbury, K.C. and Kripke, M.L. (1979): Ultraviolet-induced carcinogenesis in mice treated with silica, trypan blue or pyran copolymer. *J. Reticuloendothel. Soc., 26*, 827.
15. Noonan, F.P., DeFabo, E.C. and Kripke, M.L. (1981): Suppression of contact hypersensitivity by UV radiation and its relationship to UV-induced suppression of tumor immunity. *Photochem. Photobiol., 34*, 683.

Tumor cell xenogenization as a consequence of alterations in gene expression: High frequency induction of heritable immunogenic variants by exposure to strongly or poorly mutagenic compounds

Robert S. Kerbel, Philip Frost, Douglas A. Carlow and Bruce E. Elliott

SUMMARY

Xenogenization of tumor cells (so as to increase their immunogenicity) is usually achieved by viral infection of the cells or by treatment with haptenic chemicals. These processes lead to very short term membrane structural modifications in the form of transient insertion of the viruses, viral antigens, or chemical hapten moieties. However, profound alterations in immunogenicity can also be affected by brief treatment of neoplastic cells with mutagens *in vitro*. This brings about cell surface antigenic changes which appear to depend on an alteration in the structural properties or informational content of cellular DNA. As such, this type of induced antigenic change is passed on from one generation of cells to another, i.e., it is a heritable trait.

With regard to the latter phenomenon, we show here that: (i) although antigenic changes are indeed inherited, they are not necessarily phenotypically stable in long-term (over six months) tissue culture; (ii) immunogenic variants are produced at very high frequency after *in vitro* drug treatment, sometimes affecting over 80-90% of the cells; (iii) the underlying basis of the increased immunogenicity may be either acquisition of new tumor-specific antigens or alterations in the expression of self major histocompatibility complex (MHC) antigens; (iv) such changes can be induced by treatment with drugs which are thought to be poorly, if at all, mutagenic but which can cause gene activation as a consequence of DNA hypomethylation (e.g., 5-azacytidine); and (v) such profound alterations can also be achieved using completely non-immunogenic spontaneously occurring tumors. Furthermore, immune responses induced against the highly immunogenic variants may detect antigenic specificities present on the original untreated parent tumor cells, and this is sometimes observed even when using spontaneous non-immunogenic mammary carcinomas and immunogenic variants derived from them.

The implications of the results are discussed in terms of the controversies surrounding the immunogenic and antigenic status of neoplasms.

INTRODUCTION

In a series of papers written since 1976, Boon and his colleagues have shown that treatment of a variety of tumorigenic mouse cell lines *in vitro* with a chemical mutagen (MNNG) can lead to an extraordinarily high proportion of so-called "tum$^-$" clones (see Ref. 1 for a review). These are clones which do not grow progressively in the normal syngeneic host; either no growth is observed or transient growth occurs followed by a rapid and apparently complete regression of the tumor.[1] However, if injected into highly immunosuppressed recipients, these same clones will grow progressively and eventually kill their hosts.

The latter observation strongly implied that the tum$^-$ phenotype had an underlying immunologic basis. This was subsequently proven by the demonstration that these variants could induce powerful cytolytic T cell responses. Further analysis, using cloned T cell lines, showed that the tum$^-$ clones each possessed individually specific (i.e., polymorphic) antigenic determinants while retaining the antigen(s) present on the original untreated parent cell line. Somehow, the presence of the original antigens and the newly-induced antigens renders the cells powerfully immunogenic-virtually the equivalent of a major histocompatibility complex (MHC)-incompatible allograft.[2]

Thus, mutagenesis appears to be a surprisingly effective and easy way to bring about the process known as tumor cell "xenogenization".[3] Furthermore, in contrast to the usual conventional methods of xenogenization,[3] the mutagen-induced changes seem to reside at the level of DNA, based on the inheritability of the immunogenic phenotype.[1]

In most cases studied, immune responses induced against tum$^-$ clones have been shown to cross-react with the original parent, even if the original tumor was poorly- or non-immunogenic.[4,5] These findings have led to the exciting possibility of using these variants to explore the antigenic and immunologic status of tumors in general, and spontaneous tumors in particular.

What follows is a brief summary of our experience in studying this phenomenon and its relevance to tumor immunology. We paid particular attention to assessing the possibility that the generation of tum$^-$ clones did not depend on mutagenesis *per se* but, rather, involved epigenetic alterations leading to altered gene expression. Many of our studies utilized completely non-immunogenic spontaneous tumors to comply with the criticism of Hewitt[6,7] regarding the hazards of using strongly immunogenic tumors intentionally induced in the laboratory or long-term established tumors. Such tumors may be immunogenic but the authenticity of the immunogenicity may be highly suspect.[6,7] New findings include the observation that a poorly mutagenic drug (5-azacytidine) can induce quantitatively and qualitatively similar effects as conventional mutagens and that altered expression of self MHC antigens on the tum$^-$ cells may also serve to increase the immunogenicity of the tum$^-$ clones.

MATERIALS AND METHODS

All materials and methods have been described in detail in a series of recent publications from our laboratories[5,8–10] and will not be described here. Essentially, the experiments consisted of assessing the tumorigenic and immunogenic status of clones obtained from a variety of mouse tumor cell lines after treatment *in vitro* with mutagens such as ethylmethane sulfonate (EMS) or the DNA hypomethylating agent, 5-azacytidine. Alterations in immunogenicity were assessed by comparing the ability of the treated cells to grow in normal syngeneic and athymic nude mice, and by the induction of cytolytic T-lymphocyte (CTL) responses *in vitro*.

RESULTS

Effect of mutagen treatment on the tumorigenic properties of highly tumorigenic mouse tumor lines

Because we had repeatedly noted that certain kinds of drug- or lectin-resistant mouse tumor mutants derived *in vitro* after mutagenesis lost their ability to grow easily in normal syngeneic hosts (but not in athymic nude mice), we decided to assess the possibility that the presumptive immunologic alteration in the treated cells was due to the prior mutagen treatment.[11] This reasoning was based on the findings of Boon and his colleagues[1] discussed above.

Table 1 shows the results of our initial experiments using a variety of tumors including the TA3 mammary carcinoma, the MDAY-D2 leukemia-like line, the SS1 mammary adenocarcinoma, the SP-1 mammary carcinoma, and the P815 mastocytoma.[5] It will be noted that in the case

Table 1 Tumorigenic properties of clones derived from mutagen-treated highly tumorigenic mouse cell lines

Tumor (mouse strain)	Pretreatment	% Tum⁻ clones in syngeneic mice: no. of tum⁻ clones / total no. clones tested	Growth of tum⁻ clones in nude mice	Reference
P815 mastocytoma (DBA/2 Strain)	Nothing EMS MNNG	0/16 (0%) 3/10 (33%)	Yes	9
TA3 mammary carcinoma (A/J Strain)	EMS	21/22 (95%)	Yes	9
MDAY-D2 "leukemia-like" tumor (DBA/2)	Nothing EMS MNNG	17/17 (0%) 1/53 0/27 (0%)	Yes	9
SP-1 mammary adenocarcinoma (CBA)	EMS EMS	2/6 (33%) 6/14 (43%)	Yes	10
SS-1 mammary adenoacanthoma (BALB/C)	EMS MNNG	not cloned: whole population non-tumorigenic in BALB/C mice	Yes	9

Tumor cells were treated *in vitro* with 360 μg/ml EMS for 2 hours or 3 μg/ml MNNG for 1 hour or left untreated. The cells were then cloned and a large number of independent clones from each tumor (10^6 cells) was injected s.c. into the appropriate syngeneic mouse strain. The mice were then monitored and scored for growth or no growth (tum⁻) of solid tumors at the site of inoculation.[8–10]

of TA3, a very high proportion of the clones lost their tumorigenic ability; in the case of SS1, so many of the cells apparently became highly immunogenic that the entire uncloned cell population actually acquired the tum⁻ phenotype. In contrast, the proportion of tum⁻ clones was far lower with P815 and MDAY-D2, but in the case of P815 still significant compared to the untreated cloned controls. All of the tum⁻ clones obtained from any particular tumor grew readily in nude athymic mice.

Enhanced immunogenicity of tum⁻ clones

We sought direct evidence that the tum⁻ clones derived from any particular tumor were in fact more immunogenic. We tested the ability of such clones to stimulate specific CTL responses *in vitro*. An example of the results obtained using the SS1 spontaneous adenocarcinoma is shown in Table 2. Syngeneic BALB/c mice were immunized with the parent line or a MNNG-induced tum⁻ clone. The spleen cells were harvested three weeks later and restimulated *in vitro* with various mitomycin C-treated tumor cells.[5] There were three noteworthy observations: (i) the untreated SS1 cells were unable to induce a CTL response, which is in agreement with Hewitt's contention[6,7] that spontaneous tumors are usually non-immunogenic; (ii) the tum⁻ clones induced high levels of CTL activity; (iii) perhaps most significantly, the CTL activity triggered using an SS1 tum⁻ clone could also kill the uncloned untreated SS1 parent cells. Thus the latter cells appear to possess a tumor antigen (i.e., they are 'antigenic') despite being unable to induce an immune response (i.e., they are non-immunogenic).

Phenotypic instability of the tum⁻ phenotype

In subsequent studies we noted that most tum⁻ clones gradually reverted to a tum⁺ (tumorigenic) phenotype after several weeks or months in culture.[5,9] An example of this is shown in Fig. 1. Thus, although the tum⁻ phenotype is clearly inherited, it is not necessarily stable over long periods of time.

Table 2 Induction of CMC responses by EMS- or MNNG-treated SS1 tumor cells*

In vivo 1st immunization	*In vitro* 2nd immunization	Target and % of CMC		
		SS1	SS1-E	SS1-N
1	1	4	NT**	NT
E	E	100	100	100
E	N	100	100	100
E	1	100	100	100
N	N	19±0.6†	40±2.0	30±3.1
N	E	7±1.2	32±0.9	24±0.4
N	1	18±1.4	43±1.3	27±1.3

* Five BALB/c mice were given injections of 5×10^5 SS1-E, SS1-N, or SS1 cells s.c. on Day 0. On Day 14, the spleen cells were harvested, pooled, and placed in culture with mitomycin C-treated SS1, SS1-E, or SS1-N cells. Five days later, the spleen cells were used as effectors (at a 50:1 effector to target ratio) against SS1, SS1-E, and SS1-N targets in an 18-h release assay. SS1-E and SS1-N refer to cells treated once with either EMS (E) or MNNG (N).[5]

** NT: not tested.

† Mean±SD.

Effects of 5-azacytidine on the tumorigenic and immunologic properties of the treated cells

It is now widely known that drugs which are effective in causing DNA hypomethylation can cause drastic alterations in gene expression leading to equally drastic alterations in phenotypic expression.[12–14] The best known of these drugs is 5-azacytidine[12]; treatment of tumor cell populations with this drug can often lead to 10-20%, or even more, of the cells acquiring an altered behavior with respect to a particular trait, e.g., expression of a certain enzyme[15] or sensitivity to a certain hormone.[16] Because mutagens can also cause DNA hypomethylation,[17–19] we reasoned that the results obtained with EMS or MNNG on the massive conversion of tum$^+$ cells to a tum$^-$ phenotype could be due to DNA hypomethylation, thereby leading to the activation of dormant genes coding for

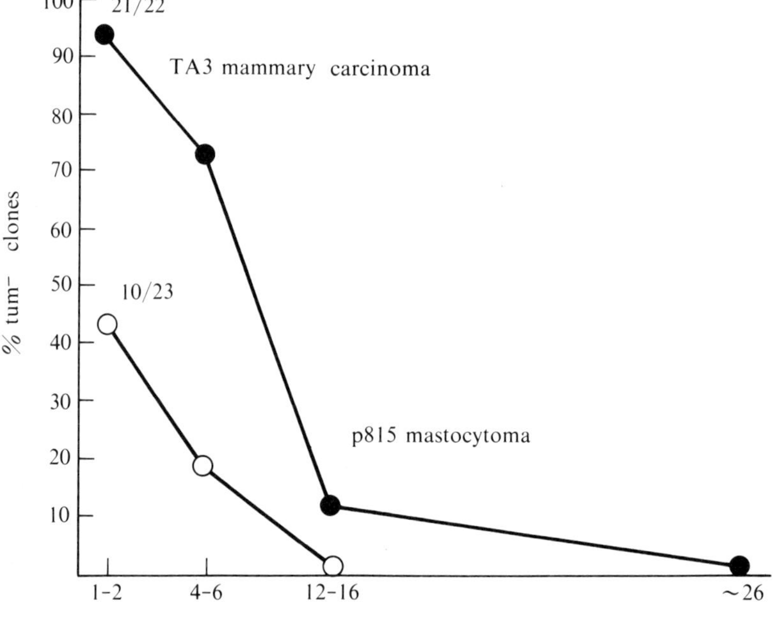

Fig. 1 Phenotypic drift of the tum$^-$ phenotype.
In one experiment, after EMS pretreatment and cloning of the TA3 mammary, we tested 22 clones and found 21 to be non-tumorigenic in A strain mice. We examined these 22 clones after they had been maintained in culture for a further 4-6 weeks, 12-16 weeks, or 26 weeks. All eventually re-acquired a tum$^+$ phenotype. Similarly, after EMS treatment of P815 mastocytoma cells, 10 of 23 clones were non-tumorigenic when first tested in DBA/2 mice. Within 26 weeks these 10 tum$^-$ clones re-acquired the tum$^+$ phenotype.

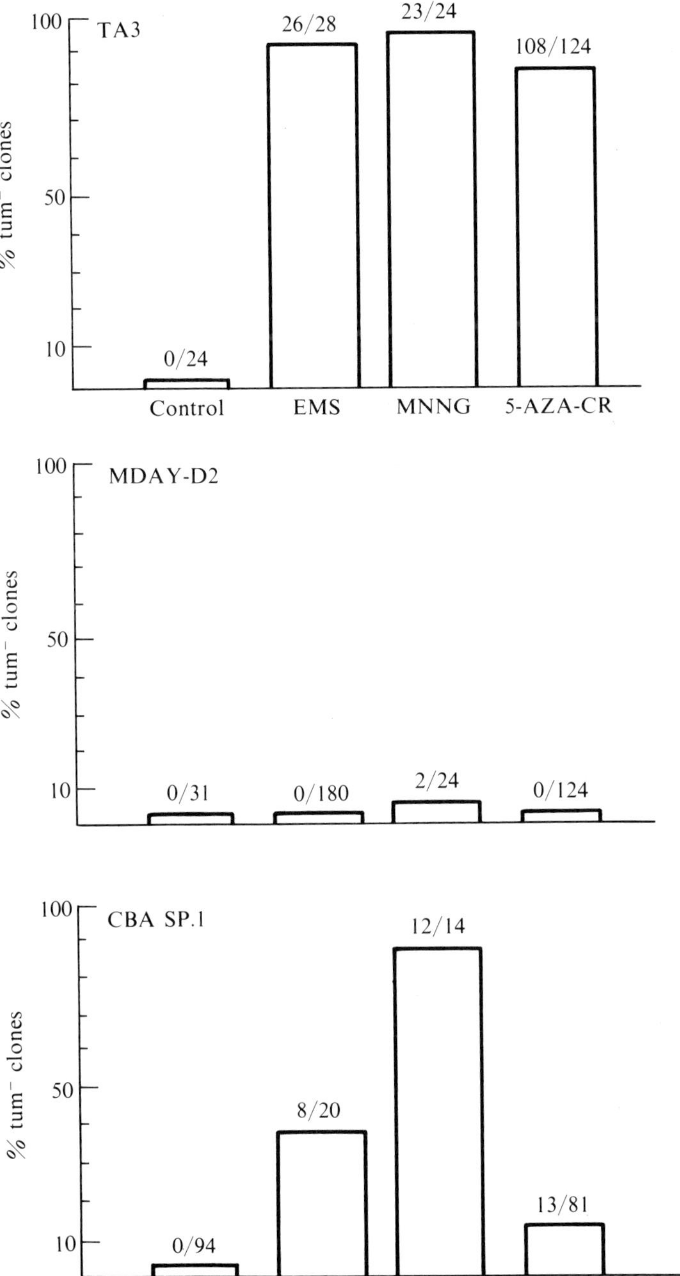

Fig. 2 Frequency of tum$^-$ variants after EMS, MNNG, or 5-azacytidine treatment.
Three different mouse tumor lines (TA3, MDAY-D2, CBA SP.1) were pretreated with EMS or MNNG (for details see Table 1) or 1 to 4 μM 5-azacytidine (5-aza-CR).[8–10]

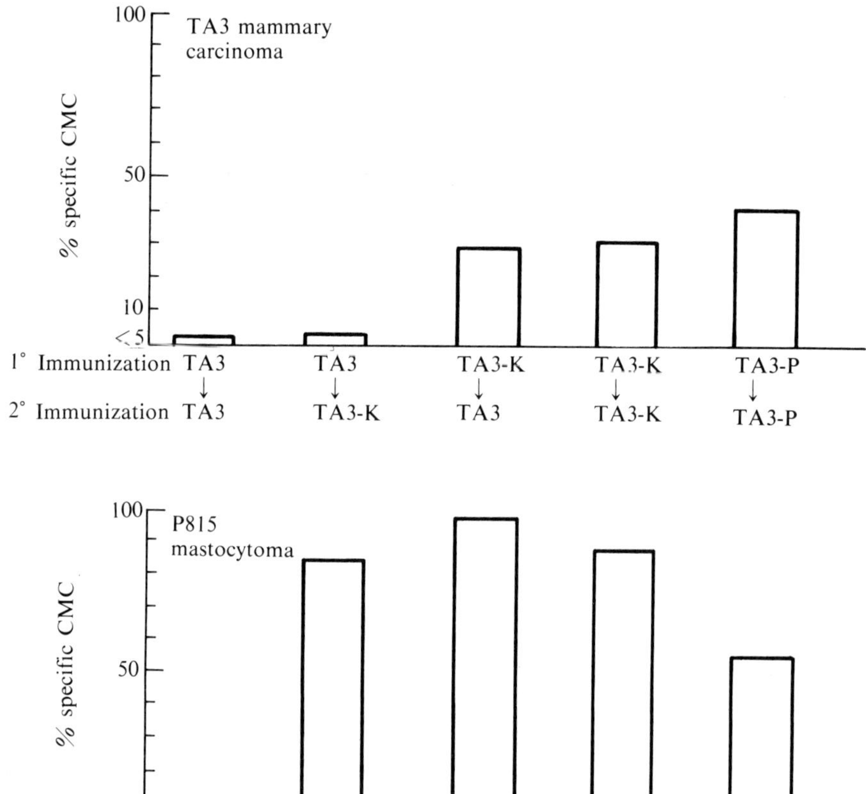

Fig. 3 Cell mediated cytotoxicity (CMC) generated by 5-azacytidine selected tum⁻ clones.

Levels of specific T cell-mediated cytotoxicity induced in the spleens of mice given injections of TA3 mammary carcinoma cells or TA3 tum⁻ clones induced with 5-azacytidine (upper figure); or given injections of P815 mastocytoma cells or P815 tum⁻ clones induced with 5-azacytidine (lower figure), are shown. Mice were first immunized (1° immunization) by a subcutaneous injection of 10^5 or 10^6 cells of the indicated tumor line. The spleens were removed and disassociated into a single cell suspension and the cells reimmunized (2° immunization) *in vitro* with the indicated tumor line or tum⁻ clone (designated by letter). The stimulator tumor cells were pretreated with mitomycin-C beforehand and assayed against tumor cells labeled with the isotope Indium 111. The target cells were either the TA3 parent line (upper graph) or the P815 line (lower graph). Levels of specific lysis were calculated using standard procedures.

potential tumor-specific antigens.[8–10]

We therefore tested the affects of 5-azacytidine on our tumor lines to determine whether it was an effective tum$^-$-inducing agent.[8] Various tumor lines were treated with 3 or 4 μM 5-azacytidine for 24 hours and cloned; a number of clones were then injected into appropriate syngeneic mice, or nude athymic mice. 5-Azacytidine was indeed effective in inducing tum$^-$ clones[8–10] (Fig. 2). These, like the mutagen-induced tum$^-$ clones, grew in nude mice; furthermore, they were usually capable of inducing strong CTL responses *in vitro* (Fig. 3), in contrast to the parent tumor counterparts. Despite the apparent ease with which 5-azacytidine can induce tum$^-$ clones, we found it was a poor mutagen when it was compared with EMS in its ability to induce single (point) gene mutations at a number of defined loci in the same tumor lines we used for our *in vivo* tumorigenicity studies.[8,9] We also found that most tum$^-$ clones were phenotypically unstable[8–10] in that they eventually acquired a tum$^+$ phenotype, usually within several months of being maintained in culture. It will also be noted from Fig. 3 that CTLs stimulated against a tum$^-$ clone could kill cells from the parental tum$^+$ line, even though it was poorly, if at all, immunogenic. One exception to this was found with the CBA Spl tumor: tum$^-$ variants of CBA Spl were poor stimulators of CTL activity even though they failed to grow in normal CBA mice but grew in nude mice (Carlow and Elliott, unpublished observations).

Cell surface antigenic changes in tum clones obtained after 5-azacytidine or mutagen treatment

As summarized earlier, Boon[1] and ourselves[5] have found evidence for new unique polymorphic tumor antigenic specificities on mutagen-derived tum$^-$ clones. However, immunogenicity (in so far as recognition by CTL is concerned) usually requires recognition of both 'self' class I MHC antigens (called H-2 antigens in the mouse and HLA in man) in conjunction with the specific foreign antigenic determinant.[20] Therefore, altered (i.e., elevated) levels of class I MHC antigens could conceivably be one explanation for the acquisition of high grade tumor cell immunogenicity in some of the mutagen- or 5-azacytidine-treated tum$^-$ clones. Indeed, Elliott and his colleagues[10] have found serological evidence for elevated levels of H-2D (but not H-2K) antigens in tum$^-$ clones obtained from the CBA Spl mammary carcinoma, a low class I MHC-expressing tumor.[10] Reversion of the tum$^-$ clones to a tum$^+$ phenotype was accompanied by a return to the wild-type low level H-2 antigen expression (data not shown here).

DISCUSSION

Our results confirm those of Boon in clearly showing that brief treatment of tumor cells with mutagenic chemicals *in vitro* can result in a massive conversion of the cells to an extraordinarily high grade immunogenic phenotype. As the experiments described above show virtually identical results are obtained when the same tumor lines are treated with a drug (5-azacytidine) which is weakly, if at all, mutagenic when compared with EMS (a known potent mutagen). As 5-azacytidine is a strong inducer of DNA hypomethylation, a process which can "turn-on" previously silent genes,[12–14] the simplest and most straightforward explanation of these results is that a heritable alteration in gene expression occurred in a very high proportion of the drug-treated cells. This could occur as a consequence of induced hypomethylation in otherwise silent genes that code for cell surface determinants which can act as tumor-specific antigens.

Another possibility, for which evidence has in fact been obtained in Elliott's laboratory,[10] is that the level of class I (or class II) MHC antigens is altered so as to make T cell recognition of the tumor antigens far more efficient and effective. This mechanism may be particularly relevant for classes of tumors expressing very low, even non-detectable, levels of MHC antigens. As most types of epithelial cells have very low quantities of class I MHC antigens,[21] tumors derived from such cells (i.e., carcinomas) would not be expected to induce significant tumor-specific CTL immune responses, because they too would be low MHC-expressing entities. Hence, 5-azacytidine treatment of such cells (in contrast to leukemias or mesenchymally-derived tumors which arise from cells which usually express abundant cell surface MHC class I molecules) might result in increased levels of MHC antigen expression, as has been suggested by Carlow et al.[10] Clearly, this could render the cells immunogenic provided they also possess a set of tumor-specific antigens. This is summarized diagrammatically in Fig. 4.

Thus, our results not only point out a new way of efficiently creating xenogenized tumor subpopulations of extraordinary immunogenicity, but they also underscore the subtleties and complexities of the tumor cell immunogenic (and antigenic) phenotypes. Quite clearly, a tumor cell population, even if it arose spontaneously and displayed no evidence of immunogenicity, could nevertheless possess tumor specific antigens (i.e., be "antigenic"). The fact that the antigenicity does not translate to immunogenicity could be a reflection of a lack of additional distinct tumor antigenic epitopes (which could bring about a helper effect in inducing a CTL response) or, alternatively, of a lack of expression of the

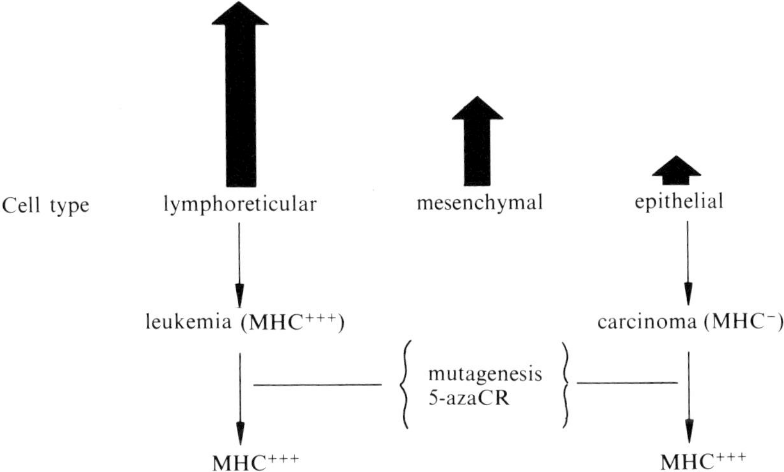

Fig. 4 Level of Class I MHC expression.
Diagrammatic representation of the possible contrasting effects of 5-azacytidine treatment (or treatment with a mutagen such as EMS) on the level of MHC class I antigen expression on tumors having different cellular (histological) origins. As leukemias are derived from lymphoreticular cells, most of which normally express high levels of class I MHC antigens,[21] tumors derived from such cells would also express high levels of the antigens, i.e., the genes encoding these antigens would be quite active, and treatment with a hypomethylating agent would not be expected to alter this high level expression. In contrast, carcinomas derived from epithelial cells, which often express very low levels of class I MHC antigens,[21] would also have low levels of these antigens. There is in fact evidence for this.[21–23] In these cases, 5-azacytidine (or mutagen) pretreatment could in theory alter (i.e., increase) levels of the MHC class I antigens. Provided such tumors have tumor-specific antigens, this could convert the cells from a non-immunogenic to an immunogenic state, as T cells require both "self" MHC antigens and specific antigens on target cells in order to mediate specific recognition of the antigen.[20]

relevant self MHC antigens that are so vital in most T cell recognition processes. In any case, like those previously published by Boon's group,[4] our results show that tum^- mutants can be obtained from completely non-immunogenic tumors of spontaneous origin and that, in at least some cases, uncloned CTLs directed against such tum^- mutants can specifically kill the untreated non-immunogenic parent cells. Thus the non-immunogenic parent cells sometimes, though not necessarily always, do appear to possess a tumor-specific antigen(s) despite their non-immunogenic status.

Although these possibilities will not be easy to sort out, the results previously described by Boon[1] and here[8–10] should provide a promising and illuminating approach to studying the problem, especially when it is combined with the new techniques of molecular genetics.

ACKNOWLEDGEMENTS

We would like to express our thanks to Mrs. Beverley Fluhrer for her excellent secretarial assistance. The work summarized here was supported by grants from the National Cancer Institute of Canada, and the Medical Research Council of Canada (to RSK and BEE), the U.S. Public Health Service (CA28060) and the Veterans Administration (to PF). RSK and BEE are Research Associates of the National Cancer Institute of Canada.

REFERENCES

1. Boon T. (1983): Antigenic tumor cell variants obtained with mutagens. *Adv. Cancer Res.*, *39*, 121.
2. Frost, P. and Kerbel, R.S. (1983): On a possible epigenetic mechanism(s) of tumor cell heterogeneity. The role of DNA methylation. *Cancer Metastasis Reviews*, *2*, 375.
3. Kobayashi, H. (1979): Viral xenogenization of intact tumor cells. *Adv. Cancer Res.*, *30*, 279.
4. Van Pel A. and Boon, T. (1982): Protection against a nonimmunogenic mouse leukemia by an immunogenic variant obtained by mutagenesis. *Proc. Natl. Acad. Sci. USA*, *79*, 4718.
5. Frost, P., Kerbel, R.S., Bauer, E., Tartamella-Biondo, R. and Cefalu, W.(1983): Mutagen treatment as a means for selecting immunogenic variants from otherwise poorly immunogenic malignant murine tumors. *Cancer Res.*, *43*, 125.
6. Hewitt, H.B. (1979): A critical examination of the foundations of immunotherapy for cancer. *Clin. Radiol.*, *30*, 361.
7. Hewitt, H.B., (1982): Animal tumor models and their relevance to human tumor immunology. *Journal of Biological Response Modifiers*, *1*, 107.
8. Frost, P., Liteplo, R.G., Donaghue, T.P. and Kerbel, R.S. (1984): Selection of strongly immunogenic "tum" variants from tumors at high frequency using 5-azacytidine. *J. Exp. Med.*, *159*, 1491.
9. Kerbel, R.S., Frost, P., Liteplo, R., Carlow, D.A. and Elliott, B.E. (1984): Possible epigenetic mechanisms of tumor progression: induction of high-frequency heritable but phenotypically unstable changes in the tumorigenic and metastatic properties of tumor cell populations by 5-azacytidine treatment. *J. Cell. Physiol. Suppl.*, *3*, 87.
10. Carlow, D., Kerbel, R.S., Feltis, T. and Elliott, B.E. (1984): Altered H-2 expression in non-tumorigenic variants derived from a non-immunogenic CBA/J spontaneous mammary adenocarcinoma. *J. Natl. Cancer Inst.*, submitted for publication.
11. Kerbel, R.S., Dennis, J.W., Lagarde, A.E. and Frost, P. (1982): Tumor progression in metastasis: an experimental approach using lectin resistant tumor variants. *Cancer Metastasis Reviews*, *1*, 99.
12. Ehrlich, M. and Wang, R.Y.-H. (1981): 5-Methylcytosine in eukaryotic DNA. *Science*, *212*, 1350.

13. Hattman, S. (1981): DNA methylation. In: *The Enzymes, Vol. 14, Chapter 25*, p. 517. Editor: P.D. Boyer. Academic Press, New York.
14. Jones, P.A. and Taylor, S.M. (1980): Cellular differentiation, cytidine analogs and DNA methylation. *Cell*, *20*, 85.
15. Harris, M. (1982): Induction of thymidine kinase in enzyme-deficient Chinese hamster cells. *Cell*, *29*, 483.
16. Gasson, J.C., Ryden, T. and Bourgeois, S. (1983): Role of *de novo* DNA methylation in the glucocorticoid resistance of a T-lymphoid cell line. *Nature*, *302*, 621.
17. Salas, C.E., Pfohl-Leszkowicz, A., Lang, M.C. and Dirheimer, G. (1979): Effect of modification by N-acetoxy-N-2-acetylaminofluorene on the level of DNA methylation. *Nature*, *278*, 71.
18. Boehm, T.L.J. and Drahovsky, D. (1983): Alteration of enzymatic methylation of DNA cytosines by chemical carcinogens: A mechanism involved in the initiation of carcinogenesis. *J. Natl. Cancer Inst.*, *71*, 429.
19. Lieberman, M.W., Beach, L.R. and Palmiter, R.D. (1983): Ultraviolet radiation-induced metallothionein-1 gene activation is associated with extensive DNA demethylation. *Cell*, *35*, 207.
20. Bevan, M.J. (1977): Cytotoxic T-cell response to histocompatibility antigens: the role of H-2. *Cold Springs Harbor Symposia on Quantitative Biology*, Vol. 41, 519.
21. Klein, J. (1975): *Biology of the Mouse Histocompatibility-2 Complex*. Springer Verlag, New York.
22. Whitwell, H.L., Hughes, H.P.A., Moore, M. and Ahmed, A. (1984): Expression of major histocompatibility antigens and leucocyte infiltration in benign and malignant human breast disease. *Br. J. Cancer*, *49*, 161.
23. Rowe, D.J. and Beverley P.C.L. (1984): Characterisation of breast cancer infiltrates using monoclonal antibodies to human leucocyte antigens. *Br. J. Cancer*, *49*, 149.

Monoclonal antibody 791T/36 for tumour detection and drug targeting

Michael J. Embleton

SUMMARY

Monoclonal antibody 791T/36 was raised initially against human osteogenic sarcoma cells but reacts also against a number of unrelated tumour lines. It localises specifically in xenografts of human tumours which express 791T/36-defined antigen, and has been used successfully for radioimmunodetection of osteogenic sarcoma and colorectal carcinoma in patients.

When conjugated to cytotoxic drugs it can direct the action of the drug specifically against cells expressing the antigen, while minimizing toxicity against non-antigenic cells *in vitro*. Some conjugates have exhibited therapeutic properties against osteogenic sarcoma xenografts *in vivo*, without the toxicity associated with free drug at equivalent doses. Antibody 791T/36 is thus a candidate for targeting drugs to human tumours.

INTRODUCTION

The development of the hybridoma technique for producing monoclonal antibodies[1] has proved invaluable in many areas of immunology, and particularly so in human tumour immunology. Hitherto the application of immunology to human tumours has been limited to relatively unsuccessful attempts to boost host immunity to the tumour, or the use of xenogeneic antisera against widespread tumour markers, e.g., carcinoembryonic antigen, for diagnosis or patient monitoring. Monoclonal antibodies can be prepared in large numbers, and after suitable screening it is possible, at least in theory, to select reagents with exquisite specificity for a given antigen and thus a high degree of tumour specificity.[2] Such antibodies can be used for immunodetection of tumours by immunoscintigraphy when labelled with appropriate radioisotopes,[3–6] and their ability to localise preferentially in tumours suggests that they could also be of use for targeting therapeutic agents. This report briefly reviews the development of monoclonal antibody 791T/36 for use in radioimmunodetection and drug targeting.

MATERIALS AND METHODS

Cell cultures

Human tumour cell lines were grown as monolayer cultures in Eagle's minimum essential medium (MEM) with 10% newborn calf serum in an atmosphere of 5% CO_2. They were harvested with 0.25% w/v trypsin and 0.5% EDTA. Hybridomas were grown in Dulbecco's modified EM (DMEM) containing 5% or 10% foetal calf serum.

Monoclonal antibody

791T/36 is an IgG2b monoclonal antibody originally raised against human osteogenic sarcoma cell line 791T; its reactivity with osteogenic sarcomas and some other tumour cell lines has been described.[7] The hybridoma was grown as an ascites line in Balb/c mice, and antibody was purified from the ascites fluid by protein A-Sepharose chromatography.[8] For immunoscintigraphy the purified antibody was labelled with ^{131}I by the iodogen method.[9]

Drug-antibody conjugates

Purified 791T/36 was conjugated directly to vindesine[10] and daunomycin,[11] and was coupled to methotrexate by a human serum albumin carrier.[12] The maximum molar ratio of drug to antibody was 6:1 in the direct conjugates, but indirect conjugates using human serum albumin (HSA) as a carrier contained up to 30 moles of methotrexate per mole antibody. All conjugates were shown by flow cytofluorimetry to retain 791T/36 antibody activity.[10–12]

Cytotoxicity tests

Cytotoxicity of drugs and conjugates was measured *in vitro* using a ^{75}Se-selenomethionine (^{75}Se-met) uptake assay as previously described.[10] Cells were plated in microtiter plates and allowed to grow exponentially in the presence of various concentrations of drug or conjugate, or following 15 minutes of exposure to the drug or conjugate and a single wash. After 24 hours, ^{75}Se was added and the cells cultured for a further 8 to 16 hours. The cells were gently washed, and incorporated radioactivity was assayed in a gamma counter. The incorporation of ^{75}Se into treated cells was expressed as a percentage of that in controls treated with culture medium alone.

Tumour xenografts

Xenografts of human tumour cells were used for radio-immunodetection studies with radiolabelled 791T/36 and for the assessment of therapeutic activity of drug-antibody conjugates. CBA mice were thymectomized and treated with cytosine arabinoside (200 mg/kg) and 9 Gy whole-body irradiation according to the method of Steel et al.[13] Xenografts were initiated by a subcutaneous inoculum of 10^6 cultured tumour cells.

Patients

Immunodetection of ^{131}I-labelled antibody was measured by immunoscintigraphy in patients with osteogenic sarcoma[4] or with primary or secondary colorectal carcinoma.[3,6]

RESULTS

Localisation of 791T/36 in xenografts

Purified antibody was labelled with ^{131}I or ^{125}I and injected intraperitoneally into immune-deprived mice bearing tumour xenografts initiated by a subcutaneous inoculum of cultured cells.[8] In control studies, mice were simultaneously given ^{125}I-labelled normal Ig instead of antibody. Mice were killed 1 to 6 days later for assessment of radioiodine uptake into various organs, including blood. Examples of the distribution of counts in organs three days after injection are shown in Table 1. Tissue-blood ratios were calculated (mean cpm per gram tissue, divided by mean cpm per gram blood) and compared for various normal tissues and osteogenic sarcoma 791T. Antibody 791T/36 was found in high concentration in 791T xenografts but background levels in normal tissues were low as judged by ^{131}I tissue-blood ratios. ^{125}I-labelled normal Ig was present at a similar low level in all tissues, including 791T tumour tissue. There was thus a clear preference for 791T on the part of the antibody.

Table 2 shows the localisation of ^{125}I-791T/36 in xenografts of other

Table 1 Localisation of 791T/36 monoclonal antibody in osteogenic sarcoma 791T xenografts

Tissue	Tissue:blood ratio* obtained with:	
	^{131}I-791T/36	^{125}I-normal mouse Ig
791T	2.85±0.25	0.40±0.07
Lung	0.47±0.27	0.42±0.07
Heart	0.37±0.14	0.35±0.14
Liver	0.26±0.07	0.22±0.10
Spleen	0.25±0.08	0.21±0.10
Kidney	0.25±0.06	0.21±0.06
Intestine	0.15±0.05	0.14±0.02

* Tissue to blood ratio=cpm per gram of tissue, divided by cpm per gram of blood. Values shown are means±standard deviations for 3 mice.

Table 2 Localisation of ^{125}I-791T/36 in different human tumour xenografts

Target tumour	Mean no. antibody binding sites per cell	^{125}I tissue:blood ratio in:	
		Tumour	Normal lung
Osteogenic sarcoma 788T	10^6	1.86±0.50	0.45±0.06
〃 〃 2 OS	2.5×10^5	1.10±0.40	0.45±0.06
Colon carcinoma HCT8	$<10^4$	0.56±0.07	0.39±0.06
Bladder carcinoma T24	10^4	0.45±0.12	0.60±0.06

tumours, compared with lung tissue from the tumour-bearing mice. Significantly increased levels were found in osteogenic sarcomas 788T and 2 OS which bind high amounts of 791T/36, but colon carcinoma HCT8 and bladder carcinoma T24 which do not express 791T/36-defined antigen did not accumulate antibody above background level.

Localisation in patients

An example of localisation of ^{131}I-791T/36 in a human osteogenic sarcoma is provided by a young patient with a tumour of the distal end of the right femur.[4] Following oral KI (60 μg 24 hours previously), she was given 200 μg of 791T/36 Ig labelled with 70 Mbq of ^{131}I intravenously. Her KI treatment was continued for two weeks. Twenty-four hours after antibody infusion, gamma camera images were acquired. Image enhancement was achieved by subtracting a blood-pool image produced after subsequent injection of ^{99m}Tc-pertechnetate ; the corrected uptake of ^{131}I into her tumour compared with adjacent tumour-free areas (tumour: non-tumour ratio) was 5:1. No ^{131}I image was seen in the left leg.[4]

Similar studies in patients with colorectal carcinoma are shown in Table 3. Twenty-three patients with primary carcinomas were imaged and

Table 3 ^{131}I-791T/36 imaging in patients with colorectal tumours

Tumour	No. of patients examined	No. of positive images	Mean tumour: non-tumour ratio*
Primary colon carcinoma	11	8	2.60:1
Primary rectal carcinoma	12	5	2.40:1
Secondary colon and rectal carcinoma	15	13	ND**
Benign colonic adenoma	4	0	0.95:1

* Tumour to non-tumour ratios were calculated by assaying tumour and adjacent normal tissue from resected specimens in a gamma counter. The means shown are for the whole group.

** ND=not determined.

of these, 13 showed positive localisation of 791T/36 within their tumour. The success rate was lower in rectal tumours compared with colon tumours because of masking by free ^{131}I in the urinary bladder. Fifteen patients with recurrent or metastatic tumours were imaged and thirteen were positive. Benign adenomas, however, gave no positive images.

Effect of drug-antibody conjugates *in vitro*

The cytotoxic drugs vindesine (VDS) and daunomycin (DAU) were conjugated directly to 791T/36, and methotrexate (MTX) was conjugated via a human serum albumin carrier (MTX-HSA-791T/36). These conjugates were tested against 791T cells and antigen-negative control cells (e. g., bladder carcinoma T24) in comparison with free drug and free antibody. Free 791T/36 was not toxic in the absence of added complement, but the effects of drugs and conjugates are shown in Table 4. The most reproducible results were obtained with VDS-791T/36 and MTX-HSA-791T/36 which were selectively toxic for 791T cells, while target cells binding little or no antibody were not affected by these conjugates. DAU-791T/36 conjugates were less consistent but some preparations showed greater toxicity for 791T than for T24. All three drugs were indiscriminately toxic in their free form for all cell lines tested.

In vivo suppression of 791T xenografts

Immunosuppressed mice bearing subcutaneous xenografts of osteogenic sarcoma 791T were given VDS-791T/36 conjugate or free VDS in seven equal intraperitoneal doses at 2 to 3 day intervals. In two separate experiments the total cumulative doses were 19 mg VDS/kg body weight

Table 4 Cytotoxicity against human tumour cells by drug-antibody conjugates and free drugs

Reagent*	Concentration	% inhibition of ^{75}Se uptake by:	
		Osteogenic sarcoma 791T**	Bladder carcinoma T24†
VDS-791T/36	40 μg/ml (VDS)	75	2
VDS	40 μg/ml	87	60
DAU-791T/36	40 μg/ml (DAU)	100	5
DAU	40 μg/ml	100	100
MTX-HSA-791T/36	40 μg/ml (MTX)	79	7
MTX	40 μg/ml	82	85

* VDS = vindesine; DAU = daunomycin; MTX = methotrexate; HSA = human serum albumin carrier.
** 791T has 10^6 antibody binding sites per cell.
† T24 has 10^4 antibody binding sites per cell.

plus 50 mg antibody/kg, and 45 mg VDS/kg plus 1.7 g antibody/kg. At these doses the conjugate significantly retarded tumour growth without ill effects on the mice.[14,15] Free VDS was tumour-inhibitory but highly toxic at these doses, which greatly exceeded the established LD_{50} of 6.3 mg/kg in mice.[16] Free antibody had no effect on the tumour.

MTX-HSA-791T/36 was also shown in one experiment to have therapeutic properties against 791T xenografts at a cumulative dose of 17.5 mg/kg MTX. Again, the conjugate was non-toxic at this dose while free MTX at 17.5 mg/kg was highly toxic to the mice.

DISCUSSION

These studies indicate that monoclonal antibody 791T/36 is able to localise specifically in an antigenic tumour in an immune-deprived animal. Lack of localisation of normal Ig and the antigenic specificity of target tumour localisation indicate that antibody targeting is due to specific antigen-antibody interaction. 791T/36 also localises within human osteogenic sarcomas and colorectal carcinomas in patients, and so has a potential role as a diagnostic agent and possibly as a targeting vehicle.

The feasibility of targeting conventional drugs with 791T/36 has been established using *in vitro* assays where drug-antibody conjugates have clearly been demonstrated to act selectively against cells which react with the antibody, while the free drug is non-selective.[10,12] The therapeutic effectiveness of such conjugates has been evaluated in pilot experiments with tumour xenografts, and preliminary findings correlate broadly with the *in vitro* experiments in that the conjugates appear to be much less toxic to normal (antigen-negative) tissues than free drug while retaining therapeutic action against the tumour. Further studies need to be carried out to refine such conjugates before their use could be contemplated in humans, but even at the present stage of development it is clear that they hold some promise of increased therapeutic efficiency over cytotoxic drugs alone.

ACKNOWLEDGEMENTS

This work was supported by the Cancer Research Campaign, London, U.K. I am indebted to my colleagues M.V. Pimm, M.C. Garnett, G.F. Rowland, R.G. Simmonds, J. Gallego, N. Armitage, P.A. Farrands and R.W. Baldwin for helping to provide data for this article, and to Mrs. B. Janes for typing the manuscript.

REFERENCES

1. Köhler, G. and Milstein, C. (1975): Continuous cultures of fused cells secreting antibody of defined specificity. *Nature (Lond.). 256*, 495.
2. Wright, G.L., Jr., (ed) (1984): Monoclonal Antibodies and Cancer, *Immunology Series Vol.23*. Marcel Dekker Inc., New York.
3. Farrands, P.A., Perkins, A.C., Pimm, M.V., Hardy, J.D., Embleton, M.J., Baldwin, R.W. and Hardcastle, J.D. (1982): Radioimmunodetection of human colorectal cancers by an anti-tumour monoclonal antibody. *Lancet (ii)*, 397.
4. Farrands, P.A., Perkins, A., Sully, L., Hopkins, J.S., Pimm, M.V., Baldwin, R.W. and Hardcastle, J.D. (1983): Localisation of human osteosarcoma by antitumour monoclonal antibody. *J. Bone Joint Surg., 65-B*, 638.
5. Epenetos, A.A., Mather, S., Granowska, M., Nimmon, C.C., Hawkins, L.R., Britton, K.E., Shepherd, J., Taylor-Papadimitriou, J., Durbin, H., Malpas, J. S. and Bodmer, W.F. (1982): Targeting of Iodine 123-labelled tumour-associated monoclonal antibodies to ovarian, breast and gastrointestinal tumours. *Lancet (ii)*, 999.
6. Armitage, N.C., Perkins, A.C., Pimm, M.V., Farrands, P.A., Baldwin, R.W. and Hardcastle, J.D. (1984): The localisation of an anti-tumour monoclonal antibody (791T/36) in gastrointestinal tumours. *Brit. J. Surg., 71*, 407.
7. Embleton, M.J., Gunn, B., Byers, V.S. and Baldwin, R.W. (1981): Antitumour reactions of monoclonal antibody against a human osteogenic sarcoma cell line. *Brit. J. Cancer, 43*, 582.
8. Pimm, M.V., Embleton, M.J., Perkins, A.C., Price, M.R., Robins, R.A., Robinson, G.R. and Baldwin, R.W. (1982): *In vivo* localisation of anti-osteogenic sarcoma 791T monoclonal antibody in osteogenic sarcoma xenografts. *Int. J. Cancer, 30*, 75.
9. Fraker, P.J. and Speck, J.C. (1978): Protein and cell membrane iodination with a sparingly soluble chloroamide, 1,3,4,6-tetrachloro-3α, 6α-diphenylglycoluril. *Biochem. Biophys. Res. Commun., 80*, 849.
10. Embleton, M.J., Rowland, G.F., Simmonds, R.G., Jacobs, E., Marsden, C.H. and Baldwin, R.W. (1983): Selective cytotoxicity against human tumour cells by a

vindesine-monoclonal antibody conjugate. *Br. J. Cancer, 47*, 43.

11. Gallego, J., Price, M.R. and Baldwin, R.W. (1984): Preparation of four daunomycin-monoclonal antibody 791T/36 conjugates with anti-tumour activity. *Int. J. Cancer, 33*, 737.
12. Garnett, M.C., Embleton, M.J., Jacobs, E. and Baldwin, R.W. (1983): Preparation and properties of a drug-carrier-antibody conjugate showing selective antibody-directed cytotoxicity *in vitro*. *Br. J. Cancer, 31*, 661.
13. Steel, G.G., Courtney, V.D. and Rostom, A.Y. (1978): Improved immunosuppression techniques for the xenografting of human tumours. *Br. J. Cancer, 37*, 224.
14. Baldwin, R.W., Embleton, M.J., Garnett, M.C., Pimm, M.V., Price, M.R., Armitage, N.A., Farrands, P.A., Hardcastle, J.D., Perkins, A. and Rowland, G. F. (1984): Application of monoclonal antibody 791T/36 for radioimmunodetection of human tumours and for targeting cytotoxic drugs. *Protides of the Biological Fluids, 31*, 775.
15. Embleton, M.J., Pimm, M.V., Garnett, M.C., Rowland, G.F., Simmonds, R.G. and Baldwin, R.W. (1984): Experience in the preparation and experimental use of immunocytostatics. *Behring Inst. Mitt., 74*, 112.
16. Todd, G.C., Gibson, W.R. and Morton, D.M. (1976): Toxicology of vindesine (desacetyl vinblastine amide) in mice, rats and dogs. *J. Toxicol. Health, 1*, 843.

Tumor cell lysis by antibody-dependent macrophage-mediated cytotoxicity using syngeneic monoclonal antibodies and its augmentation by cell-wall skeleton of *Nocardia rubra*

Ichiro Kawase, Kiyoshi Komuta, Takeshi Ogura, Hiromi Fujiwara, Toshiyuki Hamaoka and Susumu Kishimoto

SUMMARY

Four monoclonal antibodies to MH134 murine syngeneic hepatoma cells, 3H1, 7C2, 11G2 and 12A2, were produced by hybridomas constructed by fusing P3-X63-Ag8-UI murine myeloma cells with spleen cells of a C3H/HeN mouse immunized with syngeneic tumor cells. Immunodiffusion analysis with rabbit anti-mouse immunoglobulin (Ig) antisera showed that 3H1, 7C2, 11G2 and 12A2 are IgG2a, IgM, IgG1 and IgG2a respectively. Enzyme-linked immunosorbent assay (ELISA) using cells of five syngeneic tumor lines, MH134, MM102, MM46, MM48 and X5563, all derived from C3H/He strain, showed that 3H1 bound specifically to MH134 tumor cells, whereas 7C2, 11G2 and 12A2 reacted not only with MH134 but also with MM102 and MM46 tumor cells. This result strongly suggests that MH134 tumor cells display at least two kinds of tumor-associated antigens (TAA) on their cell surfaces, one expressed uniquely by MH134 tumor cells and recognized by 3H1, the other commonly shared by MH134, MM102 and MM46 tumor cells and determined by the other three monoclonal antibodies.

3H1, 11G2 and 12A2, but not 7C2, were found to be able to induce antibody-dependent cell-mediated cytotoxicity (ADCC) against MH134 tumor cells. The target specificity of ADCC induced by these monoclonal antibodies was identical with that seen using ELISA. The ability of 12A2 to induce ADCC against MH134 tumor cells was significantly stronger than that of 3H1 or 11G2. Effector cell analysis of ADCC induced by 12A2 revealed that thioglycolate-induced peritoneal macrophages of C3H/HeN mice exhibited high cytotoxicity, whereas peritoneal resident macrophages of normal mice showed low cytotoxicity. Neither normal spleen cells nor nonadherent cells obtained from thioglycolate-induced peritoneal cells mediated the cytotoxicity, indicating that the cytotoxicity is mediated by macrophages, and that stimulation of macrophages is essential for augmentation of the cytotoxicity. In preliminary experiments, peritoneal macrophages activated by cell-wall skeleton of *Nocardia rubra* (N-CWS) exhibited higher cytotoxicity against MH134 tumor cells in the presence of 12A2 than peritoneal resident macrophages. These monoclonal antibodies, derived from the syngeneic tumor immune system will contribute to the investigation of combined therapies for malignancies with monoclonal antibodies and biological response modifiers which can activate macrophages.

INTRODUCTION

Because of its possible usefulness in immunotherapy for malignancies, antibody-dependent cell-mediated cytotoxicity (ADCC) has been the subject of intensive investigation. Analysis of ADCC and application of the reaction in therapeutic trials have been hampered by the complexity and heterogeneity of the antibody populations present in conventional antisera against tumor cells. The development of monoclonal antibodies has overcome these limitations, because of their properties of defined specificity and homogeneity.

Recently, several investigators have succeeded in developing murine monoclonal antibodies which can induce ADCC against human tumor cells[1,2] or murine tumor cells.[3] Furthermore, some of them have been reported to be able to suppress the growth of tumors in BALB/c nude mice when administered *in vivo*.[4,5] However, to investigate the therapeutic efficacy of monoclonal antibodies against malignancies through ADCC, syngeneic antibodies would be more suitable than xenogeneic antibodies.

The authors have previously reported that tumor-specific transplantation resistance against syngeneic MH134 hepatoma cells is easily induced in C3H/He mice by using vaccinia virus-reactive helper T cells.[6,7] Recently, we developed hybridomas secreting monoclonal antibodies against MH134 tumor cells by fusing murine myeloma cells with spleen cells of a C3H/HeN mouse immunized with vaccinia virus-infected MH134 tumor cells. In this paper, we report that some of these monoclonal antibodies can induce ADCC against MH134 tumor cells and that the cytotoxicity is mediated by macrophages.

MATERIALS AND METHODS

Animals and tumors

C3H/HeN mice were purchased from Shizuoka Agricultural Cooperative for Experimental Animals, Kanagawa, Japan, and used at 8 to 10 weeks of age. MH134 hepatoma, MM102, MM46 and MM48 mammary carcinoma, and X5563 plasmacytoma, all derived from C3H/He strain mice, were maintained by intraperitoneal passages into syngeneic recipient mice.

Immunization procedure

C3H/HeN mice were immunized with MH134 tumor cells as reported previously.[7] Briefly, the C3H/HeN mice were injected intraperitoneally with 10^7 plaque-forming units (PFU) of vaccinia virus after being exposed to whole body irradiation at 150 R. Three or four weeks after immunization with the virus, the mice were given three intraperitoneal injections of 10^7 mitomycin C-treated, vaccinia virus-infected MH134 tumor cells, at intervals of one week. This procedure renders C3H/He mice resistant to an intraperitoneal challenge with 10^5 viable MH134 tumor cells.[7]

Antisera

C3H anti-MH134 antiserum was obtained from C3H/HeN mice immunized with MH134 tumor cells as described above. BALB/c anti-X5563 antiserum was obtained by intraperitoneal immunization of BALB/c mice with 10^7 X5563 tumor cells three times at two-week intervals. These antisera were inactivated at 56°C for 1 hour.

Fusion of immune spleen cells

Spleen cells from the immunized mice were fused with P3-X63-Ag8-U1 murine myeloma cells by polyethylene glycol (MW=3,350) (Sigma, St. Louis, Mo) and grown in HAT medium, as described elsewhere.[8]

Enzyme-linked immunosorbent assay (ELISA)

Hybridomas growing in HAT medium were selected by ELISA using a Monoab-screen P Kit (Zymed Laboratories, South San Fransisco, Calif) according to the method described in its procedure manual. Briefly, 3×10^5 target cells were suspended in 50 μl of undiluted hybridoma supernatant, antiserum diluted at 1:10, or HAT medium alone in a well of a microtiter plate (No. 76-321-05, Linbro, McLean, Va), left at room temperature for 1 hour, and then washed twice with 0.01 M phosphate buffered saline at pH 7.4 supplemented with 0.2% bovine serum albumin (0.2% BSA-PBS; Sigma). The cells treated with antibodies or medium were suspended in 50 μl of rabbit anti-mouse immunoglobulin (Ig) antiserum at a dilution of 1:200 and left at room temperature for 1 hour. After being washed three times with 0.2% BSA-PBS, the pellet was suspended in 50 μl of 0.2% BSA-PBS containing protein A-conjugated peroxidase at a dilution of 1:200, left at room temperature for 30 minutes, and washed three times with 0.2% BSA-PBS. The pellet was suspended in 100 μl citrate buffer at pH 4.2 containing 1% 2,2′-azino-di (3-ethylbenzthiazoline sulfonic acid) and 0.03% hydrogen peroxide, and incubated at 37°C for 10 minutes. Positive results were determined qualitatively by inspection, or quantitated by measuring the absorbance of the supernatant of the mixture with a photospectrometer at 420 nm after dilution of the supernatant with 2 ml of 2 mM sodium azide (Wako Pure Chemical Industries, Osaka, Japan).

ADCC effector cells

C3H/HeN mice were injected intraperitoneally with 1 ml of 10% thioglycolate (TG; Difco, Detroit, Mich). Four days after injection, peritoneal exudate cells (PEC) were obtained by lavage of the peritoneal cavities with Hanks medium (Nissui Pharmaceutical Co., Tokyo) supplemented with 5 U/ml heparin (Novo Industries, Bagsvaerd, Denmark). Peritoneal resident cells (PRC) of normal C3H/HeN mice were obtained in the same manner. These cells from three or four mice were pooled, washed twice with Hanks medium, and suspended in RPMI 1640 medium (Nissui Pharmaceutical Co.) supplemented with 10% fetal bovine serum (FBS; Filtron, Victoria, Australia), 100 units of penicillin per milliliter (Meiji Seika, Tokyo) 100 μg of streptomycin per milliliter (Meiji Seika), and 2 mM L-glutamine (Flow Laboratories, North Lyde, Australia). This medium was designated complete medium.

Unless otherwise noted, 5×10^5 PEC or PRC were added into a well of a microculture plate (No. 76-013-05, Linbro) and incubated for 2 hours at 37°C in a humidified 5% CO_2 atmosphere. After incubation, nonadherent cells were removed by repeated washings of the well with warmed 2% FBS-RPMI 1640 medium and 100 μl of complete medium was added to the well. Approximately 60% of the cells were left as adherent cells by the procedure in the cases of both TG-induced PEC and PRC. More than 92%

of the resulting adherent cells were phagocytic, as determined by phagocytosis of carbon particles. These were referred to as peritoneal exudate macrophages (PEMϕ) or peritoneal resident macrophages (PRMϕ), and used as effector cells. To obtain the nonadherent fraction of TG-induced PEC, adherent cells were removed by two consecutive 2-hour incubations of 10^7 PEC in a 60 mm dish (No. 25010, Corning, NY). The resulting nonadherent fraction contained less than 5% phagocytic cells, as determined by phagocytosis of carbon particles. The nonadherent cells were collected by centrifugation and suspended in complete medium. Spleen cells of normal C3H/HeN mice were prepared by teasing spleens in 2% FBS-RPMI 1640 medium, washed twice, and suspended in complete medium. Five hundred thousand nonadherent PEC or spleen cells in 100 μl of complete medium were seeded into a well of a microculture plate (No. 76-013-05, Linbro), and used as effector cells.

ADCC

One million target cells suspended in 1 ml of complete medium were labeled with 5 μCi of 5-[^{125}I] iodo-2′-deoxyuridine (Amersham, Buckinghamshire, U.K.) in a well of a 4-well culture plate (Nunc, Roskilde, Denmark) at 37°C for 4 hours in a humidified 5% CO_2 atmosphere, as described previously.[9] After labeling, the cells were washed three times with 2% FBS-RPMI 1640 medium and suspended in complete medium at a cell density of 10^5/ml. Sixty microliters of the cell suspension containing 6×10^3 labeled target cells was mixed with the same volume of undiluted or diluted hybridoma supernatant or antiserum and kept at 4°C for 30 minutes. One hundred microliters of the mixture containing 5×10^3 labeled target cells was added to a well containing effector cells in 100 μl of complete medium. Unless otherwise noted, the plate was incubated at 37°C for 24 hours in a humidified 5% CO_2 atmosphere. After incubation, the radioactivity of 100 μl of the supernatant was counted in a gamma counter. Percent specific cytolysis was calculated by the following formula:

$$\%\ \text{Specific cytolysis} = \frac{\text{Experimental cpm} - \text{spontaneous cpm}}{\text{Total cpm} - \text{spontaneous cpm}} \times 100$$

Spontaneous cpm, measured by incubation of target cells alone, was less than 5% of total cpm after 24 hours of incubation.

Complement-dependent cytotoxicity (CDC)

One million target cells in 0.1 ml of complete medium were labeled with 100 μCi of $Na_2{}^{51}CrO_4$ (Japan Atomic Energy Research Institute, Tokyo) for 1 hour at 37°C, washed three times, and suspended in complete medium at a cell density of 2×10^5/ml. Fifty microliters of the cell suspension was mixed with the same volume of antibody solution in a well of a microculture plate (No. 76-013-05, Linbro), and kept at 4°C for 30 minutes. The supernatant was then discarded by centrifugation and 100 μl of rabbit serum absorbed with C3H/HeN spleen cells was added at a dilution of 1:8. The plate was incubated at 37°C for 45 minutes. The ratioactivity in 50 μl of the supernatant was counted and percent specific cytolysis was calculated as described above.

Activation of peritoneal macrophages by cell-wall skeleton of *Nocardia rubra* (N-CWS)

C3H/HeN mice were injected intraperitoneally with 100 μg of N-CWS. Four days after injection, PEMϕ were obtained from these mice as described above, and used as effector cells.

RESULTS

Binding specificity of monoclonal antibodies using ELISA and CDC

In preliminary experiments using ELISA, four hybridomas were found to secrete antibodies against MH134 tumor cells constantly. After being cloned twice by limiting dilution, they were named 3H1, 7C2, 11G2 and 12A2. Immunodiffusion analysis with rabbit anti-mouse immunoglobulin (Ig) antisera (Meloy, Springfield, Va) showed that the monoclonal antibodies 3H1, 7C2, 11G2 and 12A2 were IgG2a, IgM, IgG1 and IgG2a respectively. The binding specificity of the monoclonal antibodies was determined by ELISA using cells of five syngeneic tumor lines derived from C3H/He strain mice, MH134, MM102, MM46, MM48 and X5563; the results are summarized in Fig. 1. Of the five kinds of target cells, 3H1 bound only to MH134 tumor cells. Binding of the three other monoclonal antibodies, 7C2, 11G2 and 12A2, was observed not only with MH134 but also with MM102 and MM46 tumor cells. None of these four monoclonal antibodies bound to either MM48 or X5563 tumor cells. In the CDC assay, 3H1, 7C2 and 12A2 but not 11G2 exhibited cytotoxicity against MH134 tumor cells in the presence of rabbit complement. The specificity using target cell lysis was identical to that seen using ELISA (Fig. 1).

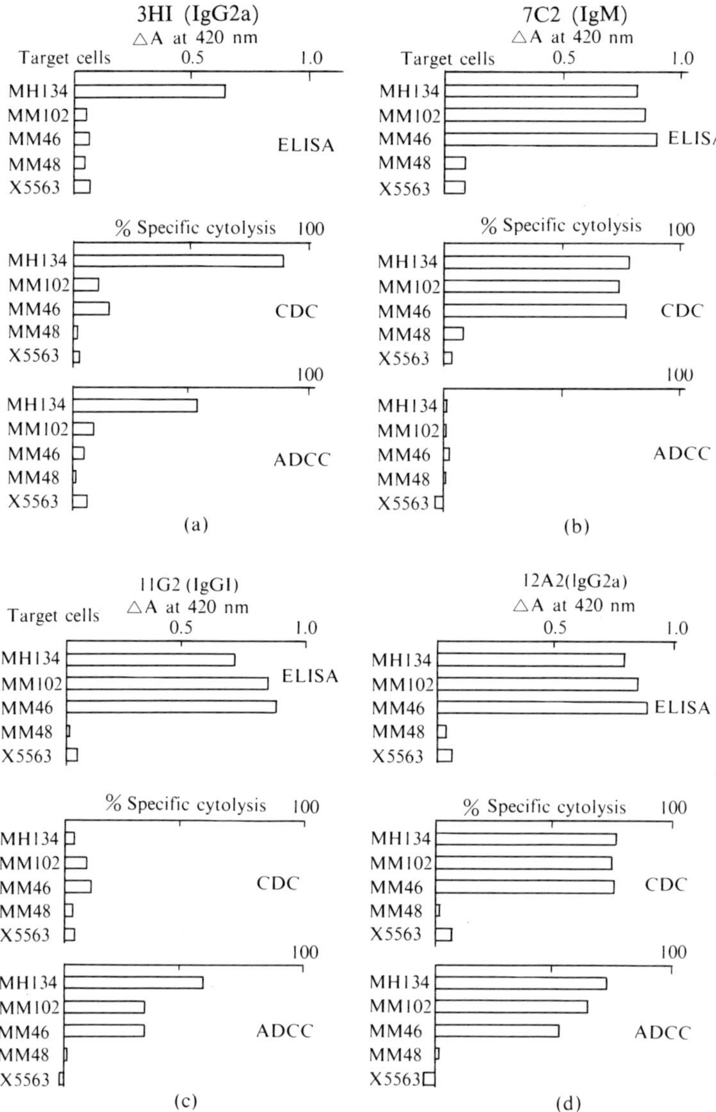

Fig. 1 In ELISA, △A is the difference between the absorbance of the supernatant at 420 nm in the reaction using monoclonal antibodies and in that using medium as the first antibody. In CDC assay, 10^4 ^{51}Cr-labeled target cells were suspended in 100 μl of hybridoma supernatant at a dilution of 1:2 and kept at 4°C for 30 minutes. The supernatant was discarded by centrifugation, and 100 μl of rabbit serum was added to the well at a dilution of 1:8. Cytotoxicity was assayed for 45 minutes. In ADCC assay, 5×10^3 ^{125}I-labeled target cells were suspended in 100 μl of hybridoma supernatant at a dilution of 1:2 and kept at 4°C for 30 minutes. The mixture was added to a well containing PEMϕ obtained from 5×10^5 TG-induced PEC. Cytotoxicity was assayed for 24 hours.

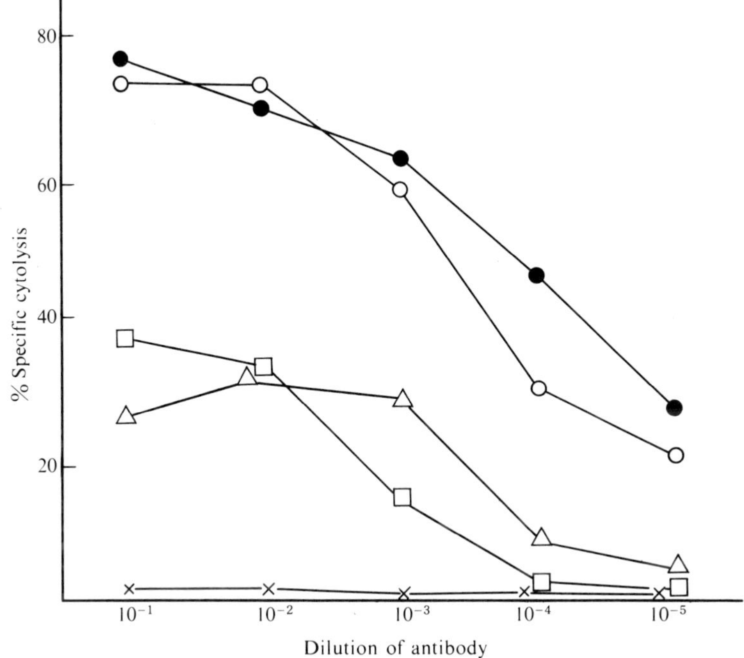

Fig. 2 ADCC was measured in the presence of hybridoma supernatant 3H1 (□—□), 7C2 (×——×), 11G2 (△——△), 12A2 (○——○) or C3H anti-MH134 antiserum (●——●) at the indicated dilutions. PEMϕ obtained from 5×10^5 TG-induced PEC were used as effector cells. Cytotoxicity was assayed for 24 hours.

Induction of ADCC against MH134 tumor cells by 12A2 monoclonal antibody

To determine whether the monoclonal antibodies could induce ADCC against MH134 tumor cells, a cytotoxicity assay against the tumor cells was performed in the presence of 12A2 using TG-induced PEMϕ as effector cells. Apparent cytotoxicity was exhibited by PEMϕ in the presence of 12A2 but not in its absence. The cytotoxicity became apparent after 8 hours of incubation and increased with prolongation of the incubation period. Cytotoxicity was also apparent when adherent cells obtained from 6.25×10^4 PEC per well were used as effector cells, and increased with an increase in the effector to target cell ratio. 12A2 did not show any cytotoxicity in the absence of PEMϕ. When the unbound antibody present in the target cell suspension was removed by centrifugation before the addition of the target cells to the effector cells, the resulting cytotoxicity was the same as that exhibited in the presence of the antibody throughout the cytotoxicity assay.

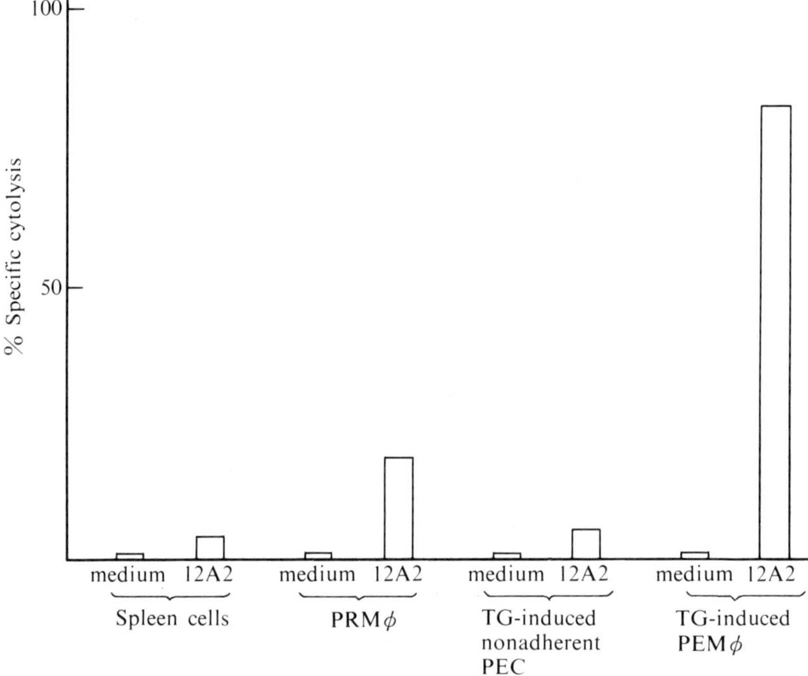

Fig. 3 Spleen cells or TG-induced nonadherent PEC (5×10^5 per well, E:T = 100:1) were seeded and used as effector cells. PRMφ and TG-induced PEMφ were obtained by repeated washings of wells containing 5×10^5 peritoneal cells. Supernatant of 12A2 hybridoma or C3H anti-MH134 antiserum was added to 5×10^3 MH134 tumor cells at a dilution of 1:2 or 1:10 respectively. Cytotoxicity was assayed for 24 hours.

Specificity of ADCC induced by the monoclonal antibodies

Using cells of the five tumor lines, target specificity of ADCC induced by the monoclonal antibodies was examined (Fig. 1a-d). 3H1 induced cytotoxicity only against MH134 tumor cells, whereas both 11G2 and 12A2 induced cytotoxicity not only against MH134 but also against MM102 and MM46 tumor cells. 7C2 did not cause cytotoxicity against cells of any tumor lines. None of these monoclonal antibodies induced ADCC against either MM48 or X5563 tumor cells.

Comparison of the ability of the monoclonal antibodies to induce ADCC

Using TG-induced PEMφ as effector cells, ADCC against MH134 tumor cells was compared among 3H1, 7C2, 11G2, 12A2 and C3H anti-MH134 antiserum at dilutions ranging from 1:10 to 1:100,000. 12A2 induced the

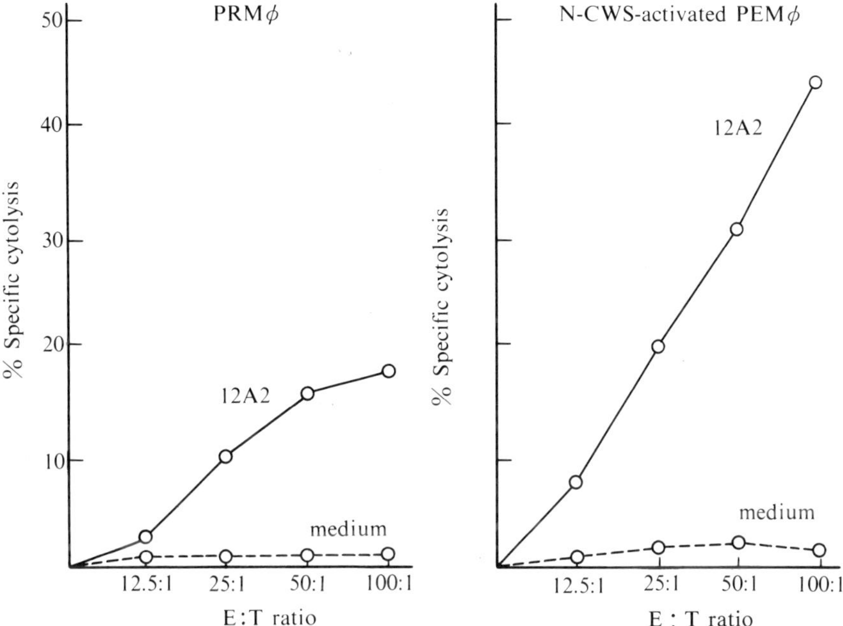

Fig. 4 ADCC was measured in the absence (○----○) or in the presence (○——○) of 12A2 hybridoma supernatant at a dilution of 1:2. Adherent cells obtained from PRC (left) or N-CWS-activated PEC (right) at a cell number ranging from 6.25×10^4 per well (E:T=12.5:1) to 5×10^5 per well (E:T=100:1) were used as effector cells. Cytotoxicity was assayed for 24 hours.

highest cytotoxicity among the four monoclonal antibodies, which was comparable to the cytotoxicity induced by the antiserum (Fig. 2). The cytotoxicity induced by 3H1 and 11G2 was significantly lower than that induced by 12A2. 7C2 did not induce cytotoxicity at any dilution.

Effector cell analysis of ADCC induced by 12A2 monoclonal antibody

Effector cells of ADCC against MH134 tumor cells induced by 12A2 were analysed by using spleen cells, PRMϕ, TG-induced PEMϕ, and TG-induced nonadherent PEC (Fig. 3). Spleen cells of normal mice did not exhibit any cytotoxicity in the presence of 12A2. PRMϕ obtained from normal mice showed low but detectable ADCC, which was, however, significantly lower than that mediated by TG-induced PEMϕ. Non-adherent cells were separated from TG-induced PEC, and their cytotoxicity against MH134 tumor cells was compared with that of TG-induced PEMϕ in the presence of 12A2. The cytotoxicity mediated by nonadherent PEC was almost negligible, while PEMϕ exhibited high cytotoxicity.

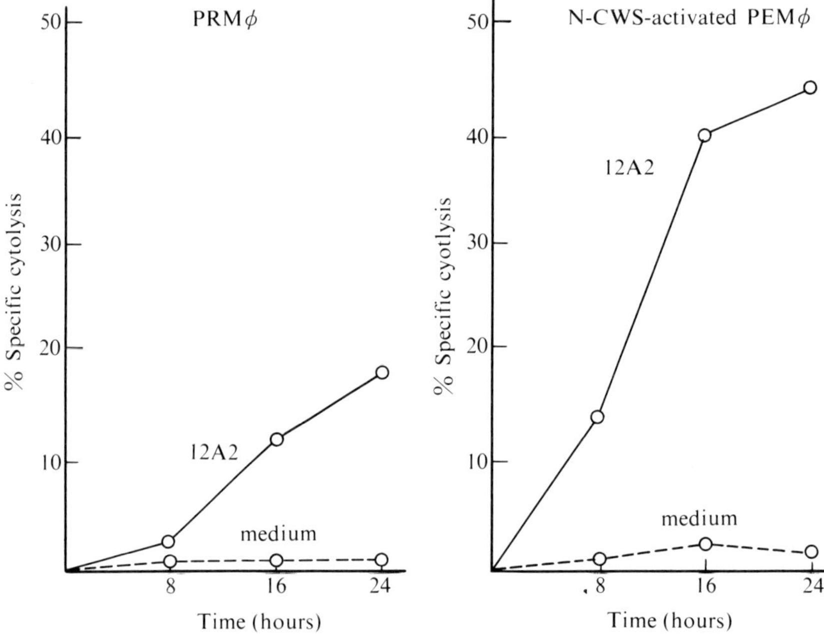

Fig. 5 ADCC was measured in the absence (○----○) or in the presence (○——○) of 12A2 hybridoma supernatant at a dilution of 1:2. Adherent cells obtained from 5×10^5 PRC (left) or 5×10^5 N-CWS-activated PEC (right) were used as effector cells. Cytotoxicity was assayed for the indicated periods.

ADCC of PEMϕ induced by N-CWS

The effect of N-CWS on the reaction was investigated by using PEMϕ induced by N-CWS. N-CWS-activated PEMϕ exhibited high cytotoxicity against MH134 tumor cells in the presence of 12A2, as compared with that shown by PRMϕ from normal mice (Figs. 4 and 5).

DISCUSSION

In this study, four hybridomas constructed by fusion of murine myeloma cells with spleen cells of C3H/HeN mice immunized with syngeneic MH134 hepatoma cells were shown to secrete monoclonal antibodies which can bind to tumor cells in an ELISA. Immunodiffusion analysis with rabbit anti-mouse Ig antisera revealed that monoclonal antibodies 3H1, 7C2, 11G2 and 12A2 were IgG2a, IgM, IgG1 and IgG2a respectively. Among cells of five syngeneic tumor lines, MH134, MM102, MM46, MM48 and X5563, all derived from C3H/He strain mice, 3H1 bound specifically to MH134 tumor cells, whereas 7C2, 11G2 and 12A2 reacted not only with MH134 but also with MM102 and MM46 tumor cells. This result strongly suggests that MH134 tumor cells possess at least two kinds of tumor-associated antigen (TAA) on their cell surfaces, one uniquely expressed by MH134 tumor cells and recognized by 3H1, the other commonly shared by MH134, MM102 and MM46 tumor cells and determined by the other three monoclonal antibodies. The latter may be a part of the MM antigen (term used by Chang et al.[10]), since MM102 and MM46 tumor cells are known to be MM antigen-positive tumor lines, while MM48 tumor cells are a negative line. These possibilities should be examined further by using cells of tumor lines other than those used in the present study. Furthermore, it will be of interest to investigate whether the antigenic determinant recognized by 3H1 shares a part of that determined by the other three monoclonal antibodies, or whether these two determinants are independently displayed.

Three of the monoclonal antibodies, the exception being 7C2, were shown to be able to induce ADCC against MH134 tumor cells using TG-induced PEMϕ as effector cells. The extent of lysis was influenced by the effector to target cell ratio, the incubation time and the amount of antibody added to the reaction mixture. It is unlikely that the cytotoxicity is mediated by complement produced by PEMϕ during the cytotoxicity assay, because 7C2 which is a IgM subclass, did not cause any cytotoxicity in the assay. The target specificity of ADCC induced by these three monoclonal antibodies was identical to that seen using ELISA.

Effector cell analysis of ADCC induced by 12A2 revealed that the cytotoxicity is mediated by the adherent fraction but not by the nonadherent fraction of TG-induced PEC. Peritoneal resident macrophages exhibited a low level of cytotoxicity. Normal spleen cells did not show any cytotoxicity in the presence of the antibody. These results indicate clearly that the cytotoxicity is mediated by macrophages, and that stimulation of macrophages is essential for augmentation of the reaction. In other words, as well as an increase in the number of receptors for the Fc portion of IgG (Fc receptors), elevated levels of phagocytic activity, membrane mobility, hydrolytic enzyme activity or other biological activities in macrophages may play an important role in the destruction of tumor cells by macrophages in the presence of antibodies. In the present study, a single intraperitoneal injection with thioglycolate was found to be enough to render peritoneal macrophages capable of exhibiting high levels of ADCC, while the stimulus was not enough to activate the cells to kill tumor cells in the absence of antibodies. Using C3H anti-MM46 antiserum, Yamasaki et al. have reported a similar phenomenon, that peritoneal macrophages of C3H/He mice can mediate ADCC against MM46 tumor cells when they are stimulated by an intraperitoneal injection with glycogen, lipopolysaccharide or *Mycobacterium bovis* BCG.[11] On the other hand, it is well known that, as well as macrophages, Fc receptor-positive lymphocytes can act as effector cells of ADCC. It is not clear why neither spleen cells nor nonadherent PEC exhibited apparent ADCC against cells of these tumor lines in the presence of monoclonal antibodies or the conventional antisera. It seems possible that Fc receptor-positive lymphocytes at an activated level may mediate the cytotoxicity.

The development of monoclonal antibodies which can induce ADCC against human tumor cells has been reported by several investigators.[1,2,5] In their reports, the cytotoxicity has been shown to be mediated by murine spleen cells or human peripheral blood mononuclear cells. However, they used these effector cells at high effector-to-target cell ratios ranging from 100:1 to 800:1 without fractionation. Therefore, the cytotoxicity shown in their studies might have been mediated not only by Fc receptor-positive lymphocytes but also by macrophages contaminating the effector cell population. More recently, Herlin and Koprowski have shown that mouse peritoneal macrophages exhibit high cytotoxicity against human tumor cells in the presence of monoclonal antibodies.[4]

Seto et al.[3] reported a similar phenomenon, that some monoclonal antibodies against MM46 tumor cells induce antibody-dependent macrophage-mediated cytotoxicity (ADMC) against the tumor cells. They developed two kinds of monoclonal antibodies with different binding specificities. One was directed to the MM antigen, which is closely associated with or identical to the Ly-6.2 alloantigen, and the other to an antigen which is restricted to MM antigen-positive tumors. In their report, monoclonal antibodies of the former group were shown to be able to induce ADMC against MM46 tumor cells. However, it is unclear whether antibodies of the latter group, antibodies which recognize a unique TAA on MM46 tumor cells, could exhibit the cytotoxicity. In contrast, the present study indicated clearly that ADMC against MH134 tumor cells was induced not only by monoclonal antibodies against a commonly shared TAA on the tumor cells (11G2 and 12A2), but also by an antibody which reacted specifically with the tumor cells (3H1).

3H1, 7C2 and 12A2 fixed rabbit complement, resulting in complement-dependent cytotoxicity whose specificity of target cell lysis was identical with that seen using ELISA or ADCC (data not shown). As expected since its isotype is IgG1, 11G2 did not fix complement. This finding suggests that complement-dependent cytotoxicity might play a role if these three monoclonal antibodies were to exhibit therapeutic effects in mice bearing MH134 hepatoma. However, these monoclonal antibodies will contribute to investigations of possible involvement of ADMC in tumor cell destruction *in vivo*, because they have different activities regarding ADMC and complement-dependent cytotoxicity, while all of them show the same target specificity.

The authors have investigated the effect of adjuvant immunotherapy with cell-wall skeleton of *Nocardia rubra* (N-CWS) for malignancies,[12] and reported that the effect of N-CWS is based mainly on activation of macrophages.[9] In preliminary experiments, mouse peritoneal macrophages activated by N-CWS exhibited low cytotoxicity against MH134 tumor cells and the cytotoxicity was significantly elevated by the addition of the monoclonal antibodies. Therefore, these monoclonal antibodies will provide important information regarding new immunotherapies for malignancies with monoclonal antibodies and biological response modifiers which can activate macrophages. Further studies are currently under way.

REFERENCES

1. Herlin, D., Herlin, M., Steplewski, Z. and Koprowski, H. (1979): Monoclonal antibodies in cell-mediated cytotoxicity against human melanoma and colorectal carcinoma. *Eur. J. Immunol., 9*, 657.
2. Imai, K., Ng, A.-K., Glassy, M.C. and Ferrone, S. (1981): ADCC of cultured human cells: Analysis with monoclonal antibodies to human melanoma-associated antigens. *Scand. J. Immunol., 14*, 369.
3. Seto, M., Takahashi, T., Nakamura, S., Matsudaira, S. and Nishizuka, Y. (1983): *In vivo* antitumor effects of monoclonal antibodies with different immunoglobulin classes. *Cancer Res., 43*, 4768.
4. Herlin, D. and Koprowski, H. (1982): IgG2a monoclonal antibodies inhibit human tumor growth through interaction with effector cells. *Proc. Natl. Acad. Sci. U.S.A., 79*, 4761.
5. Schulz, G., Bumol, T.F. and Reisfeld, R.A. (1983): Monoclonal antibody-directed effector cells selectively lyse human melanoma cells *in vitro* and *in vivo*. *Proc. Natl. Acad. Sci. U.S.A., 80*, 5407.
6. Fujiwara, H., Shimizu, Y., Takai, Y., Wakamiya, N., Ueda, S., Kato, S. and Hamaoka, T. (1984): The augmentation of tumor-specific immunity by virus-help. I. Demonstration of vaccinia virus-reactive helper T cell activity involved in enhanced induction of cytotoxic T-lymphocyte and antibody responses. *Eur. J. Immunol., 14*, 171.
7. Shimizu, Y., Fujiwara, H., Ueda, S., Wakamiya, N., Kato, S. and Hamaoka, T. (1985): The augmentation of tumor-specific immunity by virus-help. II. Enhanced induction of cytotoxic T-lymphocyte and antibody responses to tumor antigens by vaccinia virus-reactive helper T cells. *Eur. J. Immunol., 14*, 839.
8. Forster, H.K., Gudat, F.G., Girard, M.-F., Albrecht, R., Schmidt, J., Ludwig, C. and Obrecht, J.- P. (1982): Monoclonal antibody against a membrane antigen characterizing leukemic human B-lymphocytes. *Cancer Res., 42*, 1927.
9. Ogura, T., Namba, M., Hirao, F., Yamamura, Y. and Azuma, I. (1979): Association of macrophage activation with antitumor effect on rat syngeneic fibrosarcoma by *Nocardia rubra* cell-wall skeleton. *Cancer Res., 39*, 4706.
10. Chang, S., Nowinski, R.C., Nishioka, K. and Irie, R.F. (1972): Immunological studies on mouse mammary tumors. VI. Further characterization of a mammary tumor antigen and its distribution in lymphatic cells of allogeneic mice. *Int. J.*

Cancer, *9*, 409.

11. Yamazaki, M., Shinoda, H., Suzuki, Y. and Mizuno, D. (1976): Two-step mechanism of macrophage-mediated tumor lysis *in vitro*. *Gann,* *67*, 741.
12. Yamamura, Y., Ogura, T., Sakatani, M., Hirao, F., Kishimoto, S., Fukuoka, M., Takada, M., Kawahara, M., Furuse, K., Kawahara, O., Ikegami, H. and Ogawa, N. (1983): Randomized controlled study of adjuvant immunotherapy with *Nocardia rubra* cell wall skeleton for inoperable lung cancer. *Cancer Res.,* *43*, 5575.

Immune interferon induces mouse IgG2a- and IgG3-dependent cellular cytotoxicity in a human monocytic cell line (U937)

Yukio Akiyama, Michael D. Lubeck, Zenon Steplewski and Hilary Koprowski

SUMMARY

The effects of natural and recombinant human γ interferon (IFN) on mouse monoclonal antibody (MoAb)-dependent cellular cytotoxicity (ADCC) mediated by a human monocytic cell line, U937, were examined. The efficiency of different isotypes of mouse MoAb in inducing ADCC was also investigated. U937 cell-mediated ADCC against sheep or ox red blood cell targets was minimal. However, after incubation with human purified γIFN, U937 cells exhibited increased IgG2a- and IgG3-dependent lytic activity, whereas their IgG1- and IgG2b-dependent lytic activity was low. ADCC stimulated by γIFN was inhibited by protein A. The number of receptors for the Fc portion of IgG (FcR) for mouse IgG2a and IgG3 on U937 cells, as detected by IgG antibody-sensitized erythrocyte (EA7S) rosette formation, was significantly enhanced by γIFN. In contrast, FcR for mouse IgG1 and IgG2b were not detected even after γIFN stimulation. When mouse peritoneal exudate cells (PEC) were used, FcR for all IgG isotypes were easily detected, and all IgG isotypes mediated ADCC. Taken together, these results indicate that γIFN induces U937 ADCC with mouse IgG2a and IgG3, partly through augmentation of FcR expression. Recombinant γIFN showed the same effect as natural γIFN. These effects of γIFN were completely abrogated by anti-γIFN serum but not by anti-αIFN or normal rabbit serum. These findings suggest the possibility of using antitumor MoAbs of these isotypes in combination with γIFN in the immunotherapy of human cancer.

INTRODUCTION

Several murine monoclonal antibodies (MoAb) have been shown to be effective in inhibiting tumor growth,[1–4] e.g., murine MoAb against human colorectal carcinoma (CRC) cells specifically inhibit tumor growth in nude mice[3] and have been shown to depend on host macrophages for tumor cell destruction.[2] Furthermore, human macrophages as well as cultured human monocytes have been found to express receptors for the Fc portion of IgG (FcR) that cross-react strongly with murine IgG2a; such macrophages kill human CRC cells in the presence of anti-CRC MoAb *in vitro*.[5] These results suggest that FcR is important for the antibody-dependent cellular cytotoxicity (ADCC) of mononuclear phagocytes and for the tumoricidal action of MoAb.

Immune interferon (γIFN) has various biologic activities. In addition to its antiviral and antiproliferative activities, γIFN reportedly stimulates tumoricidal activity in human monocytes.[6] Furthermore, recent studies have shown that γIFN causes a dramatic increase in the expression of FcR for human monomeric IgG1 on human monocytes and on myelomonocytic human cells.[7,8]

In the present study, the authors examined whether monocyte-like U937 cells are able to mediate mouse MoAb-dependent lysis after treatment with γIFN. The efficiency of different isotypes of mouse MoAb in inducing ADCC was also compared.

MATERIALS AND METHODS

Stimulation of U937 cells

U937 cells were cultured in 24-well tissue culture plates (Costar, 3524, Cambridge, Mass) at an initial concentration of 5×10^5/ml in a total volume of 2 ml with or without γIFN at various concentrations in RPMI 1640 medium supplemented with 10% fetal bovine serum, 2 mM glutamine and 50 μg/ml gentamicin. After several hours of culture, cells were harvested and washed three times.

Interferon

Purified human γIFN was obtained from Interferon Science, Inc., New Brunswick, NJ. Human recombinant γIFN from *E. coli* was kindly supplied by Genentech, Inc., San Francisco, Calif. Rabbit antiserum against human γIFN and sheep antiserum against human αIFN were obtained from Interferon Science, Inc.

Monoclonal antibodies

IgG2a, IgG2b and IgG3 MoAbs reacting with sheep red blood cells (SRBC) were prepared by Dr. W.C. Raschke, La Jolla Cancer Research Foundation, La Jolla, Calif, and obtained through American Type Culture Collection, Rockville, Md. A MoAb (IgG1) reacting with ox red blood cells (ORBC) and cross-reactive with SRBC was established in the authors' laboratory. MoAbs were used as unconcentrated hybridoma culture supernatants.

Cytotoxicity assay

ADCC against SRBC or ORBC was quantified as described previously.[9]

IgG antibody-sensitized erythrocyte (EA7S) rosette formation

SRBC (or ORBC) were coated with equivalent amounts of antibodies to saturate binding sites and FcR were detected as described previously.[5]

RESULTS

Effect of γIFN on mouse MoAb-dependent ADCC mediated by U937 cells

The ability of various doses of purified human γIFN to enhance mouse MoAb-dependent U937 ADCC to RBC targets was tested. The ADCC activity mediated by U937 cells cultured in the absence of γIFN was usually low or barely detectable (Table 1). IFN induced a dose-dependent IgG2a- and IgG3-dependent cytotoxicity in U937 cells reaching a plateau after incubation with γIFN for 36 hours. In contrast, IgG1- and IgG2b-dependent ADCC were increased only slightly under these conditions. Since the IgG1 MoAb against ORBC also reacts with SRBC, IgG1-dependent ADCC to SRBC targets was also determined. Under these conditions, γIFN-stimulated U937 cells mediated the same level of ADCC activity against ORBC targets (data not shown). When murine

Table 1 Differential stimulation of mouse IgG-dependent lysis by γIFN-treated U937 cells*

Concentration of γIFN (units/ml)	Period of stimulation (hours)	ADCC with MoAb (%)**			
		IgG1	IgG2a	IgG2b	IgG3
0	0	0.6	0.7	−0.4	0.8
10	18	0.6	2.9	0.9	2.2
	36	1.1	4.1	0.9	3.2
	54	1.2	4.7	0.8	3.5
100	18	1.1	11.1	1.3	12.9
	36	3.3	16.7	1.6	17.8
	54	2.5	15.8	3.2	18.4
500	18	3.1	15.7	1.2	14.7
	36	4.2	22.0	2.1	21.8
	54	2.9	22.5	2.6	19.2
1,000	18	1.6	17.4	2.0	16.5
	36	3.3	23.8	3.4	23.7
	54	4.1	25.0	3.8	22.4

* U937 cells (5×10^5/ml) were incubated for various periods of time with γIFN. Cells were then assayed for ADCC against ^{51}Cr-labeled SRBC or ORBC targets at an effector to target cell ratio of 0.5:1. MoAb was used as hybridoma culture supernatant at a 1:5 dilution. Spontaneous cytotoxicity by untreated or γIFN-treated U937 cells in the absence of MoAb was not detected.

** Means of three separate experiments. Values represent percentage of specific lysis at the effector to target ratio of 0.5:1.

Table 2 Blocking by protein A of ADCC induced by γIFN*

Pretreatment	Protein A concentration (μg/ml)	ADCC with MoAb (%)**	
		IgG2a	IgG3
Medium	0	1.2	0.7
γIFN (500 units/ml)	0	20.6	21.2
	1	10.4	21.6
	5	9.4	5.2
	20	6.6	3.6
	80	4.1	2.7

* U937 cells (5×10^5/ml) were incubated for 36 hours with or without γIFN. Cells were then washed and assayed for ADCC against ^{51}Cr-labeled SRBC targets. Targets were mixed with MoAb and incubated alone or with protein A for 30 minutes before addition of effector cells. Effector to target cell ratio was 0.5:1 and MoAb were used at 1:5 dilution.

** Means of triplicate cultures.

peritoneal exudate cells (PEC) were tested for ADCC to RBC targets under the same conditions as used for U937 effector cells, IgG2a, IgG1 and IgG2b MoAbs stimulated similarly efficient RBC lysis. IgG3-dependent ADCC levels using PEC were slightly lower than ADCC mediated by IgG of other isotypes (data not shown). To determine the

Table 3 Differential enhancement expression of FcR for mouse IgG on U937 cells treated with γIFN*

Cells	Concentration of γIFN (units/ml)	Period of stimulation (hours)	EA7S rosette-forming cells (%)**			
			IgG1	IgG2a	IgG2b	IgG3
U937	0	None	— †	7.2	—	0.5
	10	12	—	18.7	—	1.3
		24	—	23.4	—	1.8
		36	—	20.7	—	1.6
	100	12	—	21.6	—	4.5
		24	—	22.2	—	4.6
		36	—	21.9	—	4.2
	1,000	12	—	24.6	—	4.1
		24	—	25.1	—	3.8
		36	—	25.6	—	3.9
Murine PEC	None	None	52.5	42.8	63.0	54.3

* U937 cells (5×10^{5}/ml) were cultured in the presence of different concentrations of γIFN. An aliquot of the cells was taken at the time points indicated, washed and tested for FcR expression by rosette formation. Thioglycolate-induced murine PEC were used as controls.

** Means of three separate experiments. Data for murine PEC are means of two separate experiments.

† —: Not detectable.

role of FcR on U937 cells in ADCC, the effect of protein A on mouse IgG2a- and IgG3-dependent ADCC was examined. γIFN-induced ADCC was inhibited by protein A in a dose-dependent manner (Table 2).

Effect of γIFN on expression of FcR for mouse IgG on U937 cells

FcR for mouse IgG2a and IgG3 were detected on 7.2% and 0.5% of the population of unstimulated U937 cells respectively, whereas FcR cross-reactive with mouse IgG1 and IgG2b were not detected (Table 3). After stimulation with γIFN, there was a steady increase in the number of rosette-forming cells for mouse IgG2a. γIFN also induced a significant increase in FcR expression for mouse IgG3; however, binding of IgG1 and IgG2b to U937 cells was not detected by this assay even after γIFN stimulation. An apparent increase of IgG2a-and IgG3-specific FcR induced by γIFN was already observed at a γIFN concentration of 10 units/ml. Kinetic studies indicated that the percentage of EA7S-rosette-forming cells reached a plateau after 12 hours of incubation. The possibility that contaminating endotoxin accounted for the stimulation of U937 cells by γIFN could be excluded, since addition of polymyxin B and lipopolysaccharide did not affect the activity of γIFN (data not shown).

Table 4 Neutralization of γIFN-induced stimulation of ADCC and FcR expression by antiserum to γIFN[a]

Pretreatment		ADCC (%)[b]		EA7S rosette-forming cells (%)	
		IgG2a	IgG3	IgG2a	IgG3
Medium		1.1	0.6	5.1	0.4
γIFN		20.5	19.6	25.0	4.3
γIFN+anti-γIFN serum	(250 units/ml)[c]	4.8	5.0	—[d]	—
	(500 units/ml)	2.0	0.4	—	—
	(1,000 units/ml)	0.5	0.3	—	—
γIFN+anti-αIFN serum	(250 units/ml)	24.0	18.8	20.6	3.6
	(500 units/ml)	23.8	23.0	21.6	3.9
	(1,000 units/ml)	23.5	17.9	22.7	3.8

[a] γIFN (500 units/ml) was neutralized with different dilutions of anti-γIFN antiserum for 45 minutes at 37°C and added to the cultures. Anti-αIFN serum was used as the control. U937 cells (5×10^5/ml) were stimulated for 36 hours before assays. In ADCC assay, the effector to target cell ratio was 0.5:1 and MoAb were used at a 1:5 dilution.

[b] Means of duplicate cultures from three separate experiments.

[c] Neutralization units.

[d] —: Not detectable.

Inhibition of γIFN-induced ADCC and FcR expression by anti-IFN serum

To identify γIFN conclusively as an enhancer of mouse MoAb-dependent lysis and FcR expression for mouse MoAb, the effect of anti-γIFN serum on γIFN-induced enhancement of ADCC and FcR expression was tested. Anti-γIFN serum treatment abolished the capacity of γIFN to induce IgG2a- and IgG3-dependent ADCC (Table 4). Furthermore, no rosette formation for IgG2a and IgG3 FcR was observed at the inducing concentration of γIFN used. Neither sheep anti-αIFN serum nor normal rabbit serum at the same concentrations inhibited the induction of ADCC and FcR expression by γIFN. The effects of recombinant γIFN were similar to those of natural γIFN (data not shown).

DISCUSSION

These experiments demonstrated that natural and recombinant γIFN stimulate a human monocytic cell line, U937, to lyse SRBC or ORBC *in vitro* in the presence of mouse MoAb. γIFN-stimulated U937 cells armed with IgG2a or IgG3 MoAb efficiently lysed target cells. The γIFN-induced enhancement of ADCC activity was accompanied by increased expression of FcR for mouse IgG2a and IgG3. FcR for mouse IgG1 and

IgG2b on U937 cells were not detected after γIFN stimulation.

Murine macrophages have at least three different FcR for mouse IgG of different isotypes.[10,11] Two different FcR for human IgG have been identified on human leukocytes.[12] A high-affinity FcR for human IgG1 is present on human monocytes but not on polymorphonuclear leukocytes (PMN), and a low-affinity FcR is present on PMN and NK/K cells but not on monocytes. Recent studies have shown that the binding of IgG1 monomers to U937 cells is detected following activation by lymphokines; enhanced expression of the low-affinity FcR was not concomitantly observed,[13] demonstrating the independent regulation of human leukocyte FcRs. Taken together, these results suggest that the human U937 cell and monocyte FcR is analogous to the mouse FcR1. In addition, γIFN-stimulated U937 cells exhibited significant FcR expression for IgG3. This finding is consistent with previous results[8] which demonstrate that IgG2a and IgG3, but not IgG1 or IgG2b, effectively compete with human IgG1 for binding to untreated and γIFN-treated human monocyte and promyelocytic cell lines.

These findings that γIFN induces FcR expression and ADCC with specificity for mouse IgG2a and IgG3 MoAb suggest the possibility of using antitumor MoAbs of these isotypes in combination with γIFN in the immunotherapy of human cancer.

ACKNOWLEDGEMENT

This research was supported by Research Grants CA10815, CA21124, CA25874 and CA37864, and NIAID Grant AI-19607.

REFERENCES

1. Badger, C.C. and Bernstein, I.D. (1983): Therapy of murine leukemia with monoclonal antibody against a normal differentiation antigen. *J. Exp. Med., 157*, 828.
2. Herlyn, D. and Koprowski, H. (1982): IgG2a monoclonal antibodies inhibit human tumor growth through interaction with effector cells. *Proc. Natl. Acad. Sci. U.S.A., 79*, 4761.
3. Herlyn, D., Steplewski, S., Herlyn, M. and Koprowski, H. (1980): Inhibition of growth of colorectal carcinoma in nude mice by monoclonal antibody. *Cancer Res., 40*, 717.
4. Young, W.W., Jr. and Hakomori, S. (1981): Therapy of mouse lymphoma with monoclonal antibodies to glycolipid: secretion of low antigenic variants *in vivo. Science, 211*, 487.
5. Steplewski, Z., Lubeck, M.D. and Koprowski, H. (1983): Human macrophages armed with murine immunoglobulin G2a antibodies to tumors destroy human cancer cells. *Science, 221*, 865.

6. Le, J., Prensky, W., Yip, Y.K., Chang, Z.L., Hoffman, T., Stevenson, H.C., Balazs, I., Sadlik, J.R. and Vilcek, J. (1983): Activation of human monocyte cytotoxicity by natural and recombinant immune interferon. *J. Immunol., 131,* 2821.
7. Guyre, P.M., Morganelli, P.M. and Miller, R. (1983): Recombinant immune interferon increases immunoglobulin G Fc receptors on cultured human mononuclear phagocytes. *J. Clin. Invest., 72*, 393.
8. Perussia, B., Dayton, E.T., Lazarus, R., Fanning, V. and Trinchieri, G. (1983): Immune interferon induces the receptor for monomeric IgG1 on human monocytic and myeloid cells. *J. Exp. Med., 158*, 1092.
9. Larrick, J.W., Fisher, D.G., Anderson, S.J. and Koren, S. (1980): Characterization of a human macrophage-like cell line stimulated *in vitro*: a model of macrophage functions. *J. Immunol., 125*, 6.
10. Diamond, B. and Yelton, D.E. (1981): A new Fc receptor on mouse macrophages binding IgG3. *J. Exp. Med., 153*, 514.
11. Unkeless, J.C. (1977): The presence of two Fc receptors on mouse macrophages: evidence from variant cell lines and differential trypsin sensitivity. *J. Exp. Med., 145*, 931.
12. Fleit, H.B., Wright, S.D., Durie, C.J., Valinsky, J.E. and Unkeless, J.C. (1984): Ontogeny of Fc receptors and complement receptor (CR3) during human myeloid differentiation. *J. Clin. Invest., 73*, 516.
13. Fleit, H.B., Wright, S.D. and Unkeless, J.C. (1982): Human neutrophil Fc receptor distribution and structure. *Proc. Natl, Acad, Sci. U.S.A., 79,* 3275.

An approach to cancer chemotherapy by application of monoclonal antibody-modified liposomes

Yoshiyuki Hashimoto

SUMMARY

Monoclonal antibody-modified liposomes containing actinomycin D were prepared by coupling SH-bearing subunits of monoclonal IgM antibody to maleimide-modified sonicated liposomes containing actinomycin D in the membrane. Actinomycin D-containing liposomes modified with a murine monoclonal antibody, 2-11-G, specific to a mouse mammary cancer, bound selectively with and killed antigen-positive cancer cells both *in vitro* and *in vivo* more efficiently than did free actinomycin D. Actinomycin D-containing liposomes modified with an anti-human bladder cancer monoclonal antibody, HBA4, also bound selectively with antigen-positive human bladder cancer cells and killed them *in vitro*.

INTRODUCTION

A monoclonal antibody recognizes an epitope present in an antigen molecule. Taking advantage of this characteristic, monoclonal antibodies against cancer cells can be used for the determination of tumor-associated antigen systems as well as for the diagnosis and therapy of cancers.

Application of monoclonal antibodies to cancer therapy has been attempted using monoclonal antibody alone or as a carrier of a toxin or anticancer agent. Several monoclonal antibody-toxin conjugates have been found to exhibit striking anticancer activity when applied locally, but they are less effective against tumors remote from the application site, probably due to inactivation of the complex before it reaches the tumor site. Conjugation of a monoclonal antibody with an anticancer agent results in increased selectivity of the agent for cancer cells, leading to an increase in the drug activity and a decrease in toxicity. However, chemical coupling of an anticancer drug with a monoclonal antibody frequently causes inactivation of the drug. In light of this, the author and his colleagues devised a more elegant method for the utilization of a monoclonal antibody as a carrier of an anticancer drug, in which liposomes containing an anticancer agent were modified with a cancer-specific monoclonal antibody.[1,2] This paper describes the methodology and the *in vitro* and *in vivo* anticancer effects of the liposomes.

METHODS AND RESULTS

Preparation of monoclonal antibody-coated liposomes

Subunits of IgM antibody (IgMs) were prepared as described previously.[1] Briefly, monoclonal IgM purified by ammonium sulfate precipitation followed by Sephacryl S-300 gel filtration was reduced with 0.05 M cystein at 23°C for 10 minutes in 0.2 M Tris-HCl buffer, pH 8.6. The products were chromatographed on a Sephacryl S-300 column which had been equilibrated with pH 6.8 phosphate buffered saline (PBS) containing 2 mM EDTA. The column was eluted with PBS-EDTA and fractions containing IgMs were collected. The yield of IgMs from IgM was usually 50% to 70%.

To couple IgMs bearing SH-groups at the Fc portion, SH-reacting maleimide groups were introduced into liposomes. N-(*m*-maleimidobenzoyl) dipalmitoylphosphatidylethanolamine (2.5 μmol), prepared from *m*-maleimidobenzoyl-N-hydroxysuccinimide ester and dipalmitoylphosphatidylethanolamine, was added to a chloroform solution containing dipalmitoylphosphatidylcholine (25 μmol) and cholesterol (17.5 μmol). The lipid mixture was evaporated *in vacuo* to obtain a dry lipid film. After addition of 5 ml of PBS, the lipid film was stirred for 10 minutes and then sonicated in a bath-type sonicator for 60 minutes. The liposome suspension was centrifuged at 10,000 g for 30 minutes to remove aggregated and large liposomes. To obtain radioactive liposomes and liposomes containing an anticancer agent, cholesteryl [1-^{14}C] oleate (3 μCi), and actinomycin D (200 μg) dissolved in chloroform respectively were added to the lipid mixture and treated as above.

The liposome suspension (4 ml) prepared was treated with IgMs solution for 60 minutes at 37°C and the excess maleimide groups were blocked by incubating the liposomes with cystein at 37°C for 30 minutes. Finally, the liposomes were purified by dextran density gradient centrifugation.[1]

Particle size of liposome preparations

Liposome preparations at each stage of purification were assayed for particle size using a submicron particle analyzer, Coulter N4 model. The liposomes in the supernatant fraction of antibody-unmodified sonicated liposomes were relatively homogeneous in size (diameter 58.5 ± 28.8 nm), whereas liposomes in the sedimented fraction consisted of heterogeneous and larger liposomes (175 ± 148 nm). The IgMs-modified liposomes purified by density gradient centrifugation were 78.1 ± 38.4 nm in diameter, which was about 150 times smaller than mouse or human erythrocytes.

In vitro targeting and cytotoxicity of actinomycin D-containing liposomes bearing antibody to tumor cells

Mouse mammary cancer cell system

A major part of this work has been reported in previous papers.[1,2] A murine monoclonal IgM antibody, 2-11-G,[3] raised against a transplantable cell line of C3H/He mouse mammary carcinoma, MM46, showed reactivity to MM46 cells but not to MM48 mammary cancer cells originated in the same mouse strain as MM46. IgMs were prepared from 2-11-G IgM antibody and coupled to maleimide-modified liposomes containing actinomycin D. The suspension of purified liposomes prepared as above contained 11 μmol of phospholipid and 20 μg of actinomycin D per milliliter.

To determine the targeting of the liposomes, radiolabeled liposomes were incubated with MM46 or MM48 cells for 60 minutes at 37°C and washed with PBS; the radioactivity of the cells was then measured. The antibody-modified liposomes bound selectively with MM46 but not with MM48 cells (Fig. 1). Binding of the liposomes was inhibited by pretreatment of MM46 cells with 2-11-G antibody, suggesting antigen-specific targeting by the antibody-modified liposomes. When the radiolabeled antibody-modified liposomes were incubated with MM46 cells for 2 hours at 37°C, the liposomes appeared on microautoradiographic observation to be internalized into the cells (Fig. 2).

To determine the cytotoxicity of the actinomycin D-containing liposomes, tumor cells were incubated with the liposomes for 60 minutes at 37°C, washed and further incubated for 12 hours. After incubation, the cells were pulsed with [^{3}H]thymidine. The antibody-modified liposomes containing actinomycin D showed much stronger cytotoxicity to MM46

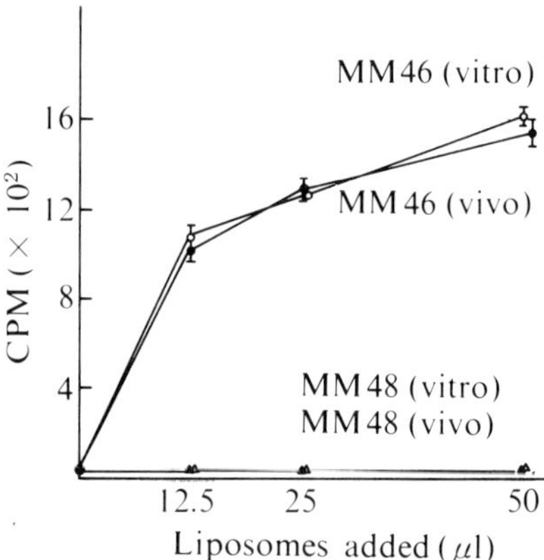

Fig. 1 Targeting of liposomes modified with subunits (IgMs) of 2-11-G IgM monoclonal antibody against mouse mammary tumor. An aliquot of ^{14}C-labeled liposome suspension was added to a suspension containing 5×10^4 tumor cells in 1 ml of medium. After incubation for 1 hour, the cells were washed; the cell-bound liposomes were then determined by measuring the radioactivity. Vitro: *in vitro* culture line; vivo: transplantation line.

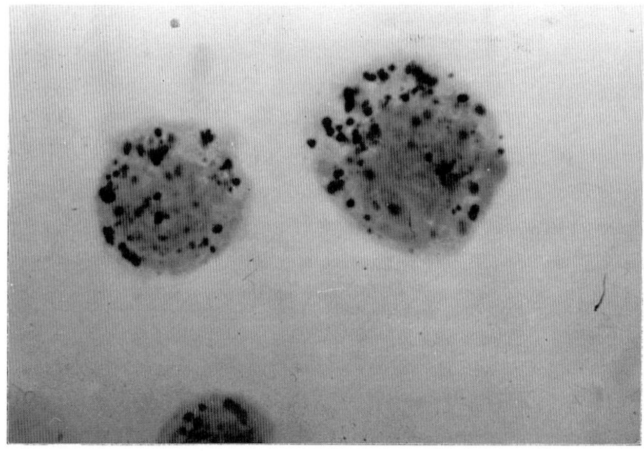

Fig. 2 Microautoradiogram of radiolabled antibody-modified liposomes bound to MM46 tumor cells.

cells than did free actinomycin D (Fig. 3). In contrast, the liposomes exerted very weak cytotoxicity to antigen-negative MM48 cells.

Human bladder cancer system

HBA4 monoclonal IgM antibody raised against a urinary bladder cancer cell line, KU-1, was found to react selectively with certain epithelial

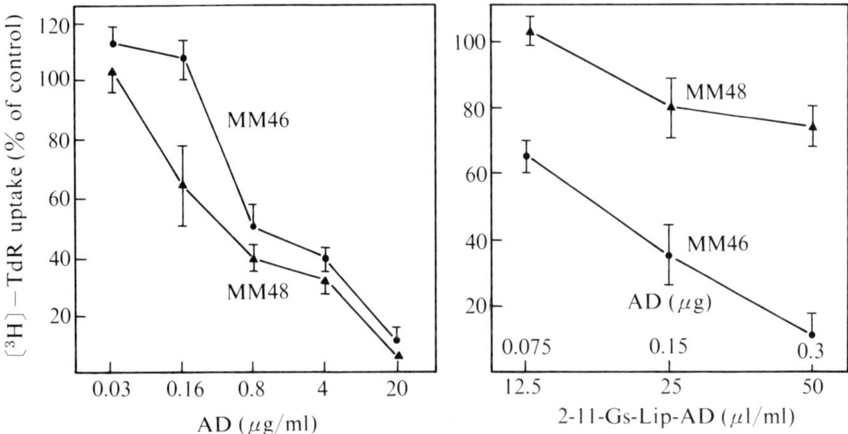

Fig. 3 Cytotoxicity of actinomycin D (AD) entrapped in 2-11-G IgMs-modified liposomes. Left, free actinomycin D; right, actinomycin D in the liposomes.

cancer cell lines including some bladder cancer lines.[4] Examination of the reactivity of HBA4 with primary bladder cancer tissues revealed that the cancer tissues from six out of nine cases showed reactivity with the antibody. Antibody-modified liposomes containing actinomycin D were prepared as described above by coupling IgMs from HBA4 antibody with maleimide-modified liposomes containing actinomycin D. The liposomes bound with and exerted a cytotoxic effect on bladder cancer cell lines (KU-1, T-24, NBT-2, and MGH-U1) bearing the HBA4-antigen but not with a fibroblast cell line, HEL (details to be reported elsewhere).

In vivo antitumor effect of actinomycin D-containing antibody-modified liposomes

The therapeutic effect of 2-11-G IgMs-modified liposomes containing various amounts of actinomycin D on MM46 or MM48 mammary cancer cells transplanted into syngeneic C3H/He mice was examined.[2] Bovine serum albumin (BSA)-modified liposomes containing actinomycin D were used as the control. One day after the transplantation of tumor cells, mice were injected with 50 μl, i.p., of a liposome preparation, free actinomycin D or 2-11-G antibody. The results are summarized in Table 1. Treatment of the mice with either free actinomycin D or 2-11-G antibody resulted in a small therapeutic effect against the MM46 tumor, but all mice died due to the tumor growth. BSA-modified liposomes containing actinomycin D prolonged survival time significantly compared with the PBS control, but all mice eventually died of the tumors. In contrast, antibody-modified liposomes containing actinomycin D

Table 1 Effect of an intraperitoneal injection of 2-11-G IgM, actinomycin D and liposome preparations on intraperitoneally-transplanted MM46 and MM48 tumors[2]

Material injected*	Dose (μg)	No. of mice dying with tumor/no. of mice tested and mean survival days of dead mice: MM46		MM48	
		5×10^4 cells			
PBS		3/3	21.0 (±2.0)†		
2-11-G IgM	60	3/3	22.3 (±3.1)		
2-11-G IgM	120	3/3	21.3 (±1.2)		
2-11-G IgM	240	3/3	27.0 (±3.0)		
PBS		6/6	21.8 (±1.2)		
Actinomycin D	1.25	6/6	22.7 (±2.0)		
Actinomycin D	2.5	6/6	23.3 (±1.9)		
Actinomycin D	5.0	6/6	23.3 (±1.5)		
PBS		6/6	21.7 (±1.4)	6/6	15.3 (±0.7)
Actinomycin D	1.25	6/6	21.9 (±2.1)	3/3	14.7 (±0.5)
Immuno-lip		3/3	21.3 (±0.7)	3/3	15.7 (±1.7)
Chemo-BSA-lip	(0.3)**	3/3	23.7 (±1.7)		
Chemo-BSA-lip	(1.0)	3/3	27.3 (±2.7)		
Chemo-immuno-lip	(0.3)	3/6	32.7 (±2.7)	3/3	15.3 (±0.6)
Chemo-immuno-lip	(0.5)	2/6	33, 36	3/3	16.7 (±3.1)
Chemo-immuno-lip	(1.0)	0/6		3/3	16.3 (±2.5)
PBS		5/5	21.6 (±1.6)		
Chemo-BSA-lip	(1.0)	5/5	27.8 (±2.1)		
Chemo-immuno-lip	(1.0)	1/5	30		
		5×10^5 cells			
PBS		5/5	20.2 (±1.2)		
Chemo-BSA-lip	(1.0)	5/5	23.8 (±1.9)		
Chemo-immuno-lip	(1.0)	2/5	25, 37		
		5×10^6 cells			
PBS		5/5	18.8 (±1.2)		
Chemo-BSA-lip	(1.0)	5/5	21.0 (±1.7)		
Chemo-immuno-lip	(1.0)	2/5	28, 36		

* Immuno-lip: actinomycin-free liposomes modified with antibody. Chemo-BSA-lip: actinomycin D-containing liposomes modified with bovine serum albumin. Chemo-immuno-lip: actinomycin D-containing liposomes modified with antibody. All liposome preparations contained 0.56 μmol phospholipid per 50 μl of preparation. Chemo-BSA-lip and chemo-immuno-lip contained 30 μg and 34 μg of protein per 50 μl of preparation respectively. All materials (50 μl of liposome preparations) were injected i.p. once one day after tumor transplantation. All surviving mice were free from tumor cells as observed by autopsy at the termination of experiments (60 to 90 days after tumor transplantation).

** Figures in parentheses in dose column indicate the dose in micrograms of actinomycin D in the injected liposomes.

† Figures in parentheses represent SD

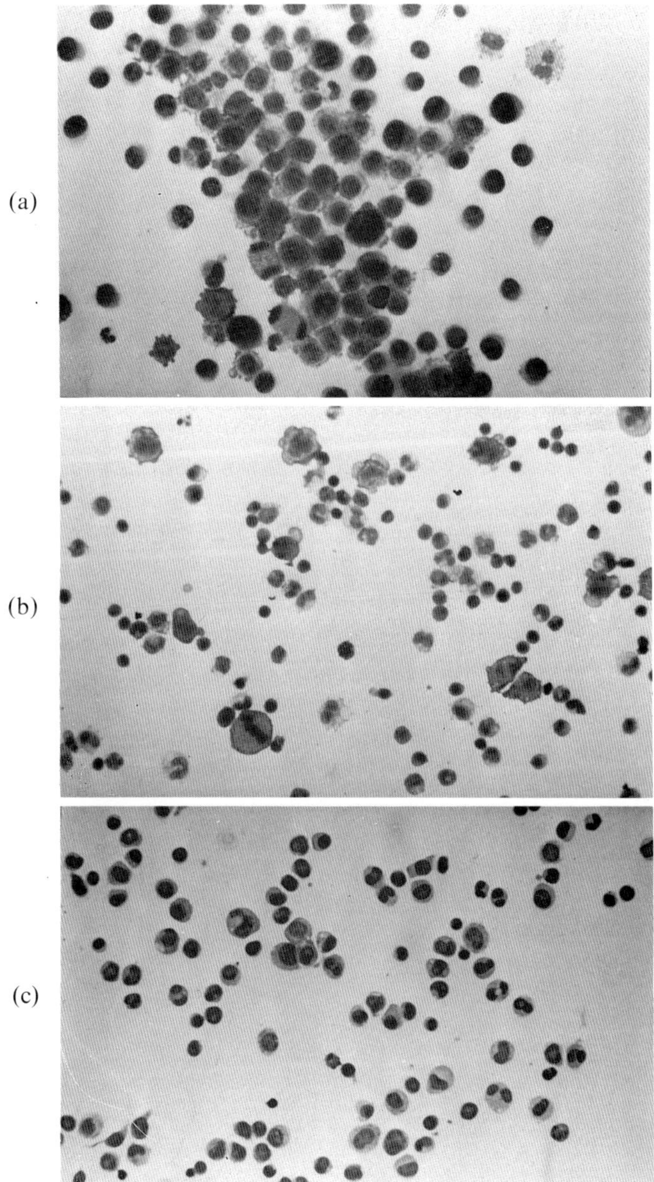

Fig. 4 Ascites figures of mice which had been transplanted with MM46 tumor cells. C3H/He mice were transplanted i.p. with 5×10^4 MM46 tumor cells; one day later, the mice were given a single i.p. injection of drug. The ascitic fluid was harvested 7 days after tumor transplantation. (a) 5 μg of free actinomycin D; the majority of the ascites cells are tumor cells. (b) 240 μg of 2-11-G IgM; a small number of tumor cells remains and a mitotic figure is seen. (c) 50 μl of 2-11-G IgMs-modified liposomes containing 1 μg of actinomycin D; all ascites cells are replaced by normal peritoneal cells and no tumor cells are present. Hematoxylin-eosin stain. $\times 100$

conferred a striking therapeutic effect on the mice transplanted with MM46 cancer cells (Fig. 4). A single injection of the liposomes (50 μl) containing 1 μg of actinomycin D resulted in a cure in mice which had been transplanted with as many as 5 $\times 10^6$ MM46 cells. However, the liposomes had no effect on MM48 tumor cells.

To investigate whether antibody-modified liposomes containing actinomycin D are also effective against tumors remote from the injection site of the drug, MM46 cells were transplanted subcutaneously and, after 4 days, when the tumor had grown to a palpable size, the mice were given an intravenous injection of the liposomes. Since the liposomes were foreign to the host, it was realized that they would bc engulfed by host phagocytes. Therefore, mice were pretreated with unmodified multilamellar liposomes one hour before injecting the antibody-modified liposomes containing 1 μg of actinomycin D. The tumor nodule decreased to an impalpable size 4 days after the liposome injection and re-grew thereafter. When the tumor nodules were resected 12 days after the treatment, the average weight of the tumors was about 50% or 60% of that of tumors in PBS-treated controls (in two experiments). When phagocytes were not blocked, the therapeutic effect of the liposomes was insignificant. Free actinomycin D (1 to 3 μg/mouse), 2-11-G antibody (100 μg/mouse) and BSA-modified liposomes containing 1 μg of actinomycin D were all ineffective in this experimental system. When phagocytes were not blocked, an injection of BSA-modified liposomes containing actinomycin D resulted in an enhancement of tumor growth, probably because liposomes were trapped in phagocytes and so decreased the macrophage-mediated anticancer activity of the host.

DISCUSSION

Both monoclonal antibody to cancer cells and liposomes are considered to be important carriers of anticancer drugs, as a drug coupled with antibody can increase the selectivity of the drug for cancer cells, and liposomes containing a drug facilitate the slower release of the drug *in vivo* and can overcome the drug resistance of cancer cells.[5] The present research demonstrated that the combined use of these two carriers increased the anticancer activity of an anticancer drug, actinomycin D, against cancer cells bearing an antigen corresponding to the antibody used for liposome modification. Although free actinomycin D showed significant cytotoxicity to MM46 cancer cells, it was ineffective against cancer cells transplanted *in vivo* even when applied locally, probably because of rapid clearance of the drug from the injection site. If the drug was included in antibody-modified liposomes, the liposomes bound selectively to antigen-bearing cancer cells and led to efficient anticancer activity by the included drug, as the mouse mammary cancer model demonstrated. For clinical use of these liposome preparations, it is critical whether the liposomes can affect tumors remote from the application site. It has generally been believed that liposomes cannot migrate through blood vessels. The present work, however, showed clearly that intravenously injected antibody-modified liposomes could carry actinomycin D to subcutaneous tumors, leading to the destruction of tumor cells or inhibition of tumor growth.

These observations have stimulated the author and his colleagues to work towards applying this method clinically. Liposomes modified with monoclonal antibody against human bladder cancers have been prepared. These liposomes, containing actinomycin D, were shown to have selective cytotoxicity to human bladder cancer cells *in vitro*. Prior to clinical application of the liposome preparation, it will be necessary to investigate its general toxicity and *in vivo* localization, and to find a method of preserving the preparation.

REFERENCES

1. Hashimoto, Y., Sugawara, M. and Endoh, H. (1983): Coating of liposomes with subunits of monoclonal IgM antibody and targeting of the liposomes. *J. Immunol. Methods, 62*, 155.
2. Hashimoto, Y., Sugawara, M., Masuko, T. and Hojo, H. (1983): Antitumor effect of actinomycin D entrapped in liposomes bearing subunits of tumor-specific monoclonal immunoglobulin M antibody. *Cancer Res., 43*, 5328.
3. Seto, M., Takahashi, T., Tanimoto, M. and Nishizuka, Y. (1982): Production of monoclonal antibodies against MM antigen: the serologic identification of MM antigen with Ly 6.2 alloantigen. *J. Immunol., 128*, 201.
4. Masuko, T., Yagita, H. and Hashimoto, Y. (1984): Monoclonal antibodies against cell surface antigens present on human urinary bladder cancer cells. *JNCI, 72*, 523.
5. Papahadjopoulos, D., Poste, G., Vall, W.J. and Biedler, J. (1976): Use of lipid vesicles as carriers to introduce actinomycin D into resistant tumor cells. *Cancer Res., 36*, 2988.

Biological response modifiers for the therapy of cancer

Ronald B. Herberman

INTRODUCTION

During the past several years, increasing attention has been devoted to the potential applications of biological response modifiers (BRMs) for therapy of patients with cancer. It has been suggested that BRMs might provide a novel approach to therapy and be an effective alternative and/or adjunct to therapy by conventional modalities such as chemotherapy, radiotherapy and surgery.

An important issue to settle here is the definition of BRMs and how this approach to the treatment of cancer overlaps with, or is different from, immunotherapy. BRMs have been defined by the Subcommittee on BRMs to the National Cancer Institute, Division of Cancer Treatment as: Those agents or approaches that modify the relationship between tumor and host by modifying the host's biological response to tumor cells with resultant therapeutic effects.[1] BRMs can essentially be placed in two main categories: (a) chemical and biological agents which can stimulate or otherwise affect the host resistance mechanisms that may be involved in the control of growth and/or metastases of tumor cells; and (b) cellular products that can have direct antitumor effects.

Predominant in the first category are immunomodulators, which could mediate their effects by activating, increasing and/or restoring reactivity of immunological effector mechanisms that are involved in resistance to tumor growth and metastasis. Immunomodulators might also act by inhibiting suppressor or other mechanisms which interfere with effective host resistance to tumors. This general category of BRMs would include chemical agents, tumor antigens, effector cells, antibodies and cytokines. Also included would be agents which increase the ability of the host to tolerate damage by chemotherapy or radiotherapy, e.g., by increasing or restoring hematopoiesis.

Included within the second main category of BRMs would be effector cells, antibodies or cytokines which have antitumor effects by: (a) direct cytotoxicity against tumor cells; (b) decreasing transformation or increasing the differentiation or maturation of tumor cells, so that they manifest reduced potential for uncontrolled growth, invasion and spread; and (c) increasing the sensitivity of tumor cells to control by host effector mechanisms.

It is apparent that many of the approaches and agents considered to be BRMs are immunological and that therefore there is much overlap with immunotherapy. It is therefore worthwhile to consider what the current status of immunotherapy is and how the approaches to therapy with BRMs hold much promise, despite the limitations of previous immunotherapeutic approaches.

During the past few years, attitudes and expectations about immunotherapy of cancer have fluctuated dramatically. A high degree of optimism as to the ability of immunologic manipulations to cure residual disease and thereby provide a major supplement to surgery and other forms of conventional therapy has largely been replaced by widespread doubts as to the value or even the potential for immunotherapy.

It seems worthwhile to reflect first on some of the reasons for the initial hopes and expectations for major therapeutic advances as a result of immunotherapy:

(1) In the 1960s and early 1970s, there was a considerable number of studies which demonstrated tumor-associated transplantation antigens on a variety of experimental tumors, primarily in inbred strains of mice. With such tumors, it was possible to induce specific resistance to autologous or syngeneic tumor growth by removal of growing tumors or by immunization with tumor cells or tumor extracts. In some cases, this resistance was rather potent, with the immunized animals able to resist challenge by large numbers of tumor cells.

(2) These *in vivo* demonstrations of effective and specific antitumor immunity were soon followed by much evidence for apparently specific cell-mediated immunity against tumor-associated antigens on such experimental tumors.[2] In addition, similar data were obtained with many human tumors, suggesting that human tumors might also have tumor-associated transplantation antigens that were immunogenic in the autologous host.

(3) Further encouragement came from the successful results of immunotherapy with various agents in some experimental tumor systems. Particular attention was focused on treatment of some transplantable tumors with the bacterial agents, *Mycobacterium bovis* (BCG) and *Corynebacterium parvum*, but some successful results were also obtained by specific immunotherapy with tumor vaccines.[3] Most impressively, immunotherapy often resulted in complete eradication of tumor and persistent immunity against subsequent tumor challenge.

(4) From several preliminary studies, it appeared that similarly successful immunotherapy could be performed on cancer patients. Of particular note were reports of significant prolongation of disease-free intervals and/or survival in patients with acute lymphocytic or myelogenous leukemia after treatment with BCG plus allogeneic irradiated tumor cells,[4] regressions of primary or metastatic skin tumors after elicitation of delayed hypersensitivity reactions by contact sensitizers or BCG applied to the tumor site,[5] and increased survival of operable lung cancer patients given intrapleural BCG shortly after surgery.[6] Most recently, much attention has been given to the antitumor effects of interferon in some cancer patients,[7] with the likely possibility that these results were mediated by stimulation of host effector mechanisms.

Despite this apparently strong basis for immunotherapy, most oncologists and even many tumor immunologists are currently quite pessimistic about clinical immunotherapy. Several possible explanations can be offered for this major change in attitude:

(1) The most immediate cause for skepticism has come from larger scale clinical immunotherapy trials, particularly several well-designed, randomized controlled trials, in which it was not possible to verify the apparent clinical benefits that were indicated in the initial studies.[8] Of particular concern has been the lack of convincing evidence for beneficial clinical results from immunotherapy with specific tumor vaccines.

(2) In addition, of fundamental concern has been the accumulating evidence against some of the basic assumptions underlying the rationale for immunotherapy:

(a) Much discussion has centered around the frequent failure to detect tumor-associated transplantation antigens on some types of tumors in experimental animals, especially spontaneous tumors.[9] Most of the earlier positive results were obtained with tumors induced by oncogenic viruses or chemical carcinogens. Since almost all human tumors are, in the absence of a clearly defined etiology, considered to be spontaneous, the negative results with spontaneous rodent tumors have often been considered to be more clinically relevant.[10]

(b) There has also been considerable evidence against a central role for immune T cells in protection against a variety of tumors. For example, the incidence of spontaneous or chemical carcinogen-induced tumors has generally been the same in nude or neonatally thymectomized mice as in euthymic mice.[11] Since thymic-dependent immunity was frequently postulated to be most important for immuno-surveillance and for general host resistance against tumors, this has raised questions about the overall role of the immune system in antineoplastic defenses. Similarly, there has been increasing evidence that what had previously been thought to be specific cytolytic T cells reactive against human tumors were actually natural effector cells, especially natural killer (NK) cells.[12]

(c) Further discouragement has come from the failure to detect consistent and clear-cut alterations in immune parameters in patients receiving immunotherapy.

The above findings have been taken by many investigators and oncologists as sufficient reasons to abandon attempts at immunotherapy. However, in addition to agreeing that the initial attitudes about immunotherapy were overly optimistic, it is the author's view that the present negativity is also an overreaction. Rather, this is an appropriate time to reconsider the premises upon which immunotherapy trials might be based and to develop a series of rational approaches to immunotherapy and other forms of biological response modification:

(1) Despite the extensive data base on some experimental animal tumor systems, there is a very wide gap between such systems and clinical situations.[13] First, almost all experimental immunotherapy studies have been performed with transplantable tumor cell lines, particularly those which were initiated at least 15 years ago. Such tumors may have normal histocompatibility antigens that are different from those expressed in current inbred strains. Closer models for human tumors would seem to be primary tumors, with immunotherapy being performed on established autochthonous tumors. In addition, although two of the basic objectives of biological response modification are to restore deficiencies in immunologic functions and to augment reactivity above existing levels, almost all of the clinical trials have employed empirically selecteed doses and schedules of administration of agents. Agents have often been given at the maximal tolerable or available doses or at arbitrary doses and schedules. Very frequently in fact, no clear hypothesis has been formulated as to the expected immunologic effect to be achieved by the immunotherapy.

(2) When a rationale for a particular immunotherapy trial has been stated, it has usually been formulated in terms of attempts to augment T cell-mediated immunity to tumor-associated transplantation antigens. Similarly, most efforts at immunologic monitoring of patients receiving immunotherapy have been focused on alterations in the numbers and functions of T cells. However, increasing evidence indicates that other types of effector cells and mechanisms may be important in resistance against tumor growth and these may not even depend on the expression of tumor-associated transplantation antigens. Such alternative immune effector mechanisms include NK cells, macrophages and possibly even granulocytes. These may all function as components of the natural cellular immune defense system, which can be activated rapidly and can react against a wide variety of tumor cells.[14,15] In addition, there is a real possibility that some of the agents in current use for immunotherapy may

also have biological response-modifying-effects other than on the immune system, e.g., alterations in the production of various cellular growth factors,[16] and therefore, as alluded to above, it is preferable to speak in terms of biological response modification rather than immunotherapy.

(3) Although it is at this time very difficult, if not impossible, to choose adequately among the various possible effector mechanisms, some hypotheses in this regard can be developed in order to formulate rational strategies for biological response modification. Prior to conducting large-scale clinical trials, it would seem essential to determine the dose and schedule for a particular agent that optimally augment for a sustained period one or more of the effector mechanisms considered important. This is of particular concern since a variety of agents may not only augment the activity of a particular immunologic function, but under some conditions also cause depression via induction of activation of suppressor cells. It should be noted that there is little reason to expect that more of a particular agent will be better. The relevant principles for immunomodulation are likely to be quite different from those that have been developed for treatment with chemotherapeutic agents, where the highest possible dose is given. One possible approach would be to determine the optimal immunomodulating dose for each of several effector functions and then set up and compare the therapeutic results of protocols based on such information. For example, one might compare the optimal schedule for augmenting macrophage cytolytic activity with that for augmenting NK or antibody-dependent cell-mediated cytotoxic (ADCC) activity. The primary concern, then, in a phase I trial with a putative biological response-modifying agent would be to carefully monitor the effects of the agent at various doses and schedules of administration. This would appear to be an obvious and straightforward approach. However, this has not tended to be the practice with agents that have been brought to the clinical level so far.

(4) It should also be noted that most previous and current phase I trials with BRMs have been performed in patients with advanced and widespread disease, in analogy with the approaches taken for initial evaluation of chemotherapeutic agents. Although studies in such patients can provide useful information about the possible toxic side effects of the agents, they are quite unlikely to provide any indications of antitumor efficacy. Although susceptibility to cure of many tumors by chemotherapy varies inversely with tumor mass[17] due to the increased likelihood of development of drug-resistant clones, drugs produce logarithmic, first-order kinetics of cytotoxicity against advanced bulky tumors as well as against small, localized tumors. In contrast, immunologically mediated antitumor effects seem mainly to be subject to a threshold, with no discernible activity against tumors beyond a certain size or degree of

tissue invasion. Most experience with animal tumor systems has indicated the limitation of effective immunotherapy or other forms of biological response modification to small tumor burdens and micrometastatic disease. Even highly immunogenic tumors have usually been shown to be insusceptible to therapy when BRMs are first given at an advanced stage of disease.[18] Thus, development of clinical protocols to evaluate the effects of BRMs on micrometastatic disease as an adjunct to surgery and/or chemotherapy or radiation therapy is more likely to provide positive results.

A major technical issue to be raised with regard to the monitoring of the effects of various agents on effector activity is the problem of substantial spontaneous fluctuation of reactivity in the assays over a period of time. Some of this may be attributed to technical variation from day to day in the assay itself, e.g., with varying susceptibility of a target cell to lysis. In addition, there may be considerable biological fluctuation in reactivity.[19]

Thus, there is a real need to carefully control the monitoring and to discriminate adequately between treatment-induced alterations and spontaneous fluctuations.

MECHANISMS OF ACTION OF BRMS

A central issue for careful consideration is the mechanism by which a BRM might induce antitumor effects. Most BRMs, even low molecular weight, chemically defined and homogeneous materials, are pleiotropic in their actions, and it is therefore necessary to gain insights into the effects most likely to be important for antitumor activity. Unfortunately, at the present time, there is no simple or straightforward way to answer this question. For example, an immunomodulator might alter the reactivity of T cells, NK cells and macrophages. One major approach would be to determine, for a particular tumor system, the relative contributions of each of these effector cells to host resistance. As noted above, although immune T cells can clearly be shown to play an important role in defense against certain types of tumors, in many other situations T cell-mediated immunity appears to play little or no significant role. In the past several years, NK cells have been shown to contribute appreciably to host resistance against a variety of experimental tumors and these effector cells appear to be particularly involved in resistance to metastatic spread of tumor cells.[15] Macrophages have also been suggested to be important effectors of host defense, and therapeutic strategies focused on activation of macrophage cytotoxic activity have been shown to have considerable therapeutic efficacy against the growth of metastases from some experimental tumors.[20] In view of the potential contributions from each of these effector cells, the immunologist is faced with the difficult problem of deciding which to make the primary focus. This decision can be facilitated, at least with experimental tumor models, by studying the effects of a particular BRM in animals that have been selectively depleted of each effector mechanism. For example, experiments can be performed on T cell-deficient nude or thymectomized mice. For studies of BRMs in NK-deficient recipients, beige mice or animals pretreated with antibodies selective for NK cells (e.g., anti-asialo GM_1) may be employed. Unfortunately, there is not at this time a satisfactorily selective treatment for depressing macrophage activity, since most macrophage-toxic agents are also inhibitory for NK activity.

Once a decision is reached as to the main mechanism of action for a given BRM, the next major issue is the determination of the protocol that would induce optimal alterations of the relevant effector mechanism. This is the primary focus for the immunopharmacology of BRMs and goes beyond an assessment of the pharmacokinetics of the agent itself, the main concern being placed on the pharmacokinetics of the alteration of the biological response. It should be noted that whereas most mechanistic studies with a BRM are focused on the alterations in reactivity after a single dose, for development of effective therapeutic protocols one needs to determine the route and schedule of administration that would produce continued alterations in reactivity over a prolonged period of time. It is not yet clear whether it would be necessary to have continuous and sustained alteration in reactivity or whether cyclic alterations would be sufficient. In any event, it seems critical to determine whether repeated administration of a BRM would lead to hyporeactivity or refractoriness to alteration. If such hyporeactivity were seen, one would anticipate the importance of understanding the basis for the refractoriness and developing protocols for avoiding or overcoming such effects.

As discussed in detail by Talmadge et al.,[21] screening studies with BRMs need to be considerably broader than the more familiar screens for chemotherapeutic agents. Before useful experiments can be performed to evaluate the therapeutic efficacy of a BRM against various experimental tumors, it is essential to adequately characterize the range of biological effects of the agent. Of particular relevance for possible therapeutic efficacy are the *in vivo* effects of a BRM on various immunologic and other biological parameters. A particular difficulty will be encountered in the evaluation of the effects of some human cytokines and most monoclonal antibodies against human tumors, which would not have the desired biological effects in experimental animal tumor systems. Special strategies would need to be developed to overcome such limitations. For agents expected to have direct antitumor effects, screening studies might be performed with human tumors growing in nude mice. However, BRMs expected to act indirectly, by altering host defense mechanisms, would require a different strategy, e.g., transfer of human effector cells as well as human tumor cells into nude mice.

EVALUATION OF INTERFERON AS A BRM

At this point, it seems useful to consider some specific examples of BRMs with potential for therapy of cancer. One very instructive example of the potential and limitations of BRMs for therapy is interferon.

Over the past several years, much attention has been focused on the potential therapeutic efficacy of various types of interferon. When clinical trials were initiated with this cytokine, the main rationale was its known ability to inhibit the proliferation of certain types of tumor cells. However, it soon became increasingly clear that interferon is a very pleiotropic agent, having the ability to act as a potent BRM, with effects on a variety of host responses as well as potential direct antitumor effects.

Despite the increasing awareness of the possible importance of such indirect biological response-modifying effects of interferon, most clinical trials that have been performed to date have centered on the frequent administration, usually daily, of the maximum amounts of interferon that were either available or were tolerated by the patients. It is quite likely that such protocols are mainly optimal for interferon's direct cytostatic antitumor activity. These protocols have had early positive therapeutic effects on some types of cancer, with partial or complete regressions being seen in patients with extensive tumor burdens who had become refractory to other forms of therapy. A substantial proportion of patients with non-Hodgkin's lymphoma, particularly nodular poorly differentiated lymphoma[22] and cutaneous T cell lymphoma,[23] and patients with hairy cell leukemia,[24] have been shown to respond to this form of therapy. However, it has been quite disappointing that most patients with other types of cancer have shown little or no therapeutic benefits from interferon administration.

One of the possible explanations for the limited therapeutic efficacy that has been seen thus far is the use of protocols for administration of interferon that are not sufficiently effective for inducing sustained alterations of other important biological effects. This possibility is supported by the experience to date in regard to the effects of the interferon protocols on NK activity. Interferon has been demonstrated to be a major factor involved in the activation of NK cells and in the augmentation of spontaneous reactivity.[25] This information, coupled with the increasing evidence for an important role of NK cells in resistance against tumors, particularly against metastases, has led to much interest in the effects of interferon administration on NK activity. Most clinical trials have now incorporated the monitoring of NK activity as a fundamental part of the study design. Unexpectedly, in view of the known ability of interferon administration to boost NK activity in mice and the early reports of sustained augmentation of NK activity in osteosarcoma patients receiving therapy with Cantell interferon α,[26] most clinical studies have revealed only transient augmentation of NK activity in patients receiving frequent high doses of various forms of interferon. For example, in a clinical trial with highly purified recombinant leukocyte interferon clone A, augmentation of NK activity was seen in very few of the patients, and about 30% of the patients receiving interferon twice daily showed NK activity depressed below the spontaneous levels measured prior to initiation of therapy.[19] The explanation for the failure of interferon to cause sustained augmentation of NK activity in cancer patients is not yet clear and is under active investigation. These results cannot be explained by a general refractoriness of the cancer patients to respond to interferon, since *in vitro* treatment of the cells of most cancer patients resulted in substantial augmentation of NK activity. Further, it appears that administration of a single dose of interferon results in augmentation in most patients. Therefore, it appears that the repeated administration of interferon results in some form of hyporeactivity. Recent studies in the author's laboratory[27] have indicated that this is not due to a decrease in the number of circulating large granular lymphocytes (LGL), which mediate NK activity, or to a decrease in the proportion of LGL which can bind to NK-susceptible target cells. Rather, it appears that the LGL develop some block in their ability to cause lysis of attached target cells and these cells are refractory to augmentation of NK activity upon *in vitro* exposure to interferon α.

A potentially useful animal model for exploring the mechanisms of this refractoriness has recently been developed. It has been found that a hybrid recombinant leukocyte interferon, A/D bgl, is able to boost mouse as well as human NK cell activity.[28] Single doses of this hybrid recombinant interferon have caused substantial augmentation of NK activity in mice, whereas repeated daily doses of this preparation have led to progressively lower NK activity, particularly in the peripheral blood.[29] Further studies to elucidate the mechanism of this refractoriness to sustained boosting of NK activity and the likely development of strategies to overcome this hyporeactivity may be helpful in designing more efficacious clinical trials. In addition, it is hoped that the extensive experience with interferon therapy will serve as a useful model for analogous attempts at therapy with other cytokines.

POTENTIAL OF MONOCLONAL ANTIBODIES FOR THERAPY OF CANCER

Monoclonal antibodies directed against tumor-associated antigens represent another promising approach to therapy. Although this technology has only been available for a few years, widespread and intensive efforts are being directed toward the development of therapeutically effective antibodies and protocols. Currently, the main challenge is to identify the parameters that are critical for *in vivo* antitumor efficacy. The central issue with monoclonal antibodies is their specificity. On the one hand, it is important for the antibodies to react well with tumor cells, preferably with high affinity, to recognize most or all neoplastic cells within a tumor and to react with metastatic lesions as well as with primary tumors. Several of the currently available monoclonal antibodies to human tumor antigens have had some problems in this regard, there being considerable heterogeneity of antigen expression on the tumor cells of a given patient.[30] Such heterogeneity would be expected to limit the therapeutic efficacy substantially. However, it is possible that some antigens might be well expressed on all clonigenic tumor cells and not on more differentiated progeny; in such a case, the ability of antibodies to eliminate the stem cells might be highly therapeutically effective.

The other key issue regarding specificity of monoclonal antibodies is the degree of reactivity with various normal cells, particularly with antigens on the cell surface. To maximize selective uptake by the tumor and to minimize toxicity, it would clearly be desirable to utilize antibodies with a high degree of specificity for tumor-associated antigens. Therefore, one critical aspect of screening of potentially useful monoclonal antibodies is the determination of their specificity for tumor cells. Substantial insight can be obtained by *in vitro* studies with tissue sections from tumors and normal tissues, utilizing an immunoperoxidase histochemical technique. However, this *in vitro* screening may not provide a sufficiently accurate indication of *in vivo* localization of the antibodies at the site of the tumor and may also fail to reveal some problems with *in vivo* binding of the antibodies to certain normal tissues.

With regard to the former issue of the degree of uptake of antibody by the tumor, very detailed information can be obtained with accessible lesions by obtaining biopsies at various times after antibody administration and examining the distribution of mouse immunoglobulins by immunoperoxidase staining. This procedure can provide direct information on the degree of coating of tumor cells with the antibody and whether some parts of the tumor are not detectably coated. Similarly, single-cell suspensions can be prepared from the biopsy material and studies performed on the coating of individual tumor cells using fluorescence flow cytometry. Such approaches provide considerably more information than is possible by radiolocalization of administered antibody coupled to a radioisotope. However, the radiolocalization technique, which has the particular advantage of also providing information about the proportion of the total antibody that actually reaches the tumor, may be more sensitive than the *in vitro* procedures just described, and can provide direct information on problems of uptake in various normal organs.

The potential toxicity of monoclonal antibodies is not yet adequately understood. One would anticipate that many of the potential difficulties would be related to lack of sufficient specificity of the antibody for tumor cells. In addition, the present generation of monoclonal antibodies that are produced in mice or rats represent some additional, particular difficulties. These antibodies that are produced in heterologous species may not discriminate tumor-associated specificities as well as human antibodies and it is hoped, as soon as the necessary technology is sufficiently developed, that human monoclonal antibodies to tumor-associated antigens can be developed. The dependence on rodents as the source of monoclonal antibodies also has the associated problem of inoculation of heterologous proteins into cancer patients. On the one hand, this might lead to some problems with induction of anaphylactic reactions, serum sickness or other immunologic manifestations of such reactivity.[31] On the other hand, the production of antibodies against mouse immunoglobulins would appear to be a major limitation to the efficacy of repeated administration of these antibodies over a prolonged period.

Another major issue appears to be the degree of antigenic modulation induced by the monoclonal antibodies. This actually appears to be a two-edged sword. On the one hand, decreased expression of the antigens recognized by a monoclonal antibody would be expected to limit the efficacy of repeated doses of the antibodies, which would probably be of particular concern with trials involving administration of antibodies alone. On the other hand, antigenic modulation or some related form of endocytosis of the antigen-antibody complexes might be a prerequisite for the toxic effects of most immunoconjugates, with the toxic moieties only having effects on tumor cells when introduced internally. Most instances of antigenic modulation that have been observed with monoclonal antibodies have been associated with leukemia and lymphoma cells. It is generally considered that solid tumors are insusceptible to antigenic modulation by monoclonal antibodies and therefore the susceptibility of solid tumors to effective therapy by immunoconjugates has been questioned. However, there are some recent indications that at least some combinations of monoclonal antibodies and solid tumors show susceptibility to toxicity by immunoconjugates. Considerable antitumor effects have been observed with a guinea pig hepatocarcinoma treated with conjugates of a monoclonal antibody with the A chain of either diphtheria toxin or abrin.[32,33] It seems necessary to screen for the particular antibody-tumor combinations which show antigenic modulation and, particularly, to demonstrate *in vitro* killing of tumor cells by the immunoconjugate. Positive results in such studies would provide considerable encouragement for use in *in vivo* therapeutic studies. This issue of antigenic modulation would not seem so important for immunoconjugates of monoclonal antibodies with radioisotopes, where delivery of radiation in the region of the tumor cells might be sufficient to cause regression of radiosensitive tumors.

In addition to the considerable potential of utilizing antibodies to deliver toxic agents to the site of tumor growth, there are several indications that administration of monoclonal antibodies alone may have antitumor effects. This might be mediated by direct cytostatic effects of the antibodies, or by complement-dependent cytolysis. However, the most likely basis for antitumor effects by monoclonal antibodies alone would be cooperation with effector cells to result in antibody-dependent cell-mediated cytotoxicity (ADCC). From available evidence, it would appear that therapeutic effects by antibodies alone will be observed mainly in situations with a relatively low tumor burden.[32,33] Lack of efficacy with more advanced disease might be related either to insufficient access of the antibody to bulky lesions or to depression of the needed effector cell mechanisms.[34,35]

A monoclonal antibody to a 250,000 molecular weight determinant associated with human malignant melanoma, 9.2.27, has been shown to have some therapeutic efficacy against human melanomas growing in nude mice.[36] These effects are presumed to be related to collaboration of the 9.2.27 antibody with either macrophages or natural killer/killer cells, the latter activity being particularly increased in nude mice. A clinical trial is currently under way in the author's Clinical Investigations Section with the 9.2.27 antibody; administration of high doses of the antibody to patients has been found to result in substantial localization in tumor sites[37] but thus far, as might be expected, no therapeutic efficacy has been observed in these patients, who all have advanced disease.

Another antibody which has been utilized in phase I clinical trials is T101, directed against a 65,000 molecular weight protein that is relatively specific for normal T cells but is expressed on B-cell as well as T-cell leukemias and lymphomas. Based on preliminary reports of some antitumor effects in a few patients,[38] a systematic clinical study has been initiated.[39] In contrast to the 9.2.27 antibody, the T101 antibody causes quite rapid modulation of the cell surface antigen. Infusion of high doses over a prolonged period led to particularly dramatic loss of antigen expression on the leukemia cells. Some transient decreases in circulating leukemia cells were seen in patients receiving lower doses, administered rapidly. Among patients with cutaneous T-cell lymphomas, several showed transient improvement in skin lesions but all responses were less than total. Although the clinical results obtained thus far with this antibody are not particularly encouraging, the ability of T101 antibody to induce rapid modulation might provide the basis for a follow-up clinical trial with the antibody conjugated to a drug, toxin, or radioisotope.

Monoclonal antibodies have also been produced against idiotypic determinants on the surface immunoglobulins of some B-cell lymphomas. Administration of relatively small amounts of such antibody to a patient has caused long-lasting regression.[40] Such antibodies provide a striking example of the potential for exquisite tumor specificity of some monoclonal antibodies and, in parallel with the early clinical studies, extensive studies are being performed with anti-idiotype monoclonal antibodies directed against mouse lymphomas. Such studies should lead to a better understanding of the mechanism for potent antitumor effects and its limitations and should help the design of more effective clinical trials. It should be noted that a major limitation of this approach is the individual specificity of the antibodies, requiring production of a new reagent for each patient. Development of effective monoclonal antibodies against determinants shared by a wide variety of tumors, at least of the same histologic type, would seem to have greater potential for large-scale therapeutic applications.

CONCLUSIONS

The author believes that the prospects for therapy of cancer by biological response modification are quite good, particularly since this offers an approach to affecting tumor cells which is substantially different from conventional chemotherapy or radiotherapy. However, in view of the rather limited success of empirical approaches with immunotherapy and other forms of biological response modification, and the unimpressive results that have been seen in patients with advanced disease, it is felt that a shift in emphasis toward more systematic and well-planned studies is needed. It will probably be necessary to develop detailed understanding of the mechanisms of action of the various BRMs, to better understand the immunoregulatory processes affected by these agents, and to develop protocols which are able to produce optimal and sustained alterations in immunologic reactivity. Since a variety of BRMs have shown considerable antitumor effects in animal tumor model systems, particularly against micrometastatic disease, which represents a major clinical problem, further research in this area may be expected to lead to significant advances in the therapy of patients with cancer.

REFERENCES

1. Mihich, E. and Fefer, A. (Eds.) (1983): Biological Response Modifiers: Subcommittee Report. *Natl. Cancer Inst. Monogr.,* (In press).
2. Herberman, R.B. (1974): Cell mediated immunity to tumor cells. In: *Advances in Cancer Research, Vol. 19,* p.207. Editors: G. Klein and S. Weinhouse. Academic Press, New York.
3. Baldwin, R.W. (1982): Manipulation of host resistance in cancer therapy. *Springer Semin. Immunopathol., 5,* 113.
4. Foon, K.A., Smalley, R.V., Riggs, C.W. and Gale R.P. (1983): The role of immunotherapy in acute myelogenous leukemia. *Archives Int. Med., 143,* 1726.
5. Klein, E., Holtermann, O.A., Helm, F., Rosner, D., Milgrom, H., Adler, S., Stoll, H.L., Case, R.W., Prior, R.L. and Murphy, G.P. (1974): Immunologic approaches to the management of primary and secondary tumors involving the skin and soft tissues: review of a ten-year program. *Transplant. Proc., 7,* 297.
6. McKneally, M.F., Maver, C.M. and Kausel, H.W. (1978): Regional immunotherapy of lung cancer using postoperative intrapleural BCG. In: *Im munotherapy of Cancer: Present Status of Trials in Man,* p.180. Editors: *W.D. Terry and D.B. Windhorst. Raven Press, New York.*
7. *Borden, E. (1979): Interferons: Rationale for clinical trials in neoplastic disease. Ann. Int. Med., 91,* 472.
8. Terry, W.D. and Rosenberg, S.A. (Eds.) (1983): *Immunotherapy of human cancer,* p. 502. Excerpta Medica, New York.
9. Hewitt, H.B., Blake, E.R. and Walder, A.S. (1976): A critique of the evidence for active host defense against cancer, based on personal studies of 27 murine tumours of spontaneous origin. *Br. J. Cancer, 33,* 241.
10. Hewitt, H.B. (1982): Animal tumor models and their relevance to human tumor immunology. *J. Biol. Resp. Modif., 1,* 107.
11. Stutman, O. (1979): Chemical carcinogenesis in nude mice: Comparison between nude mice from homozygous matings and heterozygous matings and effects of age and carcinogen dose. *J. Natl. Cancer Inst., 62,* 353.
12. Herberman, R.B. (Ed.) (1980): Natural Cell-Mediated Immunity Against Tumors, p.1321. Academic Press, New York.
13. Herberman, R.B. (1983): Counterpoint: Animal tumor models and their relevance to human tumor immunology. *J. Biol. Resp. Modif., 2,* 39.
14. Herberman, R.B. and Ortaldo, J.R. (1981): NK cells and natural defenses against cancer and microbial diseases. *Science, 214,* 24.
15. Herberman, R.B. (Ed.) (1982): NK Cells and Other Natural Effector Cells, p. 1566. Academic Press, New York.
16. Schlick, E., Bartocci, A. and Chirigos, M.A. (1982): Effect of azimexone on the bone marrow of normal and γ-irradiated mice. *J. Biol. Resp. Modif., 1,* 179.
17. Devita, V.T. (1983): The relationship between tumor mass and resistance to chemotherapy. Implications for surgical adjuvant treatment of cancer. *Cancer, 51,* 1209.

18. North, R.J., Dye, E.S., Mills, C.D. and Chandler, J.P. (1982): Modulation of antitumor immunity-immunologic approaches. *Springer Seminars in Immunopathol., 5*, 193.
19. Maluish, A.E., Ortaldo, J.R., Conlon, J.C., Sherwin, S.A., Leavitt, R., Strong, D. M., Weirnik, P., Oldham, R.K. and Herberman, R.B. (1983): Depression of natural killer cytotoxicity following in vivo administration of recombinant leukocyte interferon. *J. Immunol., 131*, 503.
20. Fogler, W.E. and Fidler, I.J. (1984): Role of macrophages in host resistance against tumors. In: *Basic and Clinical Tumor Immunology*. Editor: R.B. Herberman. Martinus Nijhoff, The Hague., (In press).
21. Talmadge, J.E., Lenz, B.F., Collins, M.S., Ulthoven, Y.-A., Schneider, M.A., Adams, J.S., Pearson, J.W., Agee, W.J., Fox, R.E. and Oldham, R.K. (1984): Tumor models to investigate the therapeutic efficacy of immunomodulators. *Behring Inst. Mitt.,* (In press).
22. Foon, K.A., Sherwin, S.A., Abrams, P.G., Longo, D.L., Fer, M.F., Stevenson, H.C., Ochs, J.J., Bottino, G.C., Schoenberger, C.S., Zeffren, J., Jaffe, E.S. and Oldham, R.K.: Recombinant leukocyte A interferon: An effective agent for the treatment of advanced non-Hodgkin's lymphoma. *N. Engl. J. Med.,* (In press).
23. Bunn, P.A., Foon, K.A., Ihde, D.C., Winkler, C.F., Zeffren, J., Sherwin, S.A. and Oldham, R.K.: Recombinant leukocyte A interferon: an active agent in advanced cutaneous T cell lymphoma. *Ann. Int. Med.,* (In press).
24. Quesada, J.R., Reuben, J., Manning, J.R., Hersh, E.M. and Gutterman, J.U. (1984): Alpha interferon for induction of remission in hairy cell leukemia. *N. Eng. J. Med., 310*, 15.
25. Herberman, R.B., Ortaldo, J.R., Djeu, J.Y., Holden, H.T., Jett, J., Lang, N.P., Rubinstein, M. and Pestka, S. (1980): Role of interferon in regulation of cytotoxicity by natural killer cells and macrophages. *Ann. NY Acad. Sci., 350*, 63.
26. Einhorn, S., Ahre, A., Blomgren, H., Johansson, B., Mellstedt, H. and Strander, H. (1982): Enhanced NK activity in patients treated by interferon-α. Relation to clinical response. In: *NK Cells and Other Natural Effector Cells*, p. 1259. Editor: R.B. Herberman. Academic Press, New York.
27. Hizuta, A., Maluish, A.E., Ortaldo, J.R. and Herberman, R.B. (1984): NK activity in patients receiving therapy with recombinant leukocyte A interferon. Editors: T. Hoshino, H.S. Koren and A. Uchida. In: *Natural Killer Activity and its Regulation*, p. 453. Excerpta Medica, Tokyo.
28. Ortaldo, J.R., Mason, A., Rehberg, E., Kelder, B., Harvey, C., Osheroff, P., Pestka, S. and Herberman, R.B. (1983): Augmentation of NK activity with recombinant and hybrid recombinant human leukocyte interferons. In: *The Biology of the Interferon System.* Editors: H. Shellekens and E. DeMaeyer. p. 535. Elsevier Science Pubs., Amsterdam.
29. Brunda, M.J. and Rosenbaum, D.: Modulation of murine natural killer cell activity *in vitro* and *in vivo* by recombinant human interferons. *J. Immunol.* In press.
30. Hand, P.H., Nuti, M., Colcher, D. and Schlom, J. (1983): Definition of antigenic heterogeneity and modulation among human mammary carcinoma cell populations using monoclonal antibodies to tumor-associated antigens. *Cancer Res.,* 43, 728.
31. Ritz, J. and Schlossman, S.F. (1982): Utilization of monoclonal antibodies in the treatment of leukemia and lymphoma. *Blood, 59*, 1.
32. Bernhard, M.I., Foon, K.A., Oeltmann, T.N., Key, M.E., Hwang, K.M., Clarke, G.C., Christensen, W.L., Hoyer, L., Hanna, M.G., Jr., and Oldham, R.K. (1983):

Guinea pig line 10 hepatocarcinoma model: characterization of monoclonal antibody and *in vivo* effect of unconjugated antibody and antibody conjugated to diphtheria toxin A chain. *Cancer Res., 43*, 4420.

33. Hwang, K.M., Foon, K.A., Cheung, P.H., Pearson, J.W. and Oldham, R.K.: Selective antitumor effect of a potent immunoconjugate composed of the A chain of abrin and monoclonal antibody to a hepatoma-associated antigen. *Cancer Res.,* (In press).
34. Rosenberg, S.A. and Terry, W.D. (1977): Passive immunotherapy of cancer in animals and man. *Adv. Cancer Res., 25*, 323.
35. Kirch, M.E. and Hammerling, U. (1981): Immunotherapy of murine leukemias by monoclonal antibody: I. Effective passively administered antibody and growth of transplanted tumor cells. *J. Immunol., 127*, 805.
36. Bumol, T.F., Wang, Q.C., Reisfeld, R.A. and Kaplan, N.O. (1983): Monoclonal antibody and an antibody-toxin conjugate to a cell surface proteoglycan of melanoma cells suppress *in vivo* tumor growth. *Proc. Natl. Acad. Sci. U.S.A., 80*, 529.
37. Schroff, R.W., Woodhouse, C.S., Foon, K.A., Oldham, R.K., Farrell, M.M., Klein, R.A. and Morgan, A.C., Jr.,: Intratumor localization of monoclonal antibody in patients with malignant melanoma treated with antibody to a 250K dalton melanoma-associated antigen. *JNCI.,* (In press).
38. Dillman, R.O., Shawler, D.L., Sobol, R.E., Collins, H.A., Beauregard, J.C., Wormsley, S.B. and Royston, I. (1982): Murine monoclonal antibody therapy in two patients with chronic lymphocytic leukemia. *Blood, 59*, 1036.
39. Foon, K.A., Bunn, P.A., Schroff, R.W., Mayer, D., Sherwin, S.A. and Oldham, R.K.: Monoclonal antibody serotherapy of chronic lymphocytic leukemia and cutaneous T cell lymphoma. In: *Monoclonal Antibodies and Cancer*. Editors: R. Dulbecco and R. Langman. Academic Press, New York., (In press).
40. Miller, R.A., Moloney, D.G., Warnke, R. and Levy, R. 1982): Treatment of B cell lymphoma with monoclonal anti-idiotype antibody. *N. Eng. J. Med., 306*, 517.

CONTRIBUTORS

CONTRIBUTORS

Numbers in parentheses indicate the pages on which authors' contributions begin.

Shigeru Abe (129)	Faculty of Pharmaceutical Sciences, Teikyo University, 1091 Suarashi, Sagamiko, Tsukui, Kanagawa 199-01 JAPAN
Yukio Akiyama (223)	The Wistar Institute of Anatomy and Biology, Thirty-Sixth Street at Spruce, Philadelphia, Pennsylvania 19104 USA Currently : Division of Basic Immunology Research, Central Research Laboratories, Ajinomoto Co., Inc., 214 Maedacho, Totsuka-ku, Yokohama 244 JAPAN
Keiko Amikura (87)	Division of Basic Immunology Research, Central Research Laboratories, Ajinomoto Co., Inc., 214 Maedacho, Totsuka-ku, Yokohama 244 JAPAN
Tadao Aoki (167)	Research Division, Shinrakuen Hospital, 1-27 Nishiariake, Niigata 950-21 JAPAN
Douglas A. Carlow (187)	Cancer Research Laboratories, Department of Pathology, Queen's University, Kingston, Ontario, CANADA K7L 3N6
Goro Chihara (116)	Division of Chemotherapy, National Cancer Center Research Institute, 5-1-1 Tsukiji, Chuo-ku, Tokyo 104 JAPAN
Bruce E. Elliott (187)	Cancer Research Laboratories, Department of Pathology, Queen's University, Kingston, Ontario CANADA K7L 3N6
Michael J. Embleton (200)	Cancer Research Campaign Laboratory, University of Nottingham, University Park, Nottingham NG7 2RD ENGLAND

Jószef Fachet (116)	Institute of Pathophysiology, Medical University, Debrecen, HUNGARY
Isaiah J. Fidler (3)	Department of Cell Biology, The University of Texas System Cancer Center, M. D. Anderson Hospital and Tumor Institute, 6723 Bertner Avenue, Houston, Texas 77030 USA
Philip Frost (187)	Department of Cell Biology, M. D. Anderson Hospital and Tumor Institute, P. O. Box HMB-173, Houston, Texas, 77030 USA
Hiromi Fujiwara (208)	Department of Oncogenesis, Institute of Cancer Research, Osaka University Medical School, 1-1-50 Fukushima, Fukushima-ku, Osaka 553 JAPAN
Hisashi Furue (151)	Department of Internal Medicine, Teikyo University, School of Medicine, 2-11-1 Kaga, Itabashi-ku, Tokyo 173 JAPAN
Robert C. Gallo (167)	Laboratory of Tumor Cell Biology, Division of Cancer Treatment, National Cancer Institute, NIH Bldg 37, Rm 6A09 Bethesda, Maryland 20205 USA
Jun-ichi Hamada (33)	Laboratory of Pathology, Cancer Institute, Hokkaido University School of Medicine, Kita 15-jo, Nishi 7-chome, Kita-ku, Sapporo 060 JAPAN
Toshiyuki Hamaoka (208)	Department of Oncogenesis, Institute of Cancer Research, Osaka University Medical School, 1-1-50 Fukushima, Fukushima-ku, Osaka 553 JAPAN
Junji Hamuro (87) (96)	Division of Basic Immunology Research, Central Research Laboratories, Ajinomoto Co., Inc., 214 Maedacho, Totsuka-ku, Yokohama 244 JAPAN
Yoshiyuki Hashimoto (231)	Department of Hygienic Chemistry, Pharmaceutical Institute, Tohoku University, Aobayama,

Sendai, Miyagi 980 JAPAN

Takao Hattori (151)
Research Institute for Nuclear Medicine and Biology, Hiroshima University, 1-2-3 Kasumi, Minami-ku, Hiroshima 734 JAPAN

Yuuichi Hattori (138)
Second Department of Anatomy, Hamamatsu University School of Medicine, 3600 Handacho, Hamamatsu, Shizuoka 431-31 JAPAN

Ronald B. Herberman (240)
Biological Therapeutics Branch, Biological Response Modifiers Program, Division of Cancer Treatment, National Cancer Institute Frederick Cancer Research Facility, Frederick, Maryland 21701 USA

Masahiro Higuchi (53)
Division of Chemical Toxicology and Immunochemistry, Faculty of Pharmaceutical Sciences, University of Tokyo, 7-3-1 Hongo, Bunkyo-ku, Tokyo 113 JAPAN

Masuo Hosokawa (25) (33)
Laboratory of Pathology, Cancer Institute, Hokkaido University School of Medicine, Kita 15-jo, Nishi 7-chome, Kita-ku, Sapporo, Hokkaido 060 JAPAN

Atsuko Imaizumi (138)
Division of Surgery, Shimizu City Hospital, 2-19 Matsubara, Shimizu, Shizuoka 424 JAPAN

Kiyoshi Ishii (74)
Third Department of Internal Medicine, University of Tokushima School of Medicine, 3-18-15 Kuramotocho, Tokushima 770 JAPAN

Makoto Ishikawa (25)
Laboratory of Pathology, Cancer Institute, Hokkaido University School of Medicine, Kita 15-jo, Nishi 7-chome, Kita-ku, Sapporo 060 JAPAN

Ichiji Ito (151)
Department of Surgery, Tokyo Metropolitan Komagome Hospital, 3-18-22 Hon-Komagome, Bunkyo-ku, Tokyo 113 JAPAN

Ichiro Kawase (62) (208)	Third Department of Internal Medicine, Osaka University Medical School, 1-1-50 Fukushima, Fukushima-ku, Osaka 553 JAPAN
Robert S. Kerbel (187)	Cancer Research Laboratories, Department of Pathology, Queen's University, Kingston, Ontario, CANADA K7L 3N6 Currently : Mount Sinai Medical Research Institute, Mount Sinai Hospital, 600 University Avenue, Toronto, Ontario, CANADA M5G 1X5
Tadashi Kimura (151)	Department of Surgery, National Medical Center Hospital, 1-21-1 Toyama, Shinjuku-ku, Tokyo 162 JAPAN
Susumu Kishimoto (62) (208)	Third Department of Internal Medicine, Osaka University Medical School, 1-1-50 Fukushima, Fukushima-ku, Osaka 553 JAPAN
Hiroshi Kobayashi (25) (33)	Laboratory of Pathology, Cancer Institute, Hokkaido University School of Medicine, Kita 15-jo, Nishi 7-chome, Kita-ku, Sapporo 060 JAPAN
Yutaka Koga (25)	Laboratory of Pathology, Cancer Institute, Hokkaido University School of Medicine, Kita 15-jo, Nishi 7-chome, Kita-ku, Sapporo 060 JAPAN
Kiyoshi Komuta (208)	Third Department of Internal Medicine, Osaka University Medical School, 1-1-50 Fukushima, Fukushima-ku, Osaka 553 JAPAN
Tatsuhei Kondo (151)	Second Department of Surgery, Nagoya University, School of Medicine, Tsurumaicho 65, Showa-ku, Nagoya 466 JAPAN
Nobuo Kondoh (96)	Life Science Laboratory, Central Research Laboratories, Ajinomoto Co., Inc., 214 Maedacho, Totsuka-ku, Yokohama 244 JAPAN

Hilary Koprowski (223) — The Wistar Institute, Thirty-Sixth Street at Spruce, Philadelphia, Pennsylvania 19104 USA

Akio Kosaka (138) — Division of Surgery, Shimizu City Hospital, 2-19 Matsubara, Shimizu, Shizuoka 424 JAPAN

Margaret L. Kripke (178) — Department of Immunology, The University of Texas System Cancer Center, M. D. Anderson Hospital and Tumor Institute, 6723 Bertner Avenue, Houston, Texas 77030 USA

Michael D. Lubeck (223) — The Wistar Institute of Anatomy and Biology, Thirty-Sixth Street at Spruce, Philadelphia, Pennsylvania 19104 USA

Michiyuki Maeda (96) — Chest Disease Research Institute, Kyoto University School of Medicine, Shogoin Kawaramachi 53, Sakyo-ku, Kyoto 606 JAPAN

Yukiko Y. Maeda (116) — Department of Oncology, The Tokyo Metropolitan Institute of Medical Sciences, 3-18-22 Honkomagome, Bunkyo-ku, Tokyo 113 JAPAN

Tomiya Masuno (62) — Third Department of Internal Medicine, Osaka University Hospital, 1-1-50 Fukushima, Fukushima-ku, Osaka 553 JAPAN

Enrico Mihich (105) — Grace Cancer Drug Center, Roswell Park Memorial Institute, New York State Department of Health, 666 Elm Street, Buffalo, New York 14263 USA

Hideo Miyakoshi (167) — Research Division, Shinrakuen Hospital, 1-27 Nishiariake, Niigata 950-21 JAPAN

Den'ichi Mizuno (129) — Faculty of Pharmaceutical Sciences, Teikyo University, 1091 Suarashi, Sagamiko, Tsukui, Kanagawa 199-01 JAPAN

Kiyoshi Morikawa (33) — Laboratory of Pathology, Cancer Institute, Hokkaido University School of Medicine, Kita 15-jo, Nishi 7-chome, Kita-ku, Sapporo 060

JAPAN

Seiji Mutsuura (44) (74)	Third Department of Internal Medicine, University of Tokushima School of Medicine, 3-18-15 Kuramotocho, Tokushima 770 JAPAN
Hiroshi Neda (15)	Fourth Department of Internal Medicine, Sapporo Medical College, Minami 1-jo, Nishi 16-chome, Chuo-ku, Sapporo 060 JAPAN
Yoshiro Niitsu (15)	Fourth Department of Internal Medicine, Sapporo Medical College, Minami 1-jo, Nishi 16-chome, Chuo-ku, Sapporo 060 JAPAN
Nobuya Ogawa (151)	Department of Pharmacology, Ehime University School of Medicine, Shitsukawa, Oaza Shigenobucho, Onsen-gun, Ehime 791-02 JAPAN
Mitsumasa Ogawara (44) (74)	Third Department of Internal Medicine, University of Tokushima School of Medicine, 3-18-15 Kuramotocho, Tokushima 770 JAPAN
Takeshi Ogura (62) (208)	Third Department of Internal Medicine, Osaka University Medical School, 1-1-50 Fukushima, Fukushima-ku, Osaka 553 JAPAN
Toshiaki Osawa (53)	Division of Chemical Toxicology and Immunochemistry, Faculty of Pharmaceutical Sciences, University of Tokyo, 7-3-1 Hongo, Bunkyo-ku, Tokyo 113 JAPAN
Makoto Rokutanda (116)	Department of Oncology, The Tokyo Metropolitan Institute of Medical Sciences, 3-18-22 Honkomagome, Bunkyo-ku, Tokyo 113 JAPAN
Mitsunori Sakatani (62)	Third Department of Internal Medicine, Osaka University Medical School, 1-1-50 Fukushima, Fukushima-ku, Osaka 553 JAPAN
Fujiro Sendo (83)	Department of Parasitology, Yamagata University School of Medicine, Nishinomae, Iida, Zao, Yamagata 990-23 JAPAN

Tsuyoshi Shiio (116)	Life Science Laboratory, Central Research Laboratories, Ajinomoto Co., Inc., 214 Maedacho, Totsuka-ku, Yokohama 244 JAPAN
Toyohiro Shirahama (74)	Third Department of Internal Medicine, University of Tokushima School of Medicine, 3-18-15 Kuramotocho, Tokushima 770 JAPAN
Hisao Sone (15)	Fourth Department of Internal Medicine, Sapporo Medical College, Minami 1-jo, Nishi 16-chome, Chuo-ku, Sapporo 060 JAPAN
Saburo Sone (44) (74)	Third Department of Internal Medicine, University of Tokushima School of Medicine, 3-18-15 Kuramotocho, Tokushima 770 JAPAN
Zenon Steplewski (223)	The Wistar Institute of Anatomy and Biology, Thirty-Sixth Street at Spruce, Philadelphia, Pennsylvania 19104 USA
Tetsuya Suga (116)	Division of Chemotherapy, National Cancer Center Research Institute, 5-1-1 Tsukiji, Chuo-ku, Tokyo 104 JAPAN
Michio Sugawara (33)	Laboratory of Pathology, Cancer Institute, Hokkaido University School of Medicine, Kita 15-jo, Nishi 7-chome, Kita-ku, Sapporo 060 JAPAN
Tetsuo Taguchi (151)	Research Institute for Microbial Diseases, Osaka University, 3-1 Yamada-oka, Suita, Osaka 565 JAPAN
Shinsuke Taki (87)	Division of Basic Immunology Research, Central Research Laboratories, Ajinomoto Co., Inc., 214 Maedacho, Totsuka-ku, Yokohama 244 JAPAN
Robert C. Y. Ting (167)	Department of Cell Biology, Biotech Research Laboratory, Rockville, Maryland 20850 USA
Eiro Tsubura (44) (74)	Third Department of Internal Medicine, University of Tokushima School of Medicine, 3-18-

15 Kuramotocho, Tokushima 770 JAPAN
Currently :
National Toneyama Hospital, 5-1-1 Toneyama, Toyonaka, Osaka 560 JAPAN

Noriko A. Uchida (116) | Department of Oncology, The Tokyo Metropolitan Institute of Medical Sciences, 3-18-22 Honkomagome, Bunkyo-ku, Tokyo 113 JAPAN

Ichiro Urushizaki (15) | Fourth Department of Internal Medicine, Sapporo Medical College, Minami 1-jo, Nishi 16-chome, Chuo-ku, Sapporo 060 JAPAN

Yoshimaru Usuda (167) | Research Division, Shinrakuen Hospital, 1-27 Nishiariake, Niigata 950-21 JAPAN

Teruhiro Utsugi (44) (74) | Third Department of Internal Medicine, University of Tokushima School of Medicine, 3-18-15 Kuramotocho, Tokushima 770 JAPAN

Naoki Watanabe (15) | Fourth Department of Internal Medicine, Sapporo Medical College, Minami 1-jo, Nishi 16-chome, Chuo-ku, Sapporo 060 JAPAN

Yuichi Yamamura (62) | Osaka University Medical School, 1-1-50 Fukushima, Fukushima-ku, Osaka 553 JAPAN

Seiko Yamasaki (87) | Division of Basic Immunology Research, Central Research Laboratories, Ajinomoto Co., Inc., 214 Maedacho, Totsuka-ku, Yokohama 244 JAPAN

Akira Yamashita (138) | Second Department of Anatomy, Hamamatsu University School of Medicine, 3600 Handacho, Hamamatsu, Shizuoka 431-31 JAPAN

Naofumi Yamauchi (15) | Fourth Department of Internal Medicine, Sapporo Medical College, Minami 1-jo, Nishi 16-chome, Chuo-ku, Sapporo 060 JAPAN

Masatoshi Yamazaki (129) | Faculty of Pharmaceutical Sciences, Teikyo University, 1091 Suarashi, Sagamiko, Tsukui, Kanagawa 199-01 JAPAN

Junji Yodoi (96)	The Institute of Immunology Research, Faculty of Medicine, Kyoto University, Yoshida-Konoecho, Sakyo-ku, Kyoto 606 JAPAN
Takashi Yoshihama (116)	Life Science Laboratory, Central Research Laboratories, Ajinomoto Co., Inc., 214 Maedacho, Totsuka-ku, Yokohama 244 JAPAN
Ryota Yoshimoto (87)	Division of Basic Immunology Research, Central Research Laboratories, Ajinomoto Co., Inc., 214 Maedacho, Totsuka-ku, Yokohama 244 JAPAN